Immunology: An Introduction

Ian R. Tizard
Texas A&M University

SAUNDERS COLLEGE PUBLISHING

Philadelphia New York Chicago
San Fransico Montreal Toronto
London Sydney Tokyo Mexico City
Rio de Janeiro Madrid

Address orders to:
383 Madison Avenue
New York, NY 10017

Address editorial correspondence to:
West Washington Square
Philadelphia, PA 19105

Text Typeface: 10/12 Baskerville
Compositor: University Graphics, Inc.
Acquisitions Editor: Michael Brown
Project Editor: Diane Ramanauskas
Copyeditor: Sarah Fitz-Hugh
Managing Editor & Art Director: Richard L. Moore
Art/Design Assistant: Virginia A. Bollard
Text Design: Caliber Design Planning, Inc.
Cover Design: Lawrence R. Didona
Production Manager: Tim Frelick
Assistant Production Manager: Maureen Iannuzzi

Cover credit: Destruction of red blood cells by macrophage (Manfred Kage © Peter Arnold, Inc.)

Library of Congress Cataloging in Publication Data

Tizard, Ian R.
   Immunology, an introduction.

   Includes bibliographies and index.

    1. Immunology. I. Title. [DNLM: 1. Immunity.
2. Immunochemistry. 3. Serology. QW 504 T625i]
QR181.T53 1983   616.07'9   83-15096
ISBN 0-03-060277-7

IMMUNOLOGY: AN INTRODUCTION   ISBN 0-03-60277-7

  56   032   9876543

CBS COLLEGE PUBLISHING
Saunders College Publishing
Holt, Rinehart and Winston
The Dryden Press

To Claire, Robert, and Fiona

Preface

The most common flaw (if I may presume to call it so) of most immunology texts is that they tend to assume too much basic knowledge on the part of their readers, who, as a result, are soon lost in the complexity of the subject. It can be argued, of course, that immunology is a complex discipline and that it does students a disservice to pretend that it is otherwise. Albert Einstein once commented that a scientific subject should be kept as simple as possible—but no simpler. I believe, however, that it should be possible to introduce the subject to students in a very simple fashion and to develop it in such a way that the reader is led to the heart of the subject while confusion is kept to a minimum. In this text, I have tried to keep to the narrow path between maximum simplification and scientific accuracy. If I have offended the immunologically competent by oversimplification, I offer no apology but hope that this minor evil will be compensated for if I succeed in arousing the interest of students in this important and exciting scientific discipline.

The second important feature of this text is its treatment of immunity to infectious disease. Immunology had its origins as a subdiscipline of microbiology—indeed, in many universities, it is still taught within microbiology departments. Perhaps it is in reaction to this practice that some immunologists have, in recent years, tended to equate immunology with lymphocytology. Many recent texts have placed too much emphasis on the unique and fascinating activities of lymphocytes while losing sight of the preeminent defensive function of the immune system.

Our knowledge of resistance mechanisms in infectious diseases has progressed steadily in recent years. Many important advances have occurred in our understanding of immunity, not only of bacteria and viruses, but also of parasitic protozoa and helminths. The most important diseases in the world today—malaria, schistosomiasis, leishmaniasis, and trypanosomiasis, for example—are currently under intense scrutiny from immunologists, and there is cause for optimism that some of these diseases may be controlled by immunological methods.

Finally, it is all too easy to present immunology as a completely plausible tale without mentioning the supporting experimental evidence. All of the information in this text has been obtained as a result of extensive laboratory investigation. In an attempt to supply this evidence, I have provided readers with a set of brief "recipes" for major immunological techniques, which are highlighted in the Contents.

While writing this book, I have received the active encouragement of many colleagues both in Guelph, Canada, and here in Texas. I owe them all my gratitude. Much of the drudgery of authorship was relieved by my most excellent typists, Betty Suehs, Linda Henderson, and Helen Corbett. Finally, this book could not have been written without the enthusiastic support of Michael Brown of Saunders College Publishing and most important, of my wife, Claire.

Ian Tizard
College Station, Texas
1983

Contents

15 Immunity at Body Surfaces   259

16 Vaccines and Vaccination   270

17 Immunity to Infection   286

1

General Principles of Immunology

The Science of Immunology

It is clear that animals such as ourselves must contend with a host of potentially dangerous microbial enemies. There are many microorganisms among the bacteria, fungi, viruses, and parasites that will readily invade the body and cause disease, and it requires "eternal vigilance" on the part of the body's defenses to protect us against these invaders. The scientific basis of our defense mechanisms is the subject of immunology.

Notwithstanding the existence of our immunological defenses, it is clear that they are not completely effective. It is almost certain, for example, that most readers of this book will have suffered from an upper-respiratory-tract infection—the common cold—within the past year or so. Indeed, you will probably recollect suffering from many such infections in previous years.

For this reason, it is not really surprising that the suggestion that one attack of an infectious disease confers resistance to subsequent attacks was not readily accepted by most people until relatively recently. Nevertheless, even in ancient times, the Greeks suspected that those individuals who survived one attack of the plague would not suffer the disease a second time. It would clearly require an act of great courage to test the hypothesis, and it is unlikely to have been widely accepted.

The Chinese first firmly established that those individuals who recovered from smallpox would not get the disease a second time. At a time when infant mortality was very high, it became accepted practice in China to infect young children with smallpox, thus saving the trouble and expense of raising them only to die from the disease when older. As experience was gained with this procedure, it was found that the least severe reactions occurred when the smallpox scabs used to transfer the disease were selected from mildly affected donors. The prevalence of adverse side affects was thus reduced to fairly low levels.

Knowledge of this technique gradually spread westward along the caravan routes of Central Asia and eventually reached Turkey. In 1718, the wife of the English ambassador in Constantinople, the remarkable Lady Mary Wortley Montagu, decided that the technique of **variolation** ("variola" is the Latin word for "smallpox") should be used on her children. Her chaplain attempted to dissuade her on the grounds that the technique worked only on Muslims and would, therefore, be ineffective in Christians. Nevertheless, her children were variolated with complete success.

News of this new technique spread rapidly to England, and it was soon employed routinely in Western Europe and the American colonies. Indeed, variolation was so successful in reducing smallpox mortality that a minor population explosion resulted, providing soldiers for the Napoleonic Wars and labor for the new factories of the Industrial Revolution.

In England, in 1774, a farmer called Benjamin Jesty, instead of using smallpox to variolate his children, substituted cowpox. It appeared to work but Jesty failed to publish his results. In 1798, a physician named Edward Jenner, learned about this use of cowpox from one of his patients and decided to investigate the matter further. He confirmed that cowpox could indeed protect against smallpox and, unlike Benjamin Jesty, published his results and received the credit for the discovery. Jenner's technique of **vaccination** ("vacca" is the Latin word for "cow"), immediately replaced variolation as the method of protection against smallpox. In 1958, the World Health Organization decided to attempt to achieve global eradication of smallpox by means of vaccination. So successful was this technique that, by 1980, smallpox had become the first infectious disease to be totally eradicated.

In spite of Jenner's observations, there was no widespread belief that the phenomenon of vaccination could be extended to other infections or that recovery from one infection could confer resistance to subsequent attacks. (Nevertheless, many unsuccessful attempts were made to use cowpox vaccine to prevent other skin disorders.)

In 1879, Louis Pasteur in France was studying the bacterium that causes fowl cholera (Now called *Pasteurella multocida*). He possessed a culture of this organism that consistently killed chickens. One afternoon, he told his assistant Charles Chamberland to infect some birds with this culture. Since it was late in the day, Chamberland decided to postpone the experiment until after the holidays. However, when the chickens were given the culture, which had remained on the bench for several weeks, they remained healthy (Fig. 1–1). Pasteur then decided to give the chickens a dose of a fresh bacterial culture. To his surprise, they survived without becoming even slightly ill. Pasteur realized immediately that this phenomenon was identical in principle to Jenner's use of cowpox. He realized that, by exposing his chickens to the aged culture of bacteria, he had protected them against disease caused by the same (or very closely related) organism.

Once this general principle was established, Pasteur found that he could apply it to other diseases. Thus, although he could not render *Bacillus anthracis* (the causal agent of anthrax) avirulent by simple aging, he could do so by growing it at an unusually high temperature over a period of time.

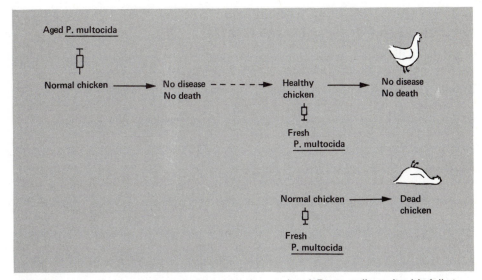

FIGURE 1–1. Pasteur's fowl cholera experiment: Aged *Pasteurella multocida* fails to kill chickens and renders them resistant to subsequent infection by fresh *P. multocida*. (From Tizard, I. Veterinary Immunology. 2nd ed. W. B. Saunders, Philadelphia, 1982. With permission.)

> **Terminology**
> **Virulence** is a measure of the disease-producing power of an organism. A highly viru-lent organism causes severe disease. An avirulent organism fails to produce disease in normal individuals.

Pasteur then showed, in a very convincing public experiment, that his heated anthrax culture would protect sheep and goats against a lethal dose of virulent anthrax. He thus clearly established the general principles of vaccination and its potential for use in protec-tion against infectious agents.

Pasteur, although remarkably successful in demonstrating the immune response and in applying his results to promoting protective immunity, had little concept of the mecha-nisms involved. It was about ten years later, in 1890, that von Behring and Kitasato in Berlin demonstrated that the protective activity induced by vaccination was found in the bloodstream. They gave the name **antibody** to the factors with this activity. Within a few years, many of the basic properties of antibodies were discovered.

In 1894, Emil Roux showed that **serum** taken from a vaccinated animal could be injected into an unvaccinated one and protect it against disease. For example, if the serum was obtained from a horse made resistant to tetanus by vaccination, and this serum was injected into a human in appropriate quantity, then the recipient was rendered resistant to tetanus for a few weeks. This technique is known as **passive immunization.**

Antibodies are exquisitely specific for the material that induces their production. Thus, in the example described above, antibodies to tetanus will protect only against teta-nus. They have no effect on any other disease.

Response to Foreign-Tissue Grafts

It was not until the development of successful surgical techniques that it became possible to transplant organs or tissues between individuals. The first attempts, however, proved immediately that living tissue, transplanted from one unrelated individual to another usu-ally survived for only a few days before dying as a result of a **rejection** process mediated by the recipient. Grafts succeeded only when donor and recipient were essentially identi-cal—when, for example, grafts were made between identical twins.

It is clear, of course, that the graft rejection mechanisms cannot have evolved for the sole purpose of frustrating surgeons. Transplantation of tissues is an entirely artificial pro-cedure that has no counterpart in nature. What, then, is the reason for the rejection process? One possible clue is the finding that individuals who have received drugs to suppress graft rejection tend to suffer from more cases of cancer (Table 19–5). This led to the suggestion that the rejection of foreign grafts reflects the existence of a system that can recognize abnor-mal cells and destroy them. These abnormal cells include not only foreign graft cells, but also cells infected by viruses, cells that are chemically altered, and cancer cells. Perhaps this form of immune response is largely directed against tumors.

When the process of graft rejection is studied, it can be shown that, unlike immunity to tetanus, the rejection process cannot be transferred from an unsensitized individual to a normal individual by means of serum. Graft rejection is not mediated by antibody but by the family of cells known as **lymphocytes.** Lymphocytes capable of causing graft rejection

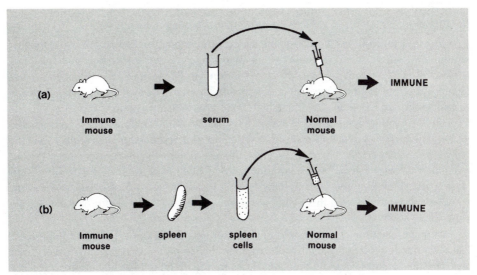

FIGURE 1-2. The difference between antibody- and cell-mediated immune responses is shown by simple transfer experiments such as these. Thus antibody-mediated immunity may be transferred to a nonimmune mouse by using serum (**A**) while cell-mediated immunity can only be transferred using viable cells (lymphocytes) such as those obtained from the spleen (**B**).

are readily obtained from the spleen, lymph nodes, or blood. The rejection of foreign tissues is, therefore, a very different type of immune reaction than that mediated by antibody (Fig. 1-2).

The Antibody-Mediated Immune Response

Antibodies are produced in small quantity following first exposure to an antigen. Foreign substances that enter the animal body and provoke the appearance of serum antibodies are called **antigens.** If an antigen gains access to an animal, then antibodies are produced that combine only with that antigen. These antibodies are not normally found in animals that have not previously encountered the inducing antigen.

A good example of such an antigen is the inactivated form of tetanus toxin called **tetanus toxoid.** The causal agent of tetanus, the bacterium *Clostridium tetani*, releases a potent protein toxin called tetanospasmin which, when it acts on nerve cells, causes clinical tetanus. If tetanus toxin is treated with formaldehyde, it loses its toxic activities but its antigenicity is unchanged. The treated material is called tetanus toxoid.

If tetanus toxoid is injected into an animal, antibodies specific for tetanus toxoid will be produced. If serum containing these antibodies is mixed with a solution of tetanus toxoid in saline, a cloudy precipitate will develop as a result of the combination between antibodies and tetanus toxoid. In addition, these antibodies bind to tetanus toxin in such a way that it can no longer bind to nerve cells and is thus rendered nontoxic. It is by means of this

neutralization process that antibodies can protect animals from the lethal effects of tetanus infection.

It is not difficult to follow the time course of antibody production following administration of a single dose of tetanus toxoid. Blood samples can be taken at intervals after vaccination. The amount of antibody in the serum can be estimated by measuring either the amount of precipitate formed on adding toxoid, or alternatively, by measuring the neutralizing ability of the serum. Both methods yield approximately similar results.

Following injection of a single dose of tetanus toxoid into an individual who has never been exposed to this antigen previously, no response is detectable for several days. This is known as the **lag period.** The more sensitive the detection method used, the shorter the lag period, but it is never less than three to four days. The level of antibodies is highest 10 to 14 days after they first appear, and then declines rapidly (Fig. 1–3). Because the amount of antibody produced during this **primary response** is small, the level of protection against tetanus is also low.

If, some time after the first, a second dose of toxoid is given to the same individual, and the antibody response is again followed, then the lag period lasts for only two or three days, and the amount of serum antibody climbs rapidly to a high level before commencing to decline slowly. This **secondary response** is specific in that it can be induced only by an antigen identical to the first. A secondary response may be provoked many months or years after first exposure to antigen, although its size does tend to decline as time passes. A secondary response may also be provoked even though the response of the animal to the first

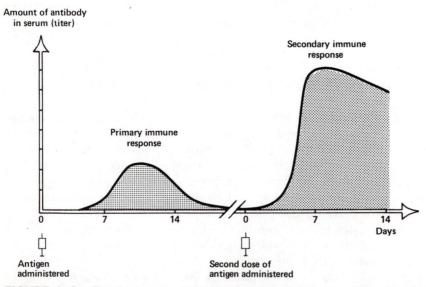

FIGURE 1–3. The time course of the immune responses to an antigen as reflected by serum antibody levels. (From Tizard, I. Veterinary Immunology. 2nd ed. W. B. Saunders, Philadelphia, 1982. With permission.)

injection of antigen was so weak as to be undetectable. We must, therefore, conclude that the antibody-forming system has the ability to "remember" previous exposure to an antigen. For this reason, the secondary immune response is sometimes known as an **anamnestic response** ("anamnesko" is the Greek word for "memory").

If a second dose of antigen is given to an individual still possessing some serum antibodies remaining after the primary immune response, then the level of these antibodies may fall for a few days before the secondary immune response gets under way. This so-called "negative phase" occurs as a result of the injected antigen binding and removing antibodies from the circulation.

A third dose of antigen given to an individual results in an immune response with an even shorter lag period and a still higher and more prolonged antibody response. However, multiple injections of antigen do not lead indefinitely to greater and greater antibody responses. The final level of antibodies achieved is well regulated and therefore tends to plateau at a constant level after repeated exposure to antigen.

The stimulation of resistance to disease through the use of repeated injections of antigen forms the basis of most current vaccination techniques. Thus tetanus toxoid is given to children in four doses. The time interval between the first three doses is eight weeks. The fourth dose is given one year after the third. Booster doses are recommended at ten-year intervals in order to maintain levels of protective antibody. The success of this procedure is demonstrated by the rapid decline in the number of cases of tetanus since vaccination was introduced (Fig. 1–4).

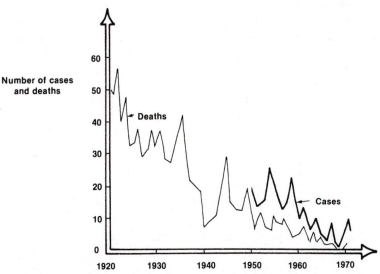

FIGURE 1–4. The progressive decline in the number of deaths and cases of tetanus in Canada from 1920 to 1970: The drop seen around 1940 is attributed to the introduction of tetanus toxoid at this time. (Used with permission of the Laboratory Centre for Disease Control, Canada.)

The Cell-Mediated Immune Response

If a skin graft is transplanted from one person to a second, unrelated individual, it will survive for about ten days. At first, the grafted skin will appear healthy, and blood vessels will connect the graft to the underlying tissues. By one week, however, the graft will become pale, begin to degenerate, and, finally, die. If not removed, it will be shed. The destruction of the graft in this way is due to a cutting off of the blood supply to the grafted skin as a result of degeneration of the connecting blood vessels. The blood-vessel degeneration is caused by lymphocytes. This slow rejection process is known as a **first-set reaction** (Fig. 1–5).

Following second exposure to a foreign graft, rejection is rapid. If a second graft from the same donor is placed on the same recipient, then the grafted skin will survive for no longer than one or two days before dying, and the underlying tissue becomes extremely red and inflamed. This rapid rejection process is known as a **second-set reaction.**

Thus we see that in the graft rejection process, the response to a first graft is relatively slow and mild. It is analogous to the primary antibody response. In contrast, the second-set reaction is rapid and very intense. It is thus similar, in these respects, to the secondary antibody response.

Graft rejection, like antibody formation, is specific in that a second-set reaction only occurs if the second graft is from the same donor as the first. The graft-rejection system also possesses a memory, since a second graft may undergo a second-set reaction many months or even years after loss of the first.

Nevertheless, as pointed out previously, there is a very basic difference between the process of graft rejection and the antibody response to tetanus toxoid. Protection against tetanus can be transferred to a normal individual using serum from an immunized one. The ability to mount a rapid second-set reaction to a graft cannot be transferred with

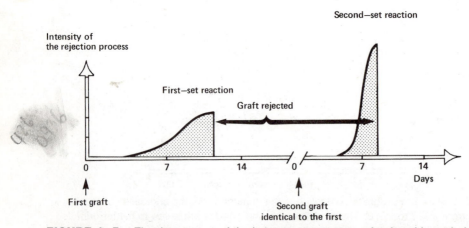

FIGURE 1–5. The time course of the immune response to a foreign skin graft: Notice the similarities between this and Figure 1–3. (From Tizard, I. Veterinary Immunology. 2nd ed. W. B. Saunders, Philadelphia, 1982. With permission.)

serum. It may, however, be transferred experimentally with a lymphocyte suspension from a sensitized donor (Fig. 1–2).

Tolerance

The immune response to tetanus toxoid and the rejection of a graft from an unrelated individual occur only because the toxoid and the graft are recognized by the body as being "foreign." This in turn implies that a mechanism exists that permits the body to distinguish between its own cells and foreign cells. Indeed healthy, normal individuals do not usually mount an immune response against self-components and are thus said to be self-tolerant. If self-tolerance breaks down, then the individual may mount an immune response against its own cells. Thus antibodies and lymphocytes may attack normal tissues and, by causing their destruction, provoke **autoimmune disease.**

It is therefore possible, under some circumstances, for the antibody- or cell-mediated immune responses to be specifically "turned-off." This may be done, for example, by giving foreign antigens to very young or fetal animals. **Tolerance** can also be provoked by giving either extremely small or extremely large doses of antigen. The unresponsiveness induced by techniques such as these may affect the cell-mediated or the antibody-mediated immune systems or both. Tolerance is specific for the inducing antigen and, like the other forms of immune response, may be boosted, only by re-exposure, to the same antigen. In the absence of this re-exposure, tolerance is gradually lost and the animal reacquires the ability to respond to this antigen. Tolerance to one antigen has no effect on the animal's ability to respond to other, unrelated antigens. The persistence of self-tolerance is therefore maintained by continuous exposure to self-antigens throughout life.

The Mechanisms of the Immune Responses (Fig. 1–6)

The immune responses may be considered to encompass two basic phenomena, namely the antibody- and the cell-mediated responses. Specific immunological tolerance is a special form of the two basic responses.

It was suggested earlier that the two basic responses serve two essentially different but complementary functions. Thus the cell-mediated responses probably reflect the existence of a self-surveillance system designed to detect and eliminate abnormal cells or cells perceived as altered. In contrast, the antibody-mediated responses are employed to protect us against non–cell-associated invaders such as the bacteria or parasites. This distinction is not absolute. Antibodies can contribute to graft rejection and to immunity against viruses, while cell-mediated immune responses can participate in resistance to many bacterial and parasitic infections.

Tolerance, on the other hand, is an essential protective mechanism that prevents an indiscriminate immune attack on normal body components.

In many ways, the immune system might be compared to a totalitarian state in which foreigners are expelled, citizens who conform are tolerated, but those who "deviate" are

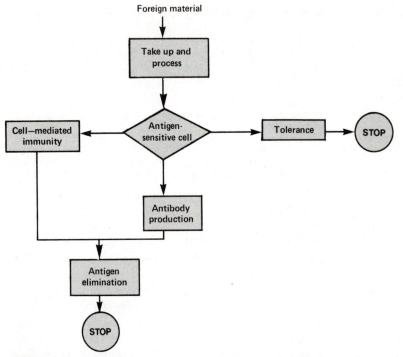

FIGURE 1–6.   A simple flow diagram shows the essential features of the immune responses. (From Tizard, I. Veterinary Immunology. 2nd ed. W. B. Saunders, Philadelphia, 1982. With permission.)

eliminated. While this analogy must not be pursued too far, it is clear that such regimes possess a number of characteristics. These include border police to repel outsiders and an internal police force that keeps the populace under surveillance and eliminates dissidents at the first trace of dissent. States of this type usually require an identification system so that foreigners not possessing the necessary identification features are readily detected and dealt with.

Similarly, when antigen enters the body, it must be trapped and processed. If it is recognized as being "not-self," presumably by an antigen-sensitive cell that has the ability to discriminate such matters, then this information must be processed in such a way that an immune response is triggered, and the foreign material eliminated. Thus an essential, very basic requirement of the immune systems is specificity. This specificity is required in order to prevent inappropriate responses to "self-antigens." The biological basis of specificity is described in the next chapter.

Sources of Additional Information

Books

There are, of course, a large number of immunology texts presently available. These approach the subject from a number of different, and sometimes innovative approaches. Some of the most important of these innovative texts include:

Bellanti, J. A. Immunology II. W. B. Saunders Company, Philadelphia, 1978. This text gives a slightly different approach to basic immunology and its clinical applications.

Clark, W. R. The Experimental Foundations of Modern Immunology. John Wiley and Sons, New York, 1980. This book makes extensive use of experimental examples.

Hood, L. E., Weissman, I. L., and Wood, W. B. Immunology. Benjamin Cummings, Menlo Park, CA, 1978. A text that views immunology within a broader biological context.

Playfair, J. H. L. Immunology at a Glance. Blackwell Scientific Publications, Oxford, 1979. A book of diagrams dealing with specific immunologic topics.

Series

As with textbooks, many publishers have attempted to produce a series of review texts in immunology. These include Advances in Immunology (Academic Press, New York), Immunological Reviews (Munksgaard, Copenhagen), and Progress in Allergy (S. Karger, Basel).

One of the most successful enterprises in this area is the publication of *Immunology Today,* by Elsevier North-Holland, Amsterdam. This is a monthly magazine highlighting recent advances and controversies in immunology. Very useful for keeping up to date.

Journals

There are a vast number of immunology journals of varying degrees of general usefulness. In writing this text, I have found that by far the most useful journal was the *Journal of Immunology,* followed by, in order, the *Journal of Experimental Medicine, Proceedings of the National Academy of Sciences, Nature, Infection and Immunity, Science, Immunology, Clinical and Experimental Immunology, New England Journal of Medicine, European Journal of Immunology, Veterinary Immunology and Immunopathology, International Archives of Allergy, Clinical Immunology and Immunopathology, Cell, Cellular Immunology,* and *Molecular Immunology.*

2

Foreign Antigens and Antigenicity

Essential Features of Antigens

In this chapter, we will discuss the features required of a substance in order for it to be recognized as foreign by the body and so provoke an immune response. It is very clear that not all foreign material is capable of stimulating an immune response. For example, stainless-steel pins and plastic prostheses are commonly implanted surgically in the body without encountering any problems from an immune response.

There are two major restrictions on the nature of antigens (agents that elicit an immune response). First, and most important, the material must be recognized as foreign. Second, because of the processing it must undergo, there are physical and chemical restrictions on the types of molecules that have the ability to stimulate the immune system. In particular, foreign molecules must be large, rigid, chemically complex, and not totally chemically inert (Table 2–1).

Factors that Govern Immune Responses

Molecular Weight In general, large foreign molecules are better antigens than small molecules. Thus, a very large molecule such as hemocyanin from invertebrates (6,700,000 daltons) is a very potent antigen. Serum albumin (60,000 daltons) is a good antigen, but is also well capable of provoking tolerance, while angiotensin (1031 daltons) is a very poor antigen. The record for minimal antigenic size is held by p-azobenzene-arsonate-trityrosine (750 daltons), which has been used to provoke antibodies in guinea pigs and rabbits. (However, you will see in the subsequent discussion on haptens that very small molecules can bind to large proteins so that the resulting complex becomes antigenic.)

Complexity In general, the more complex an antigen is, the better antigen it is. For example, starch and simple repetitive polysaccharides are poorly antigenic, but complex bacterial lipopolysaccharides are good immunogens. Similarly, complex proteins, such as the serum proteins, are better antigens than large repeating polymers, such as the lipids, carbohydrates, and nucleic acids.

Structural Stability The immune system, in order to recognize foreign material, must recognize stable structures. Consequently, compounds consisting of flexible molecules are weakly antigenic. For example, gelatin, a protein well known for its structural instability (this is why it "wobbles" on a plate), is a very poor antigen unless stabilized by the incorporation of tyrosine or tryptophan molecules. Similarly flagellin, the major protein of bac-

TABLE 2–1   Essential Features of Antigenicity

Feature	Property
Size	Larger is better.
Complexity	Simple polymers are relatively poor antigens.
Stability	Structural stability is mandatory.
Degradability	Unstable or totally inert molecules are poor antigens.
Foreignness	The more "foreign" the better.

terial flagellae is structurally unstable, and its antigenicity is greatly enhanced by polymerization.

Degradability   Since immune responses are antigen-driven processes, foreign molecules, which are extremely rapidly destroyed, will not provide sufficient antigen to stimulate an immune response. Conversely, the lack of antigenicity of the large inert organic polymers such as the plastics, is related not only to their molecular uniformity, but also to their inertness. They are not degraded or processed by cells such as macrophages to a form suitable for the initiation of an immune response.

A second example demonstrating the importance of antigen processing is seen using copolymers of D-amino acids. D-amino acids do not occur naturally in mammals. As a result, they are metabolically inert and are very poor antigens. If, however, a few short peptides consisting of L-amino acids are inserted into the D-amino acid polymer, then it is converted into a good antigen. D-amino acid copolymers are very effective in inducing tolerance.

Foreignness   The cells in the immune system, whose function is to respond to antigen, are selected in such a way that they do not normally respond to self-antigens. They are, however, capable of responding to antigens that differ even in very minor respects from normal.

It is probable that the suppression of self-reactive cells and tolerance occurs as a result of the exposure of these cells to antigen at an immature stage in their development (usually early in fetal life). If they are not exposed to antigen at that time, tolerance will not develop. For example, the sperm-forming cells in the testes are separated from the rest of the body by an effective barrier. As a result, the cells of the immune system do not normally encounter sperm and are not, therefore, tolerant to sperm antigens. If the isolation of the sperm-forming cells is broken down by damage due to injury or infection, then sperm antigen may reach the bloodstream. The antigen-sensitive cells may encounter this apparently foreign antigen and so mount an immune response. The development of antisperm antibodies is a common sequel to vasectomy as a result of the leakage of sperm antigens into the tissues. On a smaller scale, the mitochondria within normal cells are not normally exposed to antigen-sensitive cells in the circulation. Consequently, when extensive cell destruction occurs, for example, following a heart attack, antimitochondrial antibodies may develop and can be detected in serum several weeks later.

The immunogenicity of a molecule also depends to a great extent on its degree of foreignness. The greater the difference between the antigen and any self-antigens an animal may possess, the greater will be any immune response provoked. For example, humans will respond more strongly to chicken serum albumin than to bovine serum albumin. It is essentially impossible to get humans to respond to human serum albumin even though derived from an unrelated human. Nevertheless, some proteins do differ between individuals of the same species, and these may therefore function as weak antigens. Examples of these are the immunoglobulin allotypes described in Chapter 5.

Antigenic Determinants

Complex foreign particles, such as bacteria, nucleated cells, or erythrocytes, can provoke an immune response, yet they are clearly composed of a complex mixture of proteins, glycoproteins, polysaccharides, lipopolysaccharides, lipids, and nucleoproteins. When we elicit an immune response against these particles, we are, in fact, observing the sum of a number of simultaneous immune responses against each of the antigenic components of these particles.

On a smaller scale, even single protein molecules can be shown to consist of a number of different antigenic components. Thus, on the surface of a large antigenic macromolecule are a number of areas recognized as foreign, against which the immune response is directed, and with which antibodies will bind. These areas are termed **antigenic determinants** or **epitopes** (Fig. 2–1).

Clearly, in a large, complex, protein molecule, not all surface areas will function as antigenic determinants. Indeed, only prominent determinants on the surface of a protein are normally recognized by the immune system, and some of these are much more immunogenic than others. Thus, mice immunized with avian lysozyme preferentially respond to a single favored determinant, and much of the remainder of the molecule is virtually nonimmunogenic. Such determinants are said to be immunodominant. In general, the number of antigenic determinants on a molecule is, as might be anticipated, directly related to its size. There is usually about one determinant for each 5000 daltons.

It is perhaps appropriate, therefore, to narrow our definition of foreignness to the recognition of those antigenic determinants not recognized as self.

How to Determine the Size of an Antigenic Determinant

A number of different techniques have been employed to determine the average size of antigenic determinants. One of the most elegant was that of Kabat. Basically this worker made antibodies to dextran, which is an α1-6–linked glucose polymer. He then used various short-chain glucose oligosaccharides to attempt to interfere with the combination between dextran and its antibodies. What he found (Fig. 2–2) was that

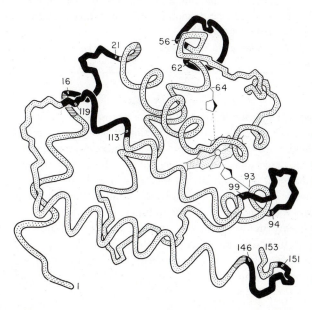

FIGURE 2–1. A schematic diagram showing the structure of sperm-whale myoglobin: The solid black portions represent segments that constitute complete antigenic determinants. The striped portions form part of the antigenic determinant with some antibodies. (From Atassi, M. Z. Immunochemistry, *12:* 435, 1975. With permission).

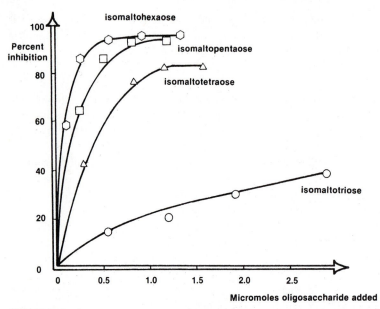

FIGURE 2–2. A demonstration of the inhibitory activities of short oligosaccharides on the ability of antidextran serum to bind to dextrose: Note that maximum inhibition is obtained with the hexaose suggesting that six isomaltose units are approximately the same size as the antigen binding site. (Reprinted with permission from Kabat [1954]. Copyright 1954 American Chemical Society.)

---

monomers and dimers of glucose were ineffective inhibitors, that trimers varied, that tetramers were consistently good inhibitors, but that for maximum inhibition, hexamers were needed. Polymers larger than the hexamer were no more effective than the hexamer. Thus, in this case, six linear glucose residues probably defined the upper size of the antigen binding site. Similar experiments using defined polypeptides indicate that antigenic determinants contain about five amino acids.

Kabat, E. A. The upper limit for the size of the human antidextran combining site. J. Immunol., 84: 82–85, 1960.

Haptens

If a small organic compound is chemically linked to a large antigenic molecule, a new surface structure is formed on the large molecule that may function as an antigenic determinant. If a protein molecule modified in this way is used to immunize an animal, then antibodies to a number of antigenic determinants will be generated. Many of these antibodies will be directed against unaltered determinants on the original antigen, but some will be directed against new antigenic determinants formed by the small organic molecule.

Small molecules or chemical groups that can be made to function as antigenic determinants in this way are called **haptens** (in Greek "aptein" means to "grasp" or "fasten") and the antigenic molecule to which they are attached is called the **carrier.**

By using haptens of known chemical structure, it has proved possible to study in great detail the interaction between antibody and antigenic determinants. For example, antibodies raised against one hapten can be tested for their ability to bind to other chemically and structurally related haptens.

By means of this simple technique, it can be shown that it makes no difference whether the hapten is chemically bound to the carrier or merely bound noncovalently. However, any alteration in the hapten structure that changes its overall three-dimensional conformation reduces its ability to bind antibodies directed against the unmodified hapten. Such alterations include changes in the charge of the hapten, changes in its size, and changes in its shape. Even such very minor chemical modifications as the difference between stereoisomers usually result in significant alterations in molecular shape and will therefore influence the combination of antibody with its hapten (Table 2–2). Since each different hapten has the ability to provoke its own specific antibodies, it is clear that animals must possess the ability to generate an extremely large variety of different antibody molecules in order to account for their ability to respond to such a vast range of potential haptens.

Protein Antigenic Determinants

As pointed out earlier, the immune responses against proteins are directed against prominent antigenic determinants on the surface of the molecules (Fig. 2-1). As with haptens, the spatial folding of the protein polypeptide chain plays a critical role in determining antigenic specificity. For example, the protein lysozyme has an intrachain disulfide bond that folds the peptide chain into a loop (Fig. 2–3). This loop peptide forms an important antigenic determinant. If this loop is removed so that the disulfide bond remains intact, then the detached loop retains its ability to combine with antibodies to lysozyme. If, however, the bond is reduced so that the loop is opened, antibodies will no longer bind to the loop.

This is a very clear demonstration that it is the conformation of a determinant and not its sequence that determines antibody specificity. Indeed, antibodies to native proteins are not usually able to bind to denatured proteins where the peptide chain conformation is drastically altered. It is, perhaps, pertinent to note here that, in order for antigens to provoke an immune response, they must be ingested and processed by cells known as macro-

TABLE 2–2 The Ability of Specific Antisera to Distinguish Between the Stereoisomeric Tartaric Acids

| | Haptens | | |
	l-Tartaric Acid	d-Tartaric Acid	m-Tartaric Acid
	COOH	COOH	COOH
	HOCH	HCOH	HCOH
	HCOH	HOCH	HCOH
Immune Sera Against	COOH	COOH	COOH
l-tartaric acid	+++	±	+
d-tartaric acid	0	+++	+
m-tartaric acid	±	0	+++

SOURCE: Landsteiner, K. The Specificity of Serological Reactions. Dover Publications, New York, 1945 (reprinted 1962).

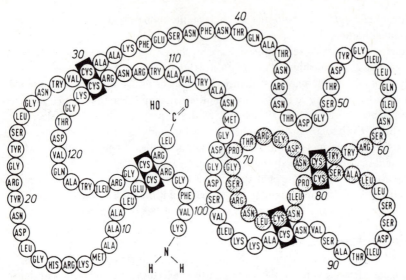

FIGURE 2–3. The amino acid sequence of lysozyme from hen egg white. The region of the "loop" peptide is shaded. This loop functions as an antigenic determinant. (From Arnon, R., and Sela, M. Proc. Natl. Acad. Sci. USA, *62:* 164, 1969. With permission).

phages (Chap. 3). Although the precise mechanisms of this processing are unclear, it is apparent from the discussion above that the conformation of protein antigens must remain unaltered for antibody formation to occur.

Mechanisms Involved in Immune Responses to Haptens and Carriers

It might well be considered that the function of a carrier molecule is merely to transport a hapten into the immune system. However, a simple experiment shows that this is not the case. A hapten linked to its carrier will provoke a primary immune response, but if it is administered a second time on an unrelated carrier protein, a secondary immune response is not provoked. A secondary immune response to a hapten will occur only if it is bound to the same carrier as in the first injection. This phenomenon is known as the **carrier effect.**

This carrier effect can be overcome if mice are first given a mixture of spleen cells, some from mice primed to the hapten and some from mice primed to the unrelated carrier (Fig. 2–4). The implication is that some form of cooperation must take place between cells responding to the hapten and cells responding to the carrier.

How to Show the Carrier Effect

A group of mice are each primed with hapten dinitrophenol (DNP) linked to the carrier protein bovine gamma globulin (BGG). They therefore make anti-DNP antibodies. These animals are then inoculated with either DNP–BGG (i.e., the same hapten and carrier), DNP on ovalbumin (DNP–OA), or with BGG alone. The only secondary

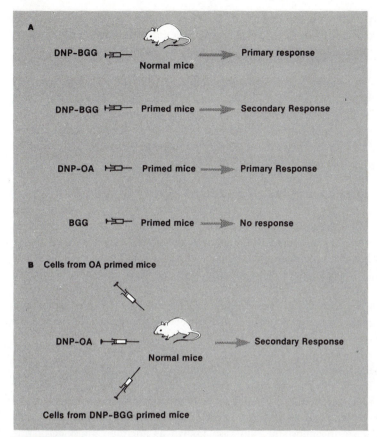

FIGURE 2–4. (**A**) The carrier effect: A secondary response to a hapten (DNP) can be obtained only if it is administered to a primed animal on the same carrier as was used in the priming dose. (**B**) The carrier effect may be overcome by administering hapten together with cells from hapten-primed (DNP–BGG [DNP-bovine gamma globulin]) and carrier-primed (OA [ovalbumin]) animals. When stimulated by DNP–OA (DNP-ovalbumin) the two cell populations cooperate to generate a secondary immune response to the hapten.

response occurs in the animals that were given the same hapten on the same carrier (Fig. 2–4).

Thus, the initiation of an immune response to a hapten-carrier conjugate (a hapten covalently linked to a carrier) requires at least two signals: One signal from the hapten and one from its carrier. This fact is really self-evident; otherwise, a hapten would be able to provoke an immune response on its own. The haptenic determinant is recognized by cells that make antibodies (the B cells; see Chap. 10) while carrier determinants are recognized by cells that either "help" the antibody response or participate in the cell-mediated immune response (the T cells). An antibody response is, therefore, hapten-specific because the B cells react to haptenic determinants. Further analysis of the immune responses to proteins indeed shows that although some determinants are recognized primarily by B cells, others are recognized by T cells. These T cells act as regulatory cells that may either "help" or "suppress" the immune responses. Since these regulatory cells are under genetic control, the net response to any antigen will differ between animals, but clearly represents the final outcome of the opposing affects of helper and suppressor influences. Nevertheless, the larger and more complex a molecule is, the more likely it will possess determinants that can provoke helper cells thereby rendering it more immunogenic. (You can find out more about helpers and suppressor determinants in Chap. 13.)

Some Practical Examples of Hapten-Carrier Conjugation In Vivo

While the concept of haptens and carrier molecules provides the basis for much of our knowledge concerning the specificity of the immune response, haptens may also be of clinical importance. For example, the antibiotic penicillin is a small molecule that is not immunogenic by itself. On being degraded within the body, however, it forms a very reactive "penicilloyl" group, which can bind to serum proteins such as albumin to form penicilloyl–protein conjugates (Fig. 2–5). The penicillin is recognized as a foreign hapten and thus provokes an immune response. Antibodies directed against the penicilloyl hapten are generated, and these may participate in penicillin allergy (Chap. 20).

A second example of naturally occurring reactive chemicals that bind to body proteins and so act as a hapten are the toxic components of poison ivy *(Rhus radicans)*. The resin of this plant, a mixture of complex catechols known as urushiol, will bind to any cells or proteins it comes into contact with. The modified cells or proteins are then regarded as foreign and attacked by lymphocytes in a manner similar to the rejection of a skin graft. The net result is a very uncomfortable skin rash known as allergic contact dermatitis (Chap. 20).

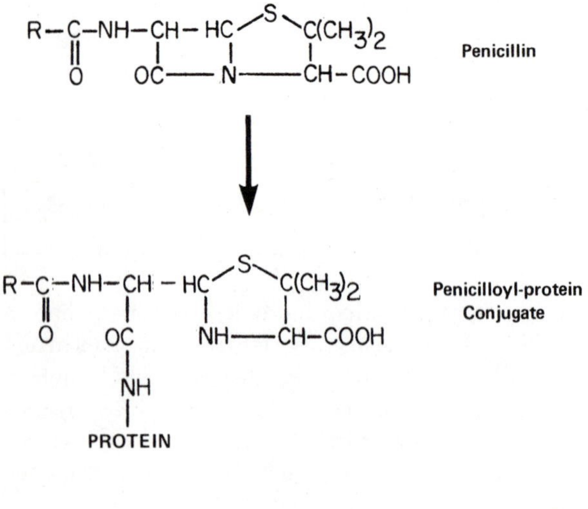

FIGURE 2–5. Penicillin can function as a hapten. In the body, penicillin can be degraded by a number of different pathways. If penicillenic acid is formed, it reacts with protein amino groups to form a penicilloyl-protein complex. At least 95% of the conjugates formed in man are of this type. (From Tizard, I. Veterinary Immunology. 2nd ed. W. B. Saunders, Philadelphia, 1982. With permission.)

Cross-Reactivity

Identical or similar antigenic determinants may sometimes be found on the surface of apparently unrelated molecules. As a result, antibody directed against one antigen may be found to react unexpectedly with antigen from an unrelated source. In addition, within a group of related animal species, the antigenic determinants on a specific protein, for example serum albumin, may differ in only minor respects. Consequently, antibodies directed against a protein in one species may also react in a detectable manner with the homologous protein in another species. Both of these phenomena are known as **cross-reactions.**

There are several good examples of cross-reactions of the first type. For example, many bacteria possess cell-wall polysaccharides in common with mammalian erythrocytes. Thus intestinal bacteria may possess blood-group substances A and B (Chap. 20), and these can be absorbed into the bloodstream. If these antigens are foreign to that individual, an immune response will be provoked. For example, blood-group substance A is foreign to an individual of blood group B. Such an individual will therefore produce anti-A in spite of never having been exposed to red blood cells of blood group A. Cross-reacting antibodies of this type are called **heterophile** antibodies.

A second example of cross-reactivity between antigens from unrelated sources is seen between the relatively avirulent bacterium *Proteus vulgaris* (Strain OX19) and the highly dangerous *Rickettsia typhi,* the cause of typhus. Because of this cross-reactivity (sometimes called the Weil-Felix reaction), it is possible to diagnose typhus simply by detecting the appearance of antibodies to *Proteus vulgaris* in serum and thus avoiding the necessity of exposing laboratory personnel to the very dangerous Rickettsia.

The second type of cross-reactivity, that between related organisms, may be demonstrated in many different biological systems. One example is the method used to detect relationships between animal species. Thus in Table 2–3, it can be shown that antisera to human serum cross-react with all great-ape sera tested and with most of the sera from Old

TABLE 2–3 Relative Amounts of Precipitate Obtained with Rabbit Antihuman Serum and Equal Amounts of Serum from Various Primates

Serum	Precipitate (%)
Human	100
Chimpanzee	130*
Gorilla	64
Orangutan	42
Cyanocephalus mormon	42
Cyanocephalus sphinx	29
Ateles (spider monkey)	29

SOURCE: Nuttall. Blood Immunity and Blood Relationship. Cambridge University Press, Cambridge, 1904.

*Loose precipitate

World monkeys. They react poorly with sera from New World monkeys and marmosets and not at all with lemur serum. Presumably, this phenomenon reflects the relationship between the antigenic determinants and is thus a useful tool in determining phylogenetic relationships.

Some Specific Groups of Antigens

While many different antigens will be described and discussed in later chapters, some general comments may be made here.

As mentioned earlier, proteins are the best antigens because of their size and structural complexity. Almost all proteins with molecular weights of greater than 1000 are antigenic, although some, such as the interferons, are of such uniform structure and so widely distributed among mammals that it is sometimes difficult to make good antisera against them. Many of the major antigens of microorganisms, such as the clostridial toxins, bacterial flagellae, virus capsids, and protozoan cell membranes are all proteins. Others include snake venoms, serum proteins, milk proteins, hormones, and even antibody molecules themselves. The cell-surface antigens responsible for self-recognition and graft rejection, known as **histocompatability antigens,** are also protein in nature (Chap. 3).

Simple polysaccharides such as starch or glycogen are not very good antigens simply because they are structurally mobile and lack complexity. However other, more complex carbohydrates, particularly if bound to proteins, may be of immunological importance. These include the major cell-wall antigens of Gram-negative bacteria, and the blood-group antigens present on erythrocytes. Many of the so-called "natural" antibodies found in the serum of unimmunized animals are directed against polysaccharide antigenic determinants and probably arise as a result of exposure to antigenic material derived from the normal intestinal flora or from food.

Lipids tend to be poor antigens because of their wide distribution, their relative simplicity, and their lack of structural stability. Nevertheless, when linked to proteins or polysaccharides, they may function as antigens.

Because of their relative simplicity and flexibility and also because they are very rapidly degraded, nucleic acids are poor antigens. Nevertheless, it is possible to produce antinucleic acid antibodies by artificially stabilizing and linking them to an immunogenic carrier. It is also noteworthy that autoantibodies to nucleic acids are a characteristic feature of several important autoimmune disorders of man and animals. The most important of these is systemic lupus erythematosus (Chap. 21).

Bacterial Antigens   Bacteria are ovoid or spherical organisms consisting of a cytoplasm containing the essential elements of cell structure surrounded by a cell membrane. The cell membrane is, in turn, covered by a cell wall that, in some bacteria, is enclosed by a capsule. From the cell there may extend flagellae and pili (Fig. 2–6).

The bacterial cytoplasm contains a complex mixture of enzymes and nucleoproteins, many of which are antigenic. Since, however, these are usually confined to the interior of the organism, they are usually less important than the surface antigens in stimulating a protective immune response.

The three major antigenic structures of the bacterial surface are the cell wall, the

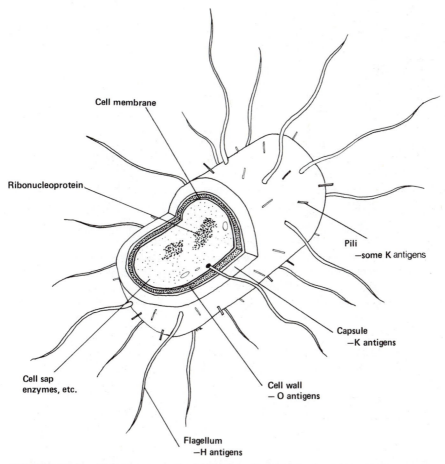

FIGURE 2-6. The structure of a bacterium showing the location of its important antigens. (From Tizard, I. Veterinary Immunology. 2nd ed. W. B. Saunders, Philadelphia, 1982. With permission.)

capsule, and the flagella. The cell wall in Gram-negative organisms is a polysaccharide–lipid–protein structure, but most of its antigenicity is associated with the polysaccharide component. This component consists of an oligosaccharide attached to a lipid (lipid A) and to a series of repeating trisaccharides (Fig. 2–7). The exact composition of these trisaccharides determines the surface antigenicity of the organism and, consequently, many bacteria are classified according to this antigenic structure. For example, the *Salmonellae* are a genus of bacteria that have been classified into about 2000 "species" on this basis. These polysaccharide antigens are called **O antigens.** O antigen number 1 is a trisaccharide with an immunodominant terminal glucose. O antigen number 2 has an immunodominant paratose, and O antigen 3 has mannose, and so on. These cell-wall antigens of Gram-negative bacteria are toxic and are thus also called **endotoxins.**

Bacterial capsules may be either polysaccharide or protein in nature. The polysac-

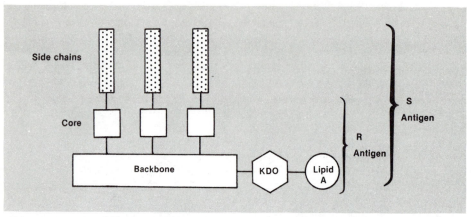

FIGURE 2–7. The basic structure of the lipopolysaccharide from the cell walls of Gram-negative bacteria. KDO is ketodexyoctonic acid. The backbone consists of repeating heptose phosphate units. The core structure consists of glucose and galactose attached to N-acetyl glucosamine. (From Tizard, I. Veterinary Immunology. 2nd ed. W. B. Saunders, Philadelphia, 1982. With permission.)

charides are usually good immunogens, possibly because they contain hexosamines, which seem to be essential for their antigenicity. These capsules serve to protect bacteria against phagocytosis (Chap. 4), and anticapsular antibodies are, therefore, protective to an infected animal. Capsular antigens are collectively known as **K antigens.**

Bacterial flagellae consist of a single protein called flagellin. Flagellin does not usually form a stable configuration unless fixed or polymerized, in which case it is a good antigen. Flagellar antigens are collectively known as **H antigens.**

Another significant group of bacterial antigens are the **exotoxins,** proteins secreted by or derived from bacteria by autolysis. The bacterial exotoxins are good antigens, being highly immunogenic and promoting the production of antibodies known as **antitoxins.** As mentioned in Chapter 1, many exotoxins, when treated with a mild protein-denaturing agent, such as formaldehyde, lose their toxigenicity but retain their antigenicity. Toxins modified in this way are known as toxoids. Toxoids as described in Chapter 1 may be used in the prevention of disease due to toxigenic organisms such as tetanus.

In syphilis, antibodies are found in serum to a complex lipid known as cardiolipin. Why this should be is unclear, but it is believed that cardiolipin is a normal tissue component (it can be extracted from heart muscle), and it probably functions as a hapten once released.

Virus Antigens   Viruses are very small, obligate intracellular organisms that generally consist of a nucleic-acid core surrounded by a layer of repeating protein subunits. This protein layer is termed the capsid and the constituent subunits are called the capsomeres (Fig. 2–8). The capsid proteins are good antigens, well capable of provoking antibodies. Some viruses may be surrounded by an antigenic envelope containing lipoprotein.

Usually viruses are not found free in the circulation but are safely hidden within cells

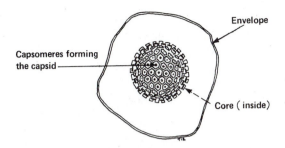

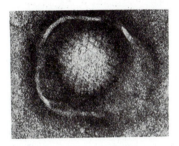

FIGURE 2-8. The structure of a typical virus ($\times$184,000) and the location of important viral antigens. (Equine herpesvirus type 1.) (Courtesy of Dr. J. Thorsen. From Tizard, I. Veterinary Immunology. 2nd ed. W. B. Saunders, Philadelphia, 1982. With permission.)

where they are protected from the unwelcome attentions of antibodies. Some viruses may, however, from within the safety of a cell, induce the production of new proteins on the surface of that cell. These proteins, functioning as antigens, may provoke an immune response against the virus-infected cell.

Cell-Surface Antigens The surface of all mammalian cells consists of a mosaic of protein molecules immersed in a fluid lipid bilayer. Most of these proteins are immunogenic when injected into an animal of another species or even into a different animal of the same species. The important cell-surface antigens may conveniently be divided into two groups. The antigens on erythrocytes are known as **blood-group antigens** and are of vital importance in blood transfusions. The antigens on nucleated cells are known as **histocompatibility antigens** and are of vital importance in the graft rejection process.

Blood-Group Antigens The earliest attempts to transfer blood between unrelated individuals usually met with disaster. The transfused cells were commonly destroyed precipitously even though the recipient had never been transfused previously. On investigation, it was found that the problem was due to the presence of naturally occurring antibodies to antigens on the red blood cells. The most important of these are the antigens of the ABO system (Chap. 20).

Histocompatibility Antigens Nucleated cells, such as leukocytes, possess many cell-surface-protein antigens, which readily provoke an immune response if transferred into a genetically different *(allogeneic)* individual of the same species. Some of these antigens are much more potent than others in provoking an immune response and are, therefore, called the major histocompatibility antigens. These antigens are of such major importance in immunology that they deserve a complete chapter of their own (Chap. 3).

Autoantigens   In some situations (not always abnormal), antibodies and sensitized lymphocytes may be produced in response to normal self-antigens. The range of identified autoantigens is large. They include hormones such as thyroglobulin; structural components such as basement membranes; complex lipids such as myelin; intracellular components such as the mitochondrial proteins, nucleic acids, or nucleoproteins; and cell-membrane antigens, especially hormone receptors. The production of these autoantibodies and the consequence of this production are discussed in detail in Chapter 21.

Some Commonly Used Antigens

The major factors used in selecting experimental antigens are that they be cheap, pure, and available in large quantity.

Bacterial lipopolysaccharide—Usually derived from *E. coli;* a thymus-independent antigen.

Bovine serum albumin—A soluble white protein of reasonable antigenicity.

Flagellin—A protein derived from the flagellae of motile salmonellae. If polymerized, it becomes thymus-independent.

Hemocyanin—A very potent antigenic protein derived from the keyhole limpet *Megathura crenulata.*

Immunoglobulin G—Derived from human blood, this protein is an excellent antigen in experimental animals.

Lysozyme—This protein is derived from egg white. Because its complete structure is well known, it is very useful for careful investigations into the functions of antigenic determinants.

Sheep erythrocytes—Plentiful and inexpensive, washed sheep erythrocytes are potent antigens and used in a wide variety of immunologic techniques. Purists make certain that the sheep are of a specific blood group in order to ensure reproducibility.

Tetanus toxoid—Formalin-treated tetanus toxin. A good antigen also used to protect against tetanus.

TGAL—A multichain synthetic antigen in which tyrosine and glutamic acid residues are attached to alanine side chains on a lysine backbone. Very useful for analyzing the immune responses to defined determinants.

Adjuvants

Under some circumstances, such as in vaccination, it may be considered desirable to enhance the normal immune response. This may be done by administering an **adjuvant** with the antigen (Table 2–4). A large variety of compounds have been employed as adjuvants, although in many cases their mode of action is unclear. The simplest adjuvants are those that function by slowing the release of antigen into the body. As described in Chapter 13, the immune system is antigen-driven. The system responds to the presence of antigen, but ceases to respond once antigen is eliminated. It is possible to slow the rate of antigen release by first mixing it with an insoluble adjuvant to form a "depot." Examples of depot-forming adjuvants include insoluble aluminium salts, such as aluminium hydroxide, aluminium phosphate, and aluminium potassium sulfate (alum). When antigen mixed with

TABLE 2–4   Some Common Adjuvants

Adjuvant	Mode of Action
Aluminium and calcium compounds such as aluminium phosphate	Form slow-release antigen depots
Oil-in-water emulsions such as Freund's complete and incomplete adjuvants	Form slow-release antigen depots. Freund's complete adjuvant makes use of the immunostimulating activities of *Mycobacterium tuberculosis*
Anaerobic corynebacteria such as *Corynebacterium parvum*	Mechanism unknown
Mycobacteria such as B.C.G. with the active fraction known as muramyl dipeptide	Promotes antigen-processing and T-cell-mediated activities
Bordetella pertussis	Acts on both T and B cells and macrophages to promote their activities
Bacterial lipopolysaccharide	B-cell stimulant
Saponin	Unknown
Lysolecithin analogues	
Vitamins A and E	
Polyanions such as dextran sulfate	
Liposomes	

one of these salts is injected into an animal, a macrophage-rich granuloma forms in the tissues. The antigen within this granuloma slowly leaks out into the body and so provides a prolonged antigenic stimulus. Antigens that normally persist for only a few days may be retained in the body for several weeks by means of this technique. Depot adjuvants such as these influence only the primary immune response and have little effect on secondary immune responses.

An adjuvant with a similar mode of action is beryllium sulfate, which also forms a local granuloma when injected with antigen and so enhances antibody formation. This adjuvant has no effect in thymectomized animals and must therefore act to stimulate T cells (Chap. 12); nevertheless, it does not influence cell-mediated immunity. Silica, kaolin, and carbon also promote antibody formation when given with antigen and probably act in a similar fashion.

An alternative method of forming a depot is to incorporate the antigen in a water-in-oil emulsion. The presence of the oil stimulates a local chronic inflammatory response and, as a result, a granuloma forms around the site of the inoculum. The antigen is slowly leached from the aqueous phase of the emulsion. Oil-emulsion droplets may also be carried to other sites through the lymphatic system. If killed tubercle bacilli *(Mycobacterium tuberculosis)* are incorporated into the water-in-oil emulsion, the resulting mixture is known as Freund's complete adjuvant (FCA) and is an extremely potent adjuvant. The active fraction of the tubercle bacilli that enhances this activity is known as muramyl dipeptide (n-acetyl-muramyl-L-alanyl-D-isoglutamine). FCA acts best when given subcutaneously or intradermally, and optimal enhancement is obtained when the antigen dose is relatively low. It acts specifically to stimulate T-lymphocyte function and therefore only enhances responses to thymus-dependent antigens (Chap. 12). FCA promotes IgG production over IgM (Chap. 6). It inhibits tolerance induction, favors delayed hypersensitivity reactions, and accelerates graft rejection as well as promotes resistance to tumors. FCA is required to induce some experimental autoimmune diseases, such as experimental allergic encephalitis and thyroiditis (Chap. 21). It also stimulates macrophages, promoting their phagocytic and cytotoxic activities.

Other bacterial products, in addition to muramyl dipeptide, also possess adjuvant activity. For example, endotoxins enhance antibody formation if given at about the same time as the antigen. They have no effect on delayed hypersensitivity, but they can break tolerance, and they have a general immunostimulatory activity, which is reflected in a non-specific resistance to bacterial infections. Endotoxins may also enhance immune reactivity by promoting **interferon** release from cells (Chap. 13). Anaerobic corynebacteria, especially *Corynebacterium parvum* (whose correct name is *Propionibacterium acnes*) promote antibody formation in a manner similar to that of the endotoxins—that is, they promote B-lymphocyte but not T-lymphocyte activity and enhance macrophage activity. As a result, they have a general immunostimulating action that leads to enhanced antibacterial and antitumor activity.

Bordetella pertussis, the cause of whooping cough in children, also has endotoxinlike activity, but in addition it causes a lymphocytosis in some species and renders rodents highly susceptible to the pharmacological agent histamine. It prolongs and enhances immunological memory and stimulates macrophage activity. *B. pertussis* may selectively enhance IgE production.

Polyribonucleotides consisting of double-stranded nucleic acids such as the copolymer of polyinosinic acid and polycytidilic acid (Poly I:C) act as stimulants of T cells, probably by functioning as interferon inducers.

Certain surface-active agents, such as sodium alginate, lanolin, lysolecithin, vitamin A, saponin, and phospholipid liposomes act on cell membranes to enhance immune reactivity. Their mode of action is unknown, but they may reduce antigen destruction within cells. Polyanions like dextran sulfate or suramin have a similar mode of action.

Compounds that act in an adjuvantlike manner are the immunoenhancing drugs, of which the most widely used is levamisole. Used originally to kill parasitic worms in animals, levamisole appears to function in a manner similar to the thymic hormone thymopoietin (Chap. 9). That is, it stimulates T-lymphocyte differentiation and the response of T lymphocytes to antigens. It also stimulates the phagocytic activities of macrophages and neutrophils. The effects of levamisole are maximal in animals with depressed T-cell function, and it has little or no effect on the immune system of normal animals. Levamisole may, therefore, be of assistance in the treatment of chronic infections and neoplastic diseases, but it may worsen diseases caused by excessive T-cell function.

Sources of Additional Information

Allison, C. A. Mode of action of immunological adjuvants. J. Res., *26:* 619–630, 1979.

Atassi, M. Z. Precise determination of the entire antigenic structure of lysozyme. Immunochemistry, *15:* 909–936, 1978.

Borek, F. Immunogenicity. Frontiers of Biology Series. Elsevier North-Holland, Amsterdam, 1972.

Kabat, E. A. Some configurational requirements and dimensions of the combining site on an antibody to a naturally occurring antigen. J. Am. Chem. Soc., *76:* 3709–3716, 1954.

Landsteiner, K. The Specificity of Serological Reactions, Harvard University Press, Cambridge, 1945.

Mitchison, N. A. The carrier effect in the secondary response to hapten-protein conjugates. II. Cellular cooperation. Eur. J. Immunol., *1:* 18–22, 1971.

Sela, M. Antigenicity: Some molecular aspects. Science, *166:* 1365–1374, 1969.

Sela, M., ed. The Antigens. Academic Press, New York, 1973.

3

Self Antigens: The Major Histocompatibility Complex

When an organ or a portion of tissue is surgically transplanted between two genetically dissimilar individuals of the same species, it usually provokes an immune response that results in the rejection and eventual destruction of the graft. The antigens on cell membranes that are recognized by the recipient as foreign and so provoke graft rejection are called **histocompatibility antigens** and these are found on all nucleated cells.

As pointed out in the first chapter, it is clear that graft rejection is not a natural phenomenon. Nevertheless, it reflects the existence of immune processes that can identify and then eliminate cells possessing histocompatibility antigens that are not recognized as self. These antigens can, therefore, be thought of as specific recognition structures. They act as identity markers for cells and, in this way, influence cell-to-cell interactions.

Each individual animal possesses its own characteristic set of histocompatibility antigens. This set is acquired by inheritance from its parents through the activities of genes that code for the histocompatibility antigens (Fig. 3–1). Studies of the graft rejection process have demonstrated that not all of the histocompatibility antigens possessed by an individual are equally important. Some are much more potent than others in provoking rapid graft rejection. These are called the major histocompatibility antigens and they are inherited together with other important antigens that influence immune responses through the activities of a complex set of genes known as the **major histocompatibility complex (MHC).**

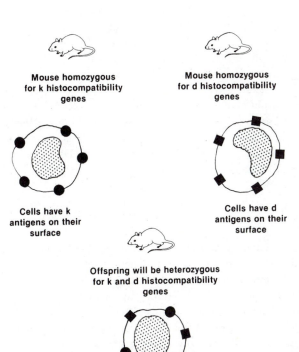

Mouse homozygous
for k histocompatibility
genes

Mouse homozygous
for d histocompatibility
genes

Cells have k
antigens on their
surface

Cells have d
antigens on their
surface

Offspring will be heterozygous
for k and d histocompatibility
genes

Cells will have both k and
d antigens on their surface

FIGURE 3–1. A simple view of the inheritance of histocompatibility antigens: Mice of the CBA/J strain have a k haplotype; mice of the DBA/2 strain have a d haplotype.

The Structure of the Major Histocompatibility Complex (MHC)

In man, the MHC is found on the short arm of chromosome 6, and in mice, it is found on chromosome 17.

Since histocompatibility antigens determine the intensity of the graft rejection process, we can think of the histocompatibility antigens as regulators of the process of graft rejection. Other genes located within the MHC can also be shown to code for proteins that regulate other types of immune responses, including antibody responses. These genes are called **immune-response (Ir) genes.** On further investigation it can be shown that these Ir genes code for protein antigens located on the surface of lymphocytes. These lymphocyte antigens are involved in the recognition of foreign antigens and it is by regulating the expression of these lymphocyte antigens that immune-response genes influence immune reactivity.

A third important class of genes found within the MHC regulates the synthesis of some components of the **complement** system (Chap. 14). (The complement system is a complex interacting set of serum proteins responsible for some aspects of protection against microbial invasion). These genes either code directly for complement proteins or alternatively, regulate their production.

The major histocompatibility complex, therefore, contains three classes of genes. First, genes that code for the production of the major histocompatibility antigens. These are called Class I antigens. Second, genes that code for lymphocyte cell-membrane proteins and thus regulate the immune response. These are called Class II antigens. Finally, there are genes that code for complement proteins. These are classified as Class III antigens. Each MHC studied so far codes for all three classes of antigens, although the number and arrangement of the genes within the complex vary widely. The collective name given to antigens produced by the MHC also varies between species. In humans, these antigens are called HLA standing for **human lymphocyte antigen,** in dogs they are called DLA, in rabbits RLA, in guinea pigs GPLA, and so on. In some species, histocompatibility antigens were identified as blood-group antigens before their role in graft rejection was recognized. In these cases, the nomenclature is anomalous. Thus, in the mouse, the MHC is called H-2, in the rat, it is called AgB or RTI, and in chickens, it is called B.

Class I Antigens

Class I antigens are protein molecules found on the surface of nucleated cells. They regulate the recognition of foreign cells and so influence graft rejection. They are coded for by three distinct gene loci in mice called K, L, and D, and by three loci in man called A, B, and C. In the human system, the Class I antigens were first identified by examining the sera of individuals who had been exposed to foreign histocompatibility antigens; for example, persons who had received multiple blood transfusions. While blood for transfusion is usually carefully matched for red-blood-cell compatibility, no effort is made to match the white blood cells. Thus, the leukocytes in transfused blood may provoke a response in recipients that is directed against their Class I HLA antigens. Alternatively, serum from women who have had many children (multiparous women) can be used, since these women may, over the course of many pregnancies, have gradually developed antibodies to paternal Class I antigens.

Antibodies against the Class I antigens can be used to "type" nucleated cells. (They are, therefore, called **serologically defined (SD) antigens.**) This is an important preliminary step in determining whether an individual will reject an organ graft such as a kidney, liver, or heart. The method used to type Class I antigens is described on page 328.

When the distribution of Class I antigens in individuals and populations and the inheritance of these individual antigens were studied, it eventually proved possible to map the precise location of their genes within the HLA complex. The genes fall into two distinct allelic groups defined by gene loci called A and B. Later, a third set of serologically defined antigens, C, was identified. The gene locus for this group lies between that of A and B.

Although the number of different antigens (alleles) identified at these three loci is still growing, it is clear that HLA-A contains about 20 different antigenic specificities, HLA-B contains about 44 specificities and HLA-C contains about 8 (Table 3–1).

Nomenclature of HLA Specificities

Each A or B antigen is numbered in the order in which it was discovered, irrespective of its locus. Thus we have A1, A2, A3, B5, B7, B8, A9, etc. If the identity of an antigen is tentative but has been discussed at a formal workshop, the suffix *w* is placed after the locus designation, for example, Aw30, Bw27, and so on.

Antigens inherited at the C locus are listed numerically, for example, Cw1, Cw2, and so on.

TABLE 3–1 The Recognized HLA Specificities (Early 1983)

HLA-A	HLA-B	HLA-C	HLA-D	HLA-DR
A1	B5	Cw1	Dw1	DR1
A2	B7	Cw2	Dw2	DR2
A3	B8	Cw3	Dw3	DR3
A9	B10, B12	Cw4	Dw4	DR4
A10	B13	Cw5	Dw5	DR5
A11	B14	Cw6	Dw6	DRw6
Aw19	B15	Cw7	Dw7	DR7
Aw23(9)	Bw16	Cw8	Dw8	DRw8
Aw24(9)	B17		Dw9	DRw9
A25(10)	B18		Dw10	DRw10
A26(10)	Bw21		Dw11	
A28	Bw22		Dw12	
A29	B27			
Aw30	Bw35			
Aw31	B37			
Aw32	Bw38			
Aw33	Bw39			
Aw34	Bw41			
Aw36	Bw42			
Aw43	Bw44-63			

The Structure of Class I Antigens

All Class I antigens identified so far have been found to be single-peptide-chain, membrane-bound glycoproteins of 45,000 daltons noncovalently linked to a molecule of a small protein called β2-microglobulin (Fig. 3–2). The single peptide chain appears to be divided into three regions each of about 100 amino acids bound together by a set of intra-chain disulfide bonds that fold the molecule into three globular units. These units are attached to the cell by a peptide that penetrates the cell membrane and extends for a short distance into the cytoplasm. These Class I molecules are tremendously heterogeneous as reflected by the large number of distinct antigenic specificities found at each locus. This variation stems from modifications in the amino-acid sequence of the region located close to the free (N-terminal) portion of the molecule. (Each amino acid chain has one end with a free amino group, the N-terminus, and the other end with a free carboxyl group, the C-terminus). The C-terminal region has many similarities to one of the regions of an immunoglobulin (antibody) molecule (Chap. 6). It is also very hydrophobic as befits that portion of the molecule attached to the lipids of the cell membrane. The β2 microglobulin molecule found associated with Class I antigens is not polymorphic but probably enhances the immunogenicity of the whole complex structure. However, β2 microglobulin is not coded for by genes in the MHC but is synthesized separately and attaches to the Class I molecules later.

The Class I molecules are usually synthesized at a greater rate than is required by the cell and, as a result, may be found in tissue fluid and serum in association with some membrane lipids. Class I antigens are found on all nucleated cells except those that are very highly differentiated, or very primitive cells in early embryonic life. They are found in highest concentration on the membranes of B cells, T cells, and macrophages. Class I antigens are absent from human erythrocytes, but they are found on mouse erythrocytes.

Class I antigens are capable of provoking a strong antibody response when an animal is exposed to foreign (**allogeneic**) cells. They have been designated, therefore, as serologically defined (SD) molecules to distinguish them from the Class II histocompatibility antigens, which must be identified by their effect on lymphocytes, and are thus called lymphocyte defined (LD) molecules. Each Class I molecule, as we might expect from its large size, bears several different antigenic determinants. Some of these have a unique specificity, as

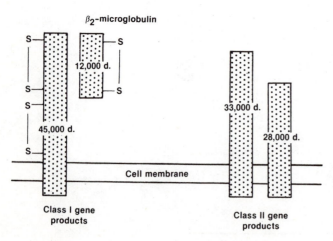

FIGURE 3–2. The basic structure of Class I and Class II histocompatibility antigens. Both have some structural resemblance to immunoglobulins (antibodies). (See also Fig. 6–11.) (From Tizard, I. Veterinary Immunology. 2nd ed. W. B. Saunders, Philadelphia, 1982. With permission.)

described above, and so are called "private" specificities. Others can be found on several different antigens and so are called "public" specificities.

Class II Antigens

When the hapten dinitrophenol (DNP) conjugated to a poly-L-lysine carrier (DNP-PLL) was injected into guinea pigs with an appropriate adjuvant it was found that some animals made antibodies to the DNP (responders) while other (nonresponders) did not.

When the nonresponder guinea pigs were bred together it was found that all their progeny were also nonresponders. On breeding the responders together, it was found that their offspring could be divided into two groups, one of responders and one of nonresponders. When nonresponders were bred with heterozygous responders, their offspring were equally divided into the two groups. Thus the response to DNP-PLL in guinea pigs is under the control of a single dominant gene, which, since it is not sex-linked, must therefore be autosomal (Table 3–2).

Further studies on these animals showed that while responders could respond to any hapten linked to PLL, nonresponders could not. This finding indicated that this gene controlled the recognition of the PLL carrier. Nonresponders could respond well to DNP linked to alternative carriers such as bovine serum albumin or ovalbumin.

A similar phenomenon also occurs in mice when the synthetic branched chain copolymer TGAL is used as an antigen (p. 26). When TGAL in Freund's complete adjuvant was injected into two strains of inbred mice known as CBA and C57Bl, the CBA mice mounted very poor antibody responses while the C57Bl mice made very good antibody responses. Crosses between the two strains made an intermediate response. Breeding studies similar to those described above for guinea pigs showed that the response to TGAL was under the control of a single gene. Since the response of mice to some other synthetic antigens was also shown to be controlled by the same gene, it was named immune response-1 (Ir-1).

When a large number of different mouse strains were tested for possession of Ir-1, it soon became obvious that it was consistently associated with certain histocompatibility antigens. (The set of histocompatibility antigens coded by an individual chromosome is known as its **haplotype** [Table 3–3]. To be precise, therefore, Ir-1 is associated with certain haplotypes.) In order to prove that Ir-1 was in fact part of the mouse MHC (called H-2), use was made of mice with a well-defined genetic background. Mice that are genetically iden-

TABLE 3–2 Response of Strain 13 and Strain 2 Guinea Pigs and Their Crosses to DNP-poly-L-lysine

Strain or Cross	Reaction*
2	+
13	−
(2 × 13) F1	+
(2 × 13) F1 × 13	50%+ 50% −
(2 × 13) F1 × 2	50%+ 50% −

*Plus sign indicates responsiveness.

TABLE 3-3 Some Important Mouse Haplotypes

Strain	Haplotype	Region of H-2 Complex			
		K	**I**	**S**	**D**
A/J	a	k	k	d	d
C57B1/10	b	b	b	b	b
CBA/J	k	k	k	k	k
B10.BYR	by1	q	k	d	b
DBA/z	d	d	d	d	d
AKM	m	k	k	k	q

The term haplotype is used to describe the set of alleles possessed by an animal. Thus the H-2 haplotype is the set of alleles within the mouse MHC. Table 3-3 shows the H-2 haplotype of some important mouse strains.

tical except for the genes within their H-2 region are called H-2 congenic. In these mice, the immune response to TGAL still varied according to the mouse's H-2 haplotype. This demonstrated that Ir-1 was in the H-2 region. It was then localized within that region by using H-2 "recombinant" mice—these are mice with known differences between their H-2 haplotypes. In this way, the Ir-1 gene was eventually found to be located between the K and S gene regions (Fig. 3–3).

A large number of other antigens have now been shown to be under Ir gene control in mice. When cells from pairs of mice that differ only at their Ir region (Ir congenic mice) are used for reciprocal immunization, the antibodies that result are directed against glycoprotein antigens found on the surface of B cells, most macrophages, dendritic cells, and a small proportion of T cells. These antigens are called Ia antigens. By careful analysis, Ia antigens may be classified into subgroups and can, therefore, be used to identify subregions within the I region. For example, the mouse I region is divided into at least four subregions, I-A, I-J, I-E, and I-C. (A reported fifth subregion, I-B, is probably an artifact.)

Clearly, the discovery that Ir genes influence the production of Ia antigens raises the question whether Ia antigens are in fact the Ir gene products. Evidence has gradually accumulated to show that this is the case. For example, antisera directed against specific Ia

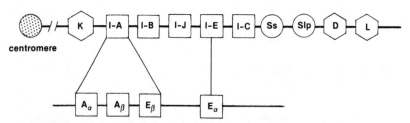

FIGURE 3–3. The structure of the H-2 gene complex in the mouse. Loci coding for Class I antigens are denoted by hexagons, loci coding for Class II antigens by squares, and loci coding for Class III antigens by circles. Three polypeptides have been shown to be coded for by genes in the I-A region and one by genes in the I-E region. Aα and Aβ chains tend to associate as do Eα and Eβ to form the classic Ia antigens. The existence of I-B is suspect as is the precise location of I-J. (See box on page 37.)

glycoproteins can be used to block the immune response to other antigens in responder animals.

Ia Antigens

Ia antigens are glycoproteins consisting of two noncovalently linked polypeptide chains, one, the α chain, has a molecular weight of 35,000 while the weight of the β chain is between 26 and 28,000 daltons, Ia antigens do not contain $\beta 2$ microglobulin (Fig. 3–2). Like the Class I molecules, Ia antigens show complex antigenic variability as well as private and public antigenic specificities. This variability appears to be restricted to the β chain, while the α chain is relatively invariant. Three distinct peptides have been identified as being coded for by I-A subregion genes, namely A_{α}, A_{β} and E_{β}. The peptide E_{α} is coded by a gene in the I-E subregion (Fig. 3–3). A_{α} and A_{β} peptides come together to make an I-A molecule, E_{α} and E_{β} peptides make an I-E molecule, while the genes in the I-J subregion code for a molecule that is not yet clearly defined.

You can read more about Ia antigens in Chapter 10 where their distribution on T lymphocytes is described, in Chapter 11 where their role in regulating the antibody response is described, and in Chapter 13, where the role of I-J coded products in suppressor-cell function is discussed.

I-J Genes

Throughout this book the reader will encounter a number of references to proteins coded for by genes in the I-J subregion. For example, these proteins have been associated with suppressor T cells and the suppressive factors derived from them. The reader could, therefore, be forgiven for believing that their existence was well established. Unfortunately, when the complete I region of the mouse MHC was cloned and characterized it was found to contain I-A and I-E subregion genes but little else. There appears to be insufficient space to code for either I-J or I-B. I-B has been under suspicion for a long time and its loss was widely anticipated but I-J has been firmly established and its loss would cause much confusion in immunological circles. It may well be that the I-J genes are uniquely different, but this remains to be demonstrated.

You can find the details in: Steinmetz, M., et al. A molecular map of the immune response region from the major histocompatibility complex of the mouse. Nature, *300:* 35–42, 1982.

Human Class II Gene Loci and Immune Response Genes

Humans, clearly, do not lend themselves to the type of breeding experiments described above for guinea pigs and mice, and it has not proved possible to directly demonstrate the occurrence of immune-response genes in man. The existence of these genes, however, has been clearly demonstrated by indirect methods.

The serological methods of tissue typing described previously identified the Class I histocompatibility antigens. There is, however, an alternative method for testing for histocompatibility by mixing the lymphocytes from two **allogeneic** individuals together in culture. Each set of lymphocytes recognizes the other set as foreign and responds by proliferation. The intensity of this proliferation is directly related to the antigenic disparity between the two individuals and can be readily measured by measuring the uptake of thymidine in the cell culture. Only dividing cells take up thymidine. If the thymidine is labelled with the radioactive isotope of hydrogen, tritium (^{3}H), then this uptake can be easily measured. The uptake of ^{3}H-thymidine is directly proportional to the amount of cell division. (Since both lymphocyte populations proliferate, the results of these mixed lymphocyte cultures are difficult to analyze unless one population is rendered incapable of responding, either by irradiation or by exposure to a cytotoxic drug such as mitomycin C.)

When mixed lymphocyte cultures (MLCs) as described above were conducted between the cells of a large number of different humans, their interrelationships and inheritance could be studied. It became clear that lymphocytes proliferate not in response to the SD histocompatibility antigens but in response to a distinct group of lymphocyte-defined (LD) antigens. Thus individuals identical at the A, B, or C loci could still give a positive MLC while, on other occasions, A-, B-, or C-dissimilar individuals failed to give a significant MLC. In man, these LD antigens are inherited through genes in a region known as D located on the centromeric side of the Class I loci (Fig. 3–4). Eight provisional D antigenic specificities have been identified in this way and labelled HLA-Dw1, HLA-Dw2, and so on.

The MLC is a much more difficult test to conduct than to the antibody-mediated cytotoxic tests. Attempts were, therefore, made to identify HLA-D antigens by serological techniques. Thus, for example, the sera of women who had several children were tested for their ability to block the mixed lymphocyte reaction between HLA-A-, B-, and C-identical lymphocytes. (Multiparous women will eventually develop antibodies against the father's histocompatibility antigens since these will be present on the fetus.) When inhibition was observed, it was assumed that antibodies were blocking a structure associated with the MLC-inducing determinants. When the patterns of this blocking activity were studied in several lymphocyte populations, they were shown not to correspond to the distribution of HLA-A, B, or C.

While these serologically defined antigens may indeed be the products of D genes, this has been difficult to prove conclusively. For this reason, the major antigens have been called DR (D-related). There are eight defined antigens in this series and is possible to show that a good correlation exists between DR and D specificities. This correlation is recognized by assigning the same numbers to related products. Thus DRw1 antisera blocks the MLC against cells bearing HLA-Dw1, and so on. DR antigens consist of three linked polypeptide chains DR$_\alpha$, DR$_\beta$ and DR$_\gamma$. DR$_\gamma$ is synthesized in excess and may be found free in serum. The α chain is closely related to the immunoglobulin-heavy chains (p. 92). DR antigens do not contain $\beta2$ microglobulin and are found mainly on B cells and macrophages. Associated with the D/Dr locus are at least two other loci. SB (Secondary B locus) located centromeric to DR, and DC located between DR and the Class III locus B/Bf. The gene products of these three loci are probably the human equivalent of mouse Ia

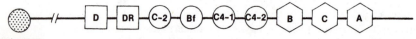

centromere

FIGURE 3–4. The arrangement of gene loci within the HLA gene complex. The Class I, II, and III loci are denoted as in Figure 3–3.

TABLE 3–4   Association Between the Presence of Certain HLA Antigens and Disease

Disease	Antigen	Frequency in Controls (%)	Frequency in Patients (%)
Ankylosing spondylitis	B27	9.4	90
Reiter's syndrome	B27	9.4	79
Rheumatoid arthritis	DRw4	28.4	70
Psoriasis	B13	4.4	18
Celiac disease	Dw3	26.3	79
Myasthenia gravis	B8	24.6	57
Systemic lupus erythematosus	B8	24.6	41
Juvenile diabetes	Dw2	25.8	0
Tuberculosis	B8	20	57
Multiple sclerosis	B35	14.6	70
"Short ragweed" allergy	Dw2	22	98

SOURCE: Svejgaard, A., et al. The HLA system: An introductory survey. S. Karger, Basel, 1979. With permission.

antigens. Thus DR antigens share sequence homology with I-E and the DC α chain is homologous with mouse I-A α chain.

In order to show that the D or DR genes function as human immune-response genes, it is necessary to resort to indirect evidence. One method is to look for associations between the D/DR phenotype and disease prevalence. If these genes do control immune responsiveness, then they would be expected to influence resistance or susceptibility to infectious or immunological diseases. Many associations, however, appear to be linked to the Class I B locus. For example, it has been found that there is a very close association between the development of the arthritic condition of the spine known as ankylosing spondylitis and possession of HLA-Bw27. Up to 90 percent of patients with ankylosing spondylitis are Bw27-positive, while only 8 percent of normal controls are. This disease appears to be related in some way to an immune response to *Klebsiella* and may, therefore, be influenced by the immune-response genes to this organism.

Other important associations between disease and histocompatibility antigens are shown in Table 3–4.

Class III Antigens

Within the major histocompatibility complex of all species investigated so far is a locus that contains genes that code for some complement components and a number of related proteins. (The complement system is described in detail in Chap. 14.)

In mice, this gene locus (called S) controls the level of a class of proteins collectively known as SS. There are two major proteins in this class. One (called SS when it was first recognized) is called C4, the fourth component of mouse complement. The other protein is called Slp. Mice that make both proteins are "SS-high." Mice that only make C4 are "SS-low." The production of Slp is sex linked in some strains of mice; that is, it is only found in males (Slp–sex-linked protein) since in these strains the Slp gene is regulated by testosterone. However, in other SS-high strains, testosterone is not a requirement and Slp is present in mice of both sexes.

The genes for C4 and Slp are discrete but closely linked and both proteins have a very similar structure. C4 and Slp are discussed in more detail in Chapter 14.

C1, C4 and C2 (three different components of the complement system) levels are also controlled by genes located within the S region. There is also a gene in this region that controls the ontogeny of the C3 receptor.

In humans, two genes have been found within the MHC that coded for what were first believed to be blood-group antigens known as Chido and Rogers (after the names of the individuals in whom they were first detected). It was subsequently shown that these antigens are plasma proteins absorbed onto red blood cells. Chido and Rogers antigens are in fact variants of the C4 molecule (C4A and C4B, respectively). This region also contains a gene locus known as Bf coding for factor B of the alternate pathway.

Other Genes that May Be Considered Part of the MHC

The MHC is, as we have seen, a region in which are grouped a number of genes that influence cell–cell interaction. The boundaries of this complex are arbitrary, however, and there are a number of genes located just outside the conventional MHC that may, with some justification, be considered part of it (Fig. 3–5). Thus, in mice, the Qa and Tla locus are found to the right of the D and L class I loci. They code for proteins found on the surface of regulatory and immature lymphocytes, respectively. These proteins each consist of a membrane-bound peptide of 44,000 daltons associated with β2 microglobulin, and both appear to be closely related to the Class I antigens. (Humans also appear to have Qa and Tla-like cell-surface antigens.) (Tla and Qa antigens are discussed further in Chap. 9.)

If we consider that the MHC functions as the genetic regulator of cell–cell interactions, it is perhaps logical to expand our ideas to consider whether it also influences animal–animal interactions. Evidence has accumulated to suggest that this is, in fact, the case. For example, mice prefer to mate with histocompatible mice when given a choice, and it can be shown that this preference is mediated through characteristic urinary odors. The precise mechanisms are unclear but this preference may be of some evolutionary consequence since a selection for histocompatibility in breeding would eventually lead to homozygosity at this locus, the advantages of which are unclear.

Arrangement of Genes within the MHC

Every mammal studied in sufficient detail has been shown to possess a major histocompatibility complex containing various arrangements of Class I, II, and III loci. In man,

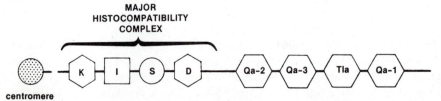

FIGURE 3–5. Four gene loci that code for cell membrane antigens of similar structure to the major histocompatibility antigens are located close to the MHC. They probably serve a similar regulatory function since they are found on lymphocyte membranes.

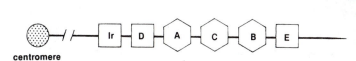

FIGURE 3–6. The probable arrangement of the canine MHC. The DLA system shows obvious similarities to the HLA and H-2 systems.

the arrangement of the HLA complex is shown in Figure 3–4, and the loci are arranged in the order II, III, and I from the centromere. In mice, by contrast, although the overall order is the same (Fig. 3–3), one class I locus (K) is moved toward the centromeric side of the complex. In dogs, another species that has been fairly well investigated, the order is II, I, II (Fig. 3–6). A class III locus has not yet been described in this species.

Sources of Additional Information

Bach, F. H., and Van Rood, J. J. The major histocompatibility complex: genetics and biology. N. Engl. J. Med., *295:* 806–813, 872–878, 927–936, 1976.

Benacerraf, B. The role of the major histocompatibility gene complex in genetic regulation of immune responsiveness. Transpl. Proc., *9:* 825–831, 1977.

Cunningham, B. A. The structure and function of histocompatibility antigens. Sci. An., *237:* 96–107, 1977.

Dausset, J., and Svejgaard, A. HLA and disease. Munksgaard, Copenhagen, 1977.

Festenstein, H., and Demant, P. Basic immunogenetics, biology and clinical relevance. Current Topics in Immunology, Vol. 9. Edward Arnold, London, 1978.

Klein, J. Biology of the Mouse Histocompatibility-2 Complex. Springer-Verlag, New York, 1975.

Makoba, M. W., et al. HLA-DR products are a subset of human Ia antigens. Nature, *301:* 531–532, 1983.

Murphy, D. B., et al. A new I subregion (I-J) marked by a locus (Ia-4) controlling surface determinants on an suppressor T lymphocytes. J. Exp. Med., *144:* 699–712, 1975.

Schreffler, D. C., and David, C. S. The H-2 major histocompatibility complex and the I immune response region: genetic variation, function and organization. Adv. Immunol., *20:* 125–195, 1975.

Svejgaard, A., et al. The HLA System: An Introductory Survey. S. Karger, Basel, 1979.

Yokoyama, K., and Nathenson, S. G. Intramolecular organization of Class I H-2 MHC antigens; localization of the alloantigenic determinants and the $\beta 2M$ binding site to different regions of the H-2K^b glycoprotein. J. Immunol., *130:* 1419–1423, 1983.

4

Cells that Trap Foreign Material

Animals must face the problem of permitting the free access of nutrients and oxygen to body tissues while, at the same time, excluding potentially dangerous foreign material. In order to solve this problem, a variety of different protective mechanisms have been developed, most of which function at body surfaces (Chap. 15). There have also developed, within the body, systems that can trap and destroy any foreign material that has succeeded in evading the outer defenses. These trapping systems act by means of cells that catch, ingest, and destroy foreign particles in a process called **phagocytosis** (from Greek words meaning "eating by cells").

The process of phagocytosis was discovered by the Russian scientist Elie Metchnikoff in 1882. He showed that mobile cells within the body cavity of starfish larvae would attempt to ingest foreign material inserted into them. He promptly suggested that this was a general phenomenon and that phagocytic cells were essential components of the defense system of all animals. Unfortunately, Metchnikoff also suggested, undiplomatically, that antibodies were only of minor importance. This suggestion, of course, provoked violent controversy, a controversy that lasted well into the twentieth century until the warring factions were reconciled by the discovery of opsonins by an Englishman called Almroth Wright in 1904. (Opsonins, antibodies that enhance phagocytosis, are discussed on p. 45).

The phagocytic cells of animals belong to two complementary systems. One system, the myeloid system, consists of rapidly acting cells that are extremely efficient at phagocytosis but which are incapable of sustained effort. These cells therefore constitute a first line of defense. The second system, the mononuclear-phagocytic system, consists of slowly acting phagocytic cells. These cells are capable of repeated phagocytosis and can process antigens in order to initiate immune responses. The mononuclear phagocytic system constitutes a second line of defense.

The Myeloid System

The predominant phagocytic cells in blood are known as polymorphonuclear neutrophil granulocytes (neutrophils, or PMNs for short). These cells are **polymorphonuclear** since their nuclei have a very irregular shape (Fig. 4–1). They are **neutrophils** since their cytoplasmic granules stain with neither acidic nor basic dyes, and they are **granulocytes** since their cytoplasm is full of granules.

Neutrophils are formed in the bone marrow; they migrate to the bloodstream where they spend about twelve hours and then enter tissues where they live for a few days before dying. They constitute about 60 to 70% of all the white cells in human blood.

The Structure of Neutrophils

Neutrophils, when suspended in blood, are round cells, about 12 to 14 μm in diameter. They possess an abundant cytoplasm, in the center of which is a complex nucleus. This nucleus consists of a series of rounded nuclear lobes joined by thinner segments. These segments usually develop as the neutrophil ages.

The cytoplasm of neutrophils contains a large number of granules, which fall into two distinct classes. Primary granules are electron-dense bodies that contain a number of important enzymes, such as myeloperoxidase and acid hydrolases. Secondary granules,

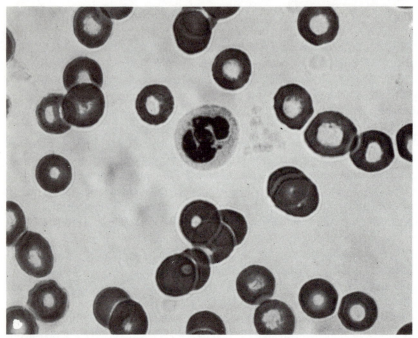

FIGURE 4–1. A neutrophil polymorphonuclear granulocyte in a blood smear. (Wright-Giemsa stain; original magnification ×1400.) (From Bellanti, J. A. Immunology II. W. B. Saunders, Philadelphia, 1979. With permission.)

which predominate in mature neutrophils, are electron-lucent bodies that contain enzymes such as alkaline phosphatase, lysozyme, and aminopeptidase (Fig. 4–2).

Neutrophils possess neither a rough endoplasmic reticulum nor a Golgi structure. Absence of these systems indicates that neutrophils can neither produce nor secrete protein. Neutrophils contain a small number of mitochondria.

Functions of Neutrophils

The major function of neutrophils is the destruction of foreign particles through the process of phagocytosis. This process is best understood by arbitrarily dividing it into several stages. It must, however, be emphasized that the phagocytic process is a continuum (Fig. 4–3).

Chemotaxis The first stage in the phagocytic process is the directed movement of neutrophils under the influence of various external chemical stimuli. This movement is called **chemotaxis.** Thus, neutrophils are attracted by many bacterial products, by factors released from damaged cells, and by the products of several reactions involving antibodies, antigens, and complement (a plasma enzyme system described in Chap. 14). Thus, by means of chemotaxis, neutrophils arrive in the vicinity of bacterial invasion, tissue damage, and immune reactions.

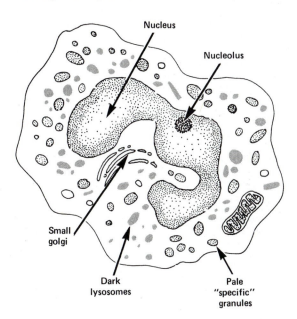

FIGURE 4-2. The basic structural features of a neutrophil polymorphonuclear granulocyte. (From Tizard, I. Veterinary Immunology. 2nd ed. W. B. Saunders, Philadelphia, 1982. With permission.)

Chemotaxis is initiated by the binding of chemoattractants to neutrophil cell membrane receptors. This binding provokes a complex series of biochémical events that include changes in ion fluxes and membrane phospholipids and the production of prostaglandins and leukotrienes. The process culminates in a local reorganization of the cytoskeleton, which causes the cells to alter their morphology and migrate along the chemotactic gradient.

Attachment   Once a neutrophil encounters a foreign particle, it must adhere firmly to it. Attachment is not a spontaneous event, since particles suspended in body fluids usually have a net negative charge (known as the zeta potential) and hence repel each other. If adherence is to take place, this zeta potential must be neutralized. One way of neutralizing the zeta potential is to coat the foreign particle with positively charged protein. A good example of such a protein is antibody. An antibody-coated particle has no net surface charge and can, therefore, come into contact with a neutrophil (Fig. 4-4). Complement proteins and the plasma protein fibronectin (see p. 59) have a similar effect. The attachment between neutrophils and antibody- or complement-coated particles is also facilitated by specific receptors for complement and antibody on the neutrophil membrane.

The process of coating a particle in order to enhance phagocytosis is known as opsonization. Material which does this coating is known as **opsonin** (the Greek word "opson" means "a sauce"; i.e., something used to make food more palatable).

A second important mechanism that facilitates attachment between a particle and a phagocytic cell is physical trapping. Normally, when a neutrophil approaches a free-floating particle, they just float apart before contact can be made. In tissues, however, particles may be trapped between neutrophils and any other surfaces and therefore be readily ingested. This process is called surface phagocytosis.

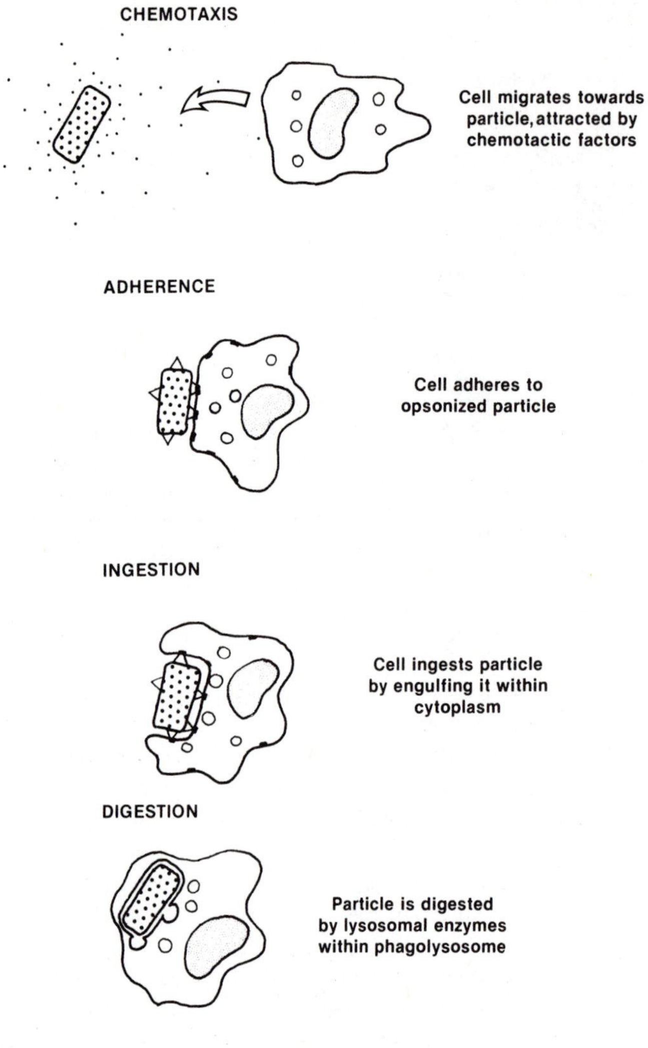

CHEMOTAXIS

Cell migrates towards particle, attracted by chemotactic factors

ADHERENCE

Cell adheres to opsonized particle

INGESTION

Cell ingests particle by engulfing it within cytoplasm

DIGESTION

Particle is digested by lysosomal enzymes within phagolysosome

FIGURE 4–3. The basic steps in the phagocytic process. (From Tizard, I. Veterinary Immunology. 2nd ed. W. B. Saunders, Philadelphia, 1982. With permission.)

Ingestion   Once a foreign particle is attached firmly to the neutrophil membrane, a series of events occurs that results in the particle being engulfed by the neutrophil. The initiating event involves binding to specific cell receptors and is followed by local membrane synthesis. The cytoplasm of the neutrophil flows over and around the particle, enclosing it completely (Fig. 4–5). The process requires the expenditure of energy and extensive changes in cytoplasmic microfilaments and microtubules. The ease with which ingestion occurs depends, in part, on the nature of the surface of the particle. For example, it is essential that the particle be more hydrophobic than the neutrophil. Highly hydrophobic bacteria such as *Mycobacterium tuberculosis* are spontaneously taken into cells with very little effort. In contrast, *Streptococcus pneumoniae,* the cause of lobar pneumonia in man, possesses a carbohydrate capsule that is very hydrophilic. As a result, this organism nor-

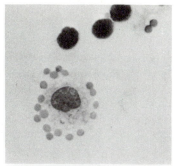

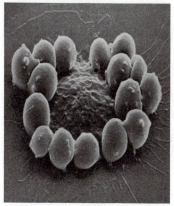

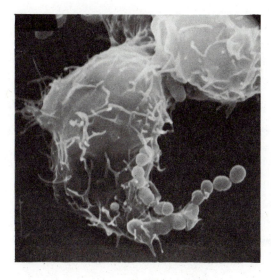

FIGURE 4-4. A light and scanning electron micrographs of guinea-pig macrophages that have been allowed to settle on a glass coverslip for one hour before fixation. They are surrounded each by a rosette of erythrocytes coated with antibody and attached to the cell through specific receptors. (Original magnification: top, ×900; bottom, × 1700.) (From Tizard, I. R., Holmes, W. L., and Parapally, N. P. J. Reticuloendothel. Soc., *16:* 225–231, 1974. With permission.)

FIGURE 4-5. A scanning electron micrograph of a neutrophil polymorphonuclear granulocyte ingesting a chain of streptococci: Note how a film of neutrophil cytoplasm appears to flow over the surface of the organism. (Original magnification ×5000).

mally resists phagocytosis. Fortunately, opsonizing antibodies and complement components render the organism hydrophobic and thus promote its engulfment.

Digestion   A particle ingested by a neutrophil finds itself in a potential cavity known as a phagosome. Here it is subject to attack through a process known as the **respiratory burst.**

The Respiratory Burst

When a particle binds to a neutrophil surface, a set of biochemical reactions is initiated that causes the cell to increase its oxygen consumption. This is known as the respiratory burst. The initiating event is a stimulation of the hexose-monophosphate shunt. This pathway converts glucose-6-phosphate to pyruvate, generating, as it does so, large quantities of reduced nicotinamide adenine dinucleotide phosphate ($NADPH_2$). When the $NADPH_2$ is converted back to NADP the recycling process generates highly toxic oxygen metabolites. These include singlet oxygen, hydrogen peroxide, hydroxyl radicals, chloramines, and aldehydes. All of these effectively kill bacteria (Fig. 4–6).

The two major enzymes involved in the generation of these oxygen metabolites are myeloperoxidase and superoxide dismutase. While their relative importance is debated, animals genetically deficient in either enzyme are highly susceptible to bacterial invasion and disease. (See p. 60). The respiratory burst is thus the major pathway of bacterial killing within phagocytic cells.

The primary granules of neutrophils contain potent hydrolytic enzymes. When a particle is ingested by a neutrophil, these granules migrate through the cytoplasm and fuse

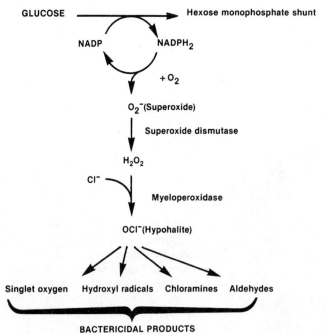

FIGURE 4–6. The respiratory-burst pathway in neutrophils: Catalase probably substitutes for myeloperoxidase in macrophages.

with the phagosome. The hydrolytic enzymes are therefore "emptied" into the phagosome where they proceed to destroy ingested bacteria. These enzymes (Table 4–1) include lysozyme, which can digest some bacterial carbohydrates, proteolytic enzymes including cathepsins, and collagenases, lipases, and ribonucleases. The action of these enzymes thus complements the activities of the respiratory burst. They are, however, probably more important in destroying dead bacteria than in killing living organisms.

The combined activities of the respiratory burst and the lysosomal enzymes is usually lethal for most organisms. But, as might be expected, variations in susceptibility are observed. Gram-positive organisms susceptible to lysozyme are rapidly destroyed. Gram-negative bacteria, such as *Escherichia coli*, persist somewhat longer, since their outer cell wall is relatively resistant to digestion. Some bacteria, such as *M. tuberculosis* and *Listeria monocytogenes* are so resistant to the lethal effects of neutrophils that they may multiply within them.

The Fate of Neutrophils

Neutrophils possess only a limited supply of energy, which they are unable to replenish. Thus, although neutrophils may be very active, they are rapidly exhausted and are usually capable of no more than a single phagocytic event. Thus, neutrophils serve as a first line of defense, rapidly moving toward and ingesting foreign material. If the neutrophils are unable to control an invading organism, a second line of defense must be called into action—the mononuclear phagocytic system. If, however, neutrophils completely eliminate

TABLE 4–1   Some Enzymes Found within the Lysosomes of Phagocytic Cells*

Enzymes acting on proteins and peptides	Cathepsins
	Collagenases
	Elastases
	Plasminogen activator
	Kininogen activator
	Acid phosphatase
Enzymes acting on lipids	Phospholipases
	Aryl sulfatase
Enzymes acting on carbohydrates	Lysozyme
	Neuraminidase
	Glucosidases
	Galactosidases
	Hyaluronidase
Enzymes acting on nucleic acids	Acid ribonuclease
	Acid deoxyribonuclease
Enzymes of the respiratory burst	Myeloperoxidase
	Superoxide dismutase
	Catalase

*More than 60 of these enzymes are known.

foreign material, there will be no stimulus and no necessity for an immune response. Thus neutrophils do not prepare antigens to stimulate the immune system.

Eosinophils

The second major cell type found within the myeloid system is the **eosinophil,** so called because its cytoplasm is rich in granules having an affinity for the acidic dye, eosin (Fig. 4–7).

Eosinophils, like neutrophils, are produced in the bone marrow. They require up to six days to mature before being released into the bloodstream where they circulate with a half-life of only 30 minutes. They then move into tissues where they have a half-life of twelve days.

Eosinophils are similar to neutrophils in that they are capable of phagocytosis and of destroying foreign particles. They are, however, less efficient in these respects than neutrophils and clearly have more specialized functions. One of these functions is to regulate inflammatory processes (Chap. 5). The other major function is to attack and destroy migrating parasitic-worm (helminth) larvae. (The larvae of many parasitic helminths undergo a tissue-migration stage usually from the intestine to the muscles or to the respiratory tract). Migrating larvae are subject to attack by both neutrophils and eosinophils. These larvae are usually many times larger than the attacking cells and hence cannot be phagocytosed. The phagocytic cells must therefore be content to adhere to the larvae and

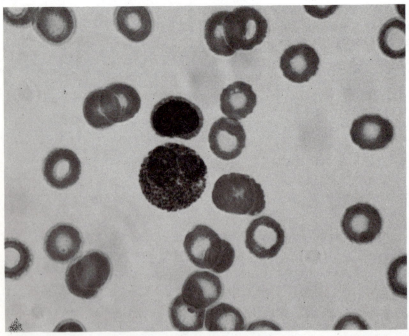

FIGURE 4–7. An eosinophil granulocyte and a lymphocyte from peripheral blood. (Wright-Giemsa stain; original magnification ×1400. (From Bellanti, J. A. Immunology II. W. B. Saunders, Philadelphia, 1979. With permission.)

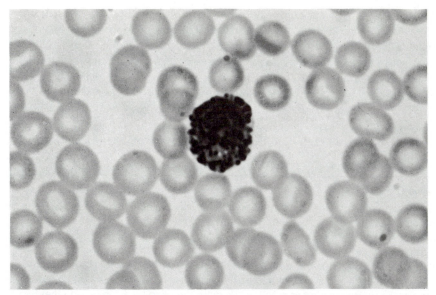

FIGURE 4–8. A basophil granulocyte from peripheral blood (Wright-Giemsa stain; original magnification ×1400): Note the intensely basophilic granules. (From Bellanti, J. A. Immunology II. W. B. Saunders, Philadelphia, 1979. With permission.)

secrete their enzymes onto the larval cuticle. The enzymes of eosinophils as well as the products of their respiratory burst appear to be especially effective in killing and disrupting these helminth larvae. This activity is very inefficient since it may cause severe damage to surrounding tissues.

Basophils

Basophils are so called because their cytoplasmic granules stain intensely with basophilic dyes, such as hematoxylin. These cells constitute only about 0.5% of blood leukocytes, and little is known about their production, distribution, or life span. They appear to be functionally related to mast cells (Chap. 20), even though they are part of the myeloid cell population (Fig. 4–8). Their granules contain vasoactive amines, such as histamine and serotonin; the presence of these substances suggests that the major function of basophils is probably the generation of acute inflammation (Chap. 5). As pointed out earlier, this inflammation is moderated by eosinophils, whose granules contain enzymes capable of neutralizing the vasoactive factors released by basophils (Fig. 20–7).

The Mononuclear Phagocytic System

Macrophages

Neutrophils are not capable of sustained phagocytic activity, they cannot process antigen in preparation for an immune response, nor can they contribute to the repair of tissue damage by removing old, dying, or damaged tissue. All of these functions are served by macrophages. Macrophages belong to the mononuclear-phagocytic system.

Immature macrophages are produced in the bone marrow and are released into the bloodstream, where they are called monocytes. Monocytes then migrate into tissues, where they become mature macrophages. When found in connective tissue, macrophages are called histiocytes. They may also be found lining the sinusoids of the liver, where they are called Kupffer cells. The macrophages of the brain are called microglia, and in the lung they are known as alveolar macrophages. Nevertheless, irrespective of their name or location, they are all considered to belong to the mononuclear-phagocytic system (Fig. 4–9).

Terminology

The German histologist Aschoff, who studied the effects of injecting colloidal dyes into animals, found that these dyes were taken up by a great variety of cell types throughout the body. These cells included populations of large mononuclear cells, associated with reticular fibers, and vascular endothelial cells throughout the body. Aschoff believed that he had discovered a new body system and called it the **reticuloendothelial system.** As this system was studied, it gradually became clear that phagocytosis was *not* the major function of many of the cells identified by Aschoff, and that his results were partially artifactual.

Nevertheless, a portion of the reticuloendothelial system does have phagocytosis as its major function. The cells with this function each have a large, single, rounded nucleus. They are collectively termed the *mononuclear-phagocytic system.*

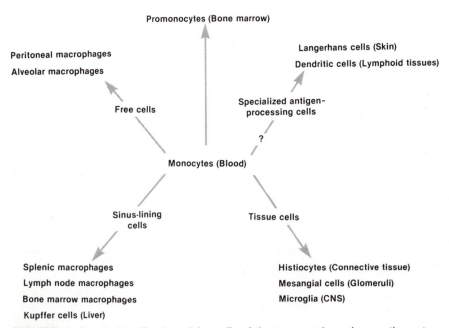

FIGURE 4–9. A classification of the cells of the mononuclear-phagocytic system.

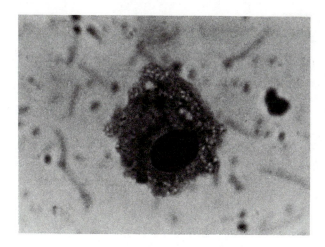

FIGURE 4–10. A typical macrophage: The small, dark dots within the cytoplasm are ingested bacteria. (Original magnification ×900). (Specimen kindly provided by Dr. B. Wilkie. From Tizard, I. Veterinary Immunology. 2nd ed. W. B. Saunders, Philadelphia, 1982. With permission.)

The Structure of Macrophages

Macrophages come in a wide variety of shapes because of their various habitats. In suspension, they are round cells about 14 to 20 μm in diameter. They possess abundant cytoplasm, at the center of which is a single, bean-shaped or indented, rounded nucleus (Figs. 4–10 and 4–11). The perinuclear cytoplasm contains a large number of lysosomes

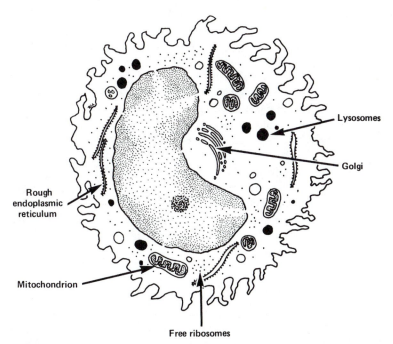

FIGURE 4–11. The major structural features of a "typical" macrophage. (From Tizard, I. Veterinary Immunology. 2nd ed. W. B. Saunders, Philadelphia, 1982. With permission.)

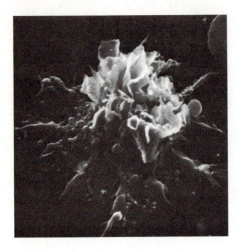

FIGURE 4–12. A scanning electron micrograph of a guinea-pig macrophage, showing the presence of extensive veil-like ruffles. Original magnification ×4000).

and mitochondria and, in contrast to neutrophils, rough endoplasmic reticulum and a Golgi apparatus. Thus macrophages can both synthesize and secrete protein. The peripheral cytoplasm is usually devoid of organelles, especially in cultured cells. In living macrophages this peripheral cytoplasm is in continuous movement, forming and reforming veil-like ruffles (Fig. 4–12). Macrophages, like neutrophils, can adhere tenaciously to glass surfaces, on which they spread by sending out thin cytoplasmic filaments. Some macrophages show variations on the basic macrophage structure. Thus monocytes have round nuclei, which elongate as the cells mature. Alveolar macrophages possess very little rough endoplasmic reticulum, but their cytoplasm tends to be full of granules. (Most macrophages derive their energy from glycolysis. The alveolar macrophage, as befits a cell living in the airways of the lung, derives its energy from aerobic metabolism).

The microglia of the central nervous system normally have rod-shaped nuclei and long thin cytoplasmic processes. These processes retract if the cell is stimulated into activity. The structure of macrophages may also alter following cell-mediated immune responses to some bacteria. These "activated" cells enlarge, and their lysosomes increase in number (Chap. 12).

In situations where foreign material persists for long periods, macrophages may accumulate in large numbers around the persistent material and present an epitheliumlike appearance on histological examination. These cells are therefore called **epithelioid cells.** On occasion, epithelioid cells may fuse together to form multinucleated giant cells in an attempt to totally enclose large particles that cannot be ingested by a single cell working alone.

Life History of Macrophages

All members of the mononuclear-phagocytic system arise from radiation-sensitive bone-marrow precursor cells called promonocytes. These precursors develop into monocytes, which enter the bloodstream where they remain for one to three days before migrating into tissues and maturing into macrophages. They constitute about 5% of the total leukocyte population in man.

Macrophages rarely divide and are thus radioresistant. Tissue macrophages are relatively long-lived cells, replacing themselves at a rate of about 1% per day unless called upon to undertake phagocytosis. In that case, their life span depends upon the nature of the phagocytosed material. If, for example, the ingested particle is easily digested by lysosomal enzymes, then the life span of the macrophage may remain unaffected. Macrophages may also have a normal life span if they ingest totally inert particles such as the colloidal carbon used in tattoos. In such cases, however, it is common for the macrophages to fuse and form giant cells in an additional attempt to eliminate the foreign material.

In some circumstances, as, for example, after the intravenous infusion of colloidal carbon (for example, India ink) macrophages may carry ingested particles to the lung or intestine and, by migrating into the bronchiolar or intestinal lumen, eliminate them from the body.

By contrast, some particles, such as inhaled asbestos particles, although readily phagocytosed, are toxic to macrophages. When released from dying cells, they are promptly rephagocytosed and thus cause continual macrophage destruction. As a result of this destruction, there is excessive release of lysosomal enzymes, extensive tissue damage, inflammation, and local fibrosis of the lung—a condition known as asbestosis.

The Functions of Macrophages

Macrophages probably have three major roles. First, they destroy foreign particles as well as dead or dying tissues through phagocytosis. Second, they process antigen for the immune response and serve to regulate the immune responses. Third, they are major secretory cells, releasing a large array of different biologically active factors into the environment.

Phagocytosis by Macrophages   The process of phagocytosis by macrophages is very similar to that described previously for neutrophils. Macrophages are chemotactically attracted to foreign material. The chemoattractants include not only bacterial products and products of antigen-antibody-complement interaction, but also factors released from dying cells, especially neutrophils (Chap. 5). Thus, not only do neutrophils lead the way to sites of invasion, but also, in dying, serve to promote macrophage accumulation.

Opsonized antigen binds to macrophages through receptors for antibody (Fc receptors) and for the third component of complement (C3). However, the antibody receptors must be triggered for ingestion to occur. The ingestion process promotes a respiratory burst, which tends to be much less intense than in neutrophils. Myeloperoxidase is usually absent from mature macrophages, but its place is probably taken by catalase. Macrophages also contain a full range of lysosomal hydrolytic enzymes.

Macrophages and Immune Stimulation   Macrophages promote the immune response in three ways. First, they present the antigen to antigen-sensitive lymphocytes in the correct physical configuration. Second, they regulate the dose of antigen that is presented to the antigen-sensitive lymphocytes, and third, they secrete immunoregulatory molecules.

If all foreign material were totally ingested and digested, there would be no necessity and no stimulus for the immune responses. It is, therefore, apparent that at least some antigen must survive in order to stimulate antigen-sensitive lymphocytes. You may recall from Chapter 2 that the antibody response is directed against conformational determinants on protein antigens. This implies that antigen must be presented to the immune system in its native form. If the fate of radiolabelled antigen is followed as it is ingested by macrophages, it is found that, although most is destroyed, a few molecules persist intact both within the macrophage cytoplasm and on its surface membrane. These molecules may remain on the macrophage surface for a very long period and act as the stimulus for the first stage of the immune response—the triggering of antigen-sensitive small lymphocytes (Chap. 11).

This form of antigen processing is a very inefficient procedure, since much of the available antigen is destroyed. Once an animal possesses serum antibodies, a second more efficient antigen-processing system is brought into play. This system involves antigen uptake by a specialized population of mononuclear cells collectively called dendritic cells. It must also be pointed out that not all macrophages can process antigen for the immune response. Antigen-processing macrophages in mice must possess the Class II histocompatibility antigens, surface glycoproteins known as Ia. Ia-positive (Ia$^+$) macrophages generally predominate in the spleen, thymus, and liver and Ia$^-$ macrophages may acquire Ia if activated. If macrophages are treated with antibodies against Ia, they lose their ability to initiate an immune response. Similarly the macrophages of newborn mice are (Ia$^-$) and, as a result, these animals are effectively immunodeficient. Only when Ia antigen appears on the macrophages of the developing animal is the ability to mount an immune response acquired.

Dendritic Cells

Scattered throughout most tissues of the body with the exception of the brain, and found in high concentrations in the skin and in the cortex of lymph nodes, is a population of macrophagelike cells called dendritic cells. These cells, known as **Langerhans cells** in skin, possess an extensive array of long, filamentous cytoplasmic processess (Fig. 4–13). Dendritic cells are nonphagocytic Ia^{+++} cells that can bind antibody to their cytoplasmic processes in such a way that it retains its ability to bind antigen (Fig. 4–14). Consequently, the cytoplasmic processes of dendritic cells can function as antigen-trapping webs. Antigen that encounters antibody on a dendritic cell process will adhere and may then persist in

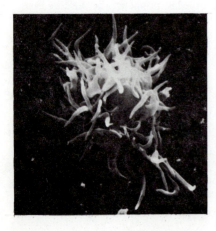

FIGURE 4–13. A scanning electron micrograph of a dendritic cell from a guinea-pig lymph node. Note the extensive cytoplasmic processes. Original magnification ×4000. (From Tizard, I. R., and Holmes, W. L. J. Reticuloendothel Soc., *17*: 333–341, 1975. With permission.)

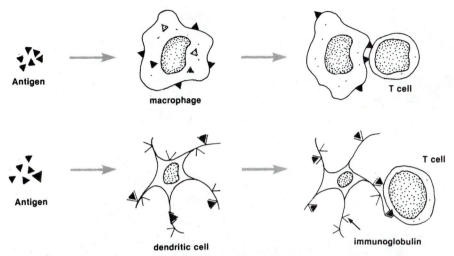

FIGURE 4–14.   Both macrophages and dendritic cells may present antigen to antigen-sensitive cells. Macrophages can do so in the absence of preexisting antibody, but they destroy much of the antigen they ingest. By contrast, dendritic cells bind antigen through membrane-bound immunoglobulin (antibody). Although dendritic cells can only present antigen in previously sensitized individuals, they are much more efficient than macrophages.

that location for months or even years. This dendritic cell-bound antigen provides a very potent stimulus for the immune response (Fig. 4–15). Since antibody is required for antigen binding by dendritic cells, these cells are only effective when stimulating a secondary immune response. Indeed, the enhanced immune response seen following a second dose of antigen is probably due, in part, to the greater efficiency of dendritic-cell processing as compared with macrophage processing. The relative antigen-binding efficiencies of the two systems may be compared by measuring the half-life of radiolabelled antigen deposited in lymph-node follicles. In unimmunized mice, this half-life is only a few hours. In immunized mice, the half-life of antigen is about eight weeks.

Macrophages as Regulators of Antigen Dose

Antigen-sensitive small lymphocytes are triggered into responding to antigen by exposure to a narrow range of antigen doses. Thus, either excessive or inadequate doses fail to provoke an immune response. Indeed by "turning off" the antigen-sensitive cells, these doses generally provoke tolerance (Chap. 13).

Macrophages appear to play a critical role in regulating the dose of antigen that is presented to antigen-sensitive cells so that they respond optimally. Antigen not processed by macrophages triggers tolerance.

Macrophages as Secretory Cells

Macrophages possess a rough endoplasmic reticulum and are, therefore, capable of synthesizing and secreting proteins. Some of these proteins are released continuously (Table

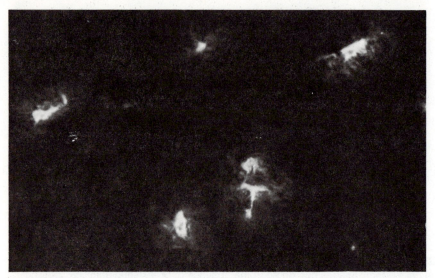

FIGURE 4–15. Ia-positive dendritic cells in rat heart. Frozen sections of heart were incubated in monoclonal anti-Ia and then with fluorescein-labelled rabbit antimouse globulin. (From Hart, D. N. J., and Fabre, J. W. J. Exp. Med., *154:* 350, 1981. With permission.)

4–2). These include the enzyme lysozyme and the complement components C2, C3, C4, and C5 (Chap. 14).

Some macrophage products are only released during the phagocytic process. These include lysosomal proteases, collagenases, elastases, plasminogen activators, and leukotrienes. These products may cause tissue damage and probably contribute significantly to the inflammatory process (Chap. 5).

TABLE 4–2   Some Secretory Products of Macrophages

Factors synthesized and secreted continuously	Lysozyme
	Complement components C2, C3, C4, C5
	Fibronectin
Factors released during phagocytosis	Plasminogen activators
	Procoagulants
	Collagenase
	Elastase
	Lysosomal proteases
	Leukotrienes
	Thromboxanes
	Thromboplastin
Regulatory factors released during immune responses	Interferon
	Interleukin 1
	Lymphocyte-activating factors
	Prostaglandins E1 and E2
	Cyclic AMP

Macrophages also secrete a mixture of products that act to regulate immune responses. These include interleukin I and other lymphocyte activators (Chap. 11), which tend to promote immune responses, plasminogen activator, which stimulates T cells, and interferon and prostaglandins, which tend to inhibit immune responses. Their net effect is, therefore, complex.

Fibronectins

Fibronectins are adhesive glycoproteins found in plasma and on cell membranes. The cell membrane fibronectin mediates cell adherence to surfaces and probably plays a role in cell–cell interaction. Plasma fibronectin, on the other hand, regulates mononuclear phagocytic cell activity. This protein functions as a "universal opsonin" by binding to a great variety of particulate material. If plasma fibronectin levels drop, such as occurs in major surgery, burns, severe trauma, or bacterial sepsis, then the clearance of particles from the blood-stream is severely reduced. Infusion of fibronectin causes clinical improvement. Thus, by regulating mononuclear phagocyte activity, this protein is a vital component of the defense system against invading microorganisms.

Defects in Phagocytosis and Antigen Processing

Neutrophil Deficiencies

Neutrophils are, of course, required to ingest and destroy the bulk of invading foreign material. If the neutrophils are either absent or ineffective, then, clearly, protection will be insufficient and affected individuals will suffer from recurrent infections.

Neutropenias

Neutrophil numbers in the blood may be reduced by drugs or by radiation, by over-whelming infections, or by some autoimmune disorders. Cytotoxic drugs and radiation cause a **neutropenia** because they are selectively toxic for rapidly dividing cells, and the neutrophil precursors of the bone marrow are, therefore, very susceptible to destruction (Table 4–3).

Severe bacterial infections are also commonly associated with a profound neutro-penia. In these cases, cause and effect are sometimes difficult to separate, since bacterial toxins may exert a suppressive influence on bone-marrow function. Autoantibodies to mye-

TABLE 4–3   Neutrophil Deficiency Syndromes

Acquired neutropenias	Autoantibody-mediated neutropenia
	Drug-induced neutropenias
	Isoimmune neutropenia of the newborn
	Neutropenia in systemic lupus erythematosus
	Feltys syndrome
Inherited neutropenias	Cyclic and noncyclic neutropenias

loid tissue also cause bone-marrow depression, while the replacement of normal bone marrow by cancer cells can lead to neutropenia—a common complication of leukemia.

Some neutropenias are inherited. They appear to fall into two distinct groups. In one group, the neutropenia occurs at periodic intervals. This cyclic neutropenia has been observed in children and dogs. The lesion, which presumably affects the myeloid precursor cells in some way, has not been well defined. Another group of inherited neutropenias are progressively unremitting. As might be anticipated, individuals suffering from cyclic neutropenia suffer from repeated episodes of recurrent infection, while those suffering from noncyclic neutropenia have a more progressive disease.

In all these neutrophil-deficiency syndromes, affected individuals suffer from recurrent infections by bacteria such as Streptococci, especially *Strep pneumoniae,* and Micrococci.

Terminology

The suffix ''-penia'' means ''a loss.'' Thus a **neutropenia** is a condition in which the number of neutrophils is reduced. A **leukopenia** is a condition in which there is a reduced number of leukocytes.

Neutrophil Dysfunction

If neutrophils are present but are not functioning correctly, the net effect will be very similar to that due to a neutropenia—namely recurrent, uncontrolled bacterial infections (Table 4–4). Clearly there are many different ways in which neutrophils can fail to function, and defects have been described involving each of the major mechanisms in phagocytosis, namely defective chemotaxis, opsonization, ingestion or digestion.

By far the most important group of neutrophil dysfunction syndromes is collectively known as chronic granulomatous disease (CGD). The commonest form of this is an X-linked (i.e., males-only) condition in which defects occur in the respiratory burst, and, as a

TABLE 4–4   Neutrophil Dysfunction Syndromes

Depressed microbicidal activity	Chronic granulomatous disease
	Myeloperoxidase deficiency
	Chediak-Higashi syndrome
	Glucose-6-phosphate dehydrogenase deficiency
Impaired opsonization	Complement deficiencies
	Antibody deficiencies
	Fibronectin deficiency
	Sickle cell disease
Impaired chemotaxis	Complement deficiencies
	Antibody deficiencies
	Wiscott-Aldrich syndrome
	Chronic mucocutaneous candidiasis
	Chediak-Higashi syndrome
	Hyperimmunoglobulin E syndrome
	Chronic granulomatous disease
	Diabetes mellitus

result, there is reduced production of bactericidal oxygen metabolites. The disease usually develops at about 1 year of age when the children begin to suffer from recurrent sepsis and multiple abscess formation (Fig. 4–16). The organisms isolated from these children include staphylococci, *E. coli*, Klebsiella species, *Serratia marcescens*, Enterobacter species, and *Proteus vulgaris*. These are all relatively weak pathogens for normal individuals.

Although it is agreed that the lesion in chronic granulomatous disease is associated with a failure of the respiratory burst, the precise nature of the defect is a matter of some dispute. It is probable that affected individuals suffer from a NADPH oxidase deficiency. This condition may be due either to an absolute deficiency or, in some cases, to production of an abnormal enzyme. As a result of this deficiency, the recycling of NADPH will be prevented and effectively result in a deficiency of NADP and a failure to produce hydrogen peroxide. NADP is involved in several other metabolic pathways in addition to the respiratory burst, including cell-membrane formation. Thus, this deficiency may also influence the stability of lysosomal membranes to the detriment of the affected individual.

The dye nitroblue tetrazolium is normally reduced by the respiratory burst enzymes to a blue precipitate from a colorless precursor. Thus, normal neutrophils exposed to this dye will develop deposits of blue precipitate in their cytoplasm. Neutrophils from CGD-

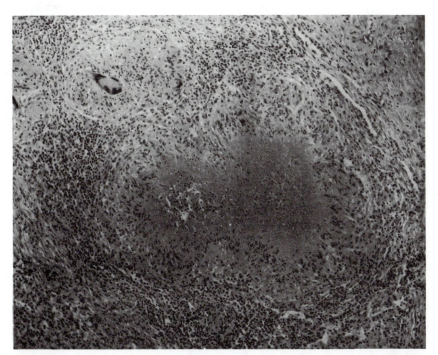

FIGURE 4–16. A photomicrograph of a granuloma from a child with chronic granulomatous disease. Note the central area of dead cells (necrosis) surrounded by inflammatory cells. A multinucleated giant cell is at the lower right (hematoxylin and eosin stain; original magnification ×120). (From Bellanti, J. A. Immunology II. W. B. Saunders, Philadelphia, 1979. With permission.)

affected children will fail to do so. This procedure thus provides a convenient aid to diagnosis.

Other inherited enzyme deficiencies that lead to neutrophil dysfunction include congenital absences of glutathione peroxidase, myeloperoxidase, superoxide dismutase, or of glucose-6-phosphate dehydrogenase.

A second interesting neutrophil dysfunction syndrome is known as the Chediak-Higashi syndrome, an inherited condition seen in cattle, mice, mink, Persian cats, tigers, killer whales, and man. The melanin granules in the skin of affected animals are unusually large. As a result, these animals have a very attractive pale-brown coat that is easily recognized. There is also a defect in lysosomal membranes, as a result of which, the neutrophil primary granules are extraordinarily large, abnormally fragile, and rupture spontaneously to cause tissue damage (Fig. 4–17). These leukocytes are defective in chemotactic responsiveness and have a reduced capacity for intracellular killing as a result of very low levels of neutral protease activity. The impairment seems to be related to abnormalities in cyclic nucleotide metabolism, since cells have an abnormal cyclic GMP/cyclic AMP ratio, and also to alterations in membrane glycosphingolipids. Chediak-Higashi animals also have a deficiency in natural-killer-cell and cytotoxic-T-cell activity.

Deficiencies of neutrophil chemotaxis may be due either to defects in the production of chemotactic factors, for example C5a, or to an intrinsic defect in the neutrophils themselves. Thus, one condition is called "lazy leukocyte" syndrome, in which neutrophils are poorly mobilized and defective in random motility. These chemotactic deficiencies are commonly associated with defects involving chromosomes 7 or 16 in man. A lactoferrin deficiency has been associated with a chemotactic defect and recurrent skin abscesses.

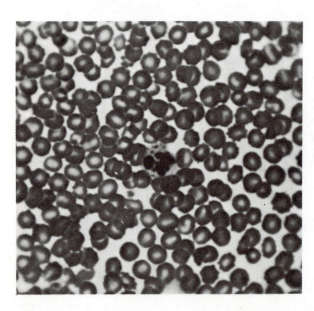

FIGURE 4–17. A neutrophil from an Aleutian mink with Chediak-Higashi syndrome. Note the abnormally large dark granules within the cell (original magnification ×750). (Specimen kindly provided by Dr. S. H. An. From Tizard, I. Veterinary Immunology. 2nd ed. W. B. Saunders, Philadelphia, 1982. With permission.)

Sources of Additional Information

Allison, A. C. Macrophage activation and nonspecific immunity. Int. Rev. Exp. Pathol., *18:* 304–346, 1978.

Babior, B. M. Oxygen-dependent microbial killing by phagocytes. N. Engl. J. Med., *298:* 659–668, 721–726, 1978.

Bainton, D. F. Sequential degranulation of the two types of polymorphonuclear leukocyte granular during phagocytosis of microorganisms. J. Cell. Biol., *58:* 249–264, 1974.

Bellanti, J. A., and Dayton, D. H. The phagocytic cell in host resistance. Raven Press, New York, 1975.

Boggs, D. R. Physiology of neutrophil proliferation, maturation and circulation. Clin. Hematol., *4:* 535–551, 1975.

Cohn, Z. A. Macrophage physiology. Fed Proc., *34:* 1725–1729, 1975.

Dannenberg, A. M. Macrophages in inflammation and infection. N. Engl. J. Med., *293:* 489–493, 1975.

Davies, P., and Bonney, R. J. Secretory products of mononuclear phagocytes: A brief review. J. Res., *26:* 37–47, 1979.

Jaffe, E. A., and Mosher, D. F. Synthesis of fibronectin by cultured human endothelial cells. J. Exp. Med., *147:* 1779–1791, 1978.

Mandel, T. E., et al. Long-term antigen retention by dendritic cells in the popliteal lymph node of immunized mice. Immunology, *43:* 353–362, 1981.

Mocking, W. G., and Golde, D. W. The pulmonary alveolar macrophage. N. Engl. J. Med., *301:* 580–587, 639–645, 1979.

Nathan, C. F., Murray, H. W., and Cohn, Z. A. The macrophage as an effector cell. N. Engl. J. Med., *303:* 622–626, 1980.

Rosenthal, A. S., Lipsky, P. E., and Shevach, E. M. Macrophage–lymphocyte interaction and antigen recognition. Fed. Proc., *34:* 1743–1748, 1975.

Rossi, F., and Patriarcha, P., eds. Biochemistry and function of phagocytes. *In* Advances in Experimental Medicine and Biology, vol. 141. Plenum Press, New York, 1982.

Wilkinson, P. C. Recognition and response in mononuclear and granular phagocytes: A review. Clin. Exp. Immunol., *25:* 355–366, 1976.

5

Inflammation

Inflammation may be described simply as the response of irritated or damaged tissues to injury. In its classic form, it is considered to have five cardinal signs: heat, redness, swelling, pain, and loss of function. All of these signs are a direct result of changes in local vascular permeability. These alterations permit the escape of electrolytes, macromolecules, and cells from blood vessels into extracellular fluid.

In acute inflammation, blood vessels dilate, and there is an increase in the redness and apparent warmth of the inflamed area. There is a local swelling caused by the escape of fluids and cells into the extravascular tissues. The pain and loss of function that accompany inflammation are due to pressure on nerve endings from the accumulation of extravascular fluid and the release of irritant chemical mediators, such as histamine and the kinins (Table 5–1).

Inflammation is of critical importance as a vital protective mechanism, since it provides a means by which protective factors, such as antibodies, complement, and phagocytic cells, which are normally confined to the bloodstream, can penetrate tissues and gain access to the sites of foreign invasion. It may, therefore, be considered to be a mechanism for focusing these immunological protective mechanisms at a localized region within tissues (Fig. 5–1).

Classification of Inflammation

Inflammation is conveniently classified according to its severity and duration (Table 5–2). This classification has the advantage that severe, recent inflammation or acute inflammation is characteristically very different from prolonged or chronic inflammation.

Acute Inflammation

Acute inflammation is the form of inflammation seen within a few hours of tissue damage or infection, at a time when there is severe redness, pain, and swelling around the damaged area (Fig. 5–2). The initial changes in an acute inflammatory response involve blood vessels. Immediately following injury, there is a transient constriction of local arterioles followed by dilation of all the local blood vessels. As a result, there is a great increase of blood flow to the area, which may last from several minutes to several hours. Eventually, the flow diminishes and gradually returns to normal. While the blood vessels are dilated, there is

TABLE 5–1 The Cardinal Signs of Inflammation

Sign	Mechanism
Redness	Capillary dilation
Swelling	Edema due to increased vascular permeability and cellular infiltration
Heat	Increased blood flow
Pain	Pressure on nerve endings due to edema and the release of pain mediators such as histamine

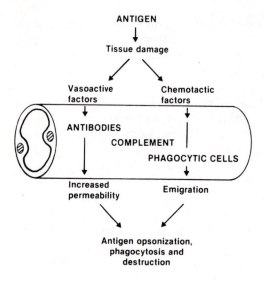

FIGURE 5-1. Inflammation may be considered to be a mechanism by which antibodies, complement, and phagocytic cells can escape into tissues and destroy invading antigen.

also an increase in vascular permeability. As a result, protein-rich plasma exudes into the tissues, where it causes local edema and swelling.

Within a few hours of the onset of these vascular changes, leukocytes (neutrophils, eosinophils, and monocytes) begin to adhere to the vascular endothelium in a process called pavementing. If the blood vessels are significantly damaged, platelets may also bind to the vessel walls and release both vasoactive and clotting factors.

After adhering to the blood-vessel walls, the leukocytes commence to migrate into the surrounding tissues through gaps between endothelial cells (Fig. 5–3). Since neutrophils and eosinophils are the most mobile of all the blood leukocytes, these cells will be the first to arrive in the tissues. Blood monocytes move more slowly and therefore arrive later. Once within tissues, the leukocytes are attracted by chemotactic factors to sites of bacterial invasion and tissue damage. There they proceed to phagocytose and destroy any foreign material and, in the case of monocytes, remove dead and dying tissue.

Changes in Vascular Permeability

Vascular permeability in acute inflammation increases in two stages. First, there is an immediate increase mediated by the release of vasoactive factors. The second phase of

TABLE 5-2　A Simple Comparison of Acute and Chronic Inflammation

Acute Inflammation	Chronic Inflammation
Vasodilitation	Few vascular changes
Increased vascular permeability leading to edema	Minimal edema
Neutrophil infiltration	Macrophage and lymphocyte infiltration
Rapid onset	Slow onset
Short duration	Prolonged reaction with eventual fibrosis

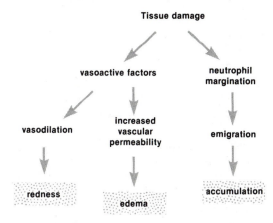

FIGURE 5-2. The basic features of acute inflammation: It is clearly characterized by redness, edema, and neutrophil accumulation.

increased vascular permeability occurs several hours after the onset of inflammation, at a time when the leukocytes are commencing to emigrate. This emigration is due to a contraction of the periendothelial cells around blood vessels, which pulls the endothelial cells apart and so permits the escape of fluid through their junctional zones.

Vasoactive Factors The major factors that increase permeability are the vasoactive amines histamine and serotonin (Table 5-3). Histamine is normally stored within mast cells and basophils (Chap. 19), and serotonin is found within platelets, tissue of the central nervous system, and the argentophil cells of the intestine. Histamine makes smooth muscle contract, causes vasodilation and increased vascular permeability, and acts on nerve endings to cause pain. Serotonin has a similar effect in laboratory rodents. It is probably only of minor importance in animals of other species.

Kinins are peptides derived from certain plasma α globulins by proteolytic enzymes. The most important kinin is called bradykinin. The kinins, like histamine, increase vascular permeability, contract smooth muscle, and produce pain. Another class of vasoactive polypeptides are the **anaphylatoxins.** These are derived from the cleavage of the α chains of two complement components C3 and C5 (see Chap. 14). They both act on blood vessels by indirectly provoking histamine release from mast cells. An important vasoactive peptide called PF/dil (permeability factor in diluted serum) is a fragment of Hageman factor. (Hageman factor is one of the most important of the blood-clotting proteins.) It activates

TABLE 5-3 Factors That Increase Vascular Permeability

Histamine
Serotonin
Leukotrienes
Prostaglandin E$_2$
Anaphylatoxins
Lymphokines
Kinins

prekallikreins, the proteolytic enzymes responsible for the generation of kinins. Presumably it is generated by damage to vascular endothelium.

The polyunsaturated fatty acid, arachidonic acid is a component of many cell-membrane phospholipids from which it is released by phospholipases. If arachidonic acid is acted on by the enzyme cyclooxygenase, then a series of cyclic endoperoxides are formed, which are known as prostaglandins. If arachidonic acid is acted on by the enzyme lipoxygenase, then it is converted to HETE's (otherwise known as hydroxy-eicosotetraenoic acids), which in turn give rise to leukotrienes.

There are many different prostaglandins (PGs) that fall into four series. The PGEs, the PGFs, the thromboxanes (PGA_2) and the prostacyclins (PGI_2). PGA_2 and PGI_2 are derived by the activities of thromboxane synthetase and prostacyclin synthetase, both of which are found in endothelial cells. The biological activities of the prostaglandins differ widely and, since many different prostaglandins are released in inflammation, the net effect may be very complex. The E prostaglandins (PGE) cause smooth-muscle relaxation and produce long-lasting vasodilation and increased vascular permeability. PGE also acts on pain receptors to increase their responses to histamine and bradykinin. The F prostaglandins (PGF) also increase vascular permeability and dilate blood vessels, but they cause smooth-muscle contraction. Thromboxanes are very unstable compounds, but they promote platelet aggregation and the release of vasoactive factors. Prostacyclins cause vascular dilation.

The leukotrienes are also a complex mixture of molecules with a great variety of biological activities. The most important are leukotriene B_4, a potent chemotactic agent, and leukotrienes C_4 and D_4 that cause increased vascular permeability. One special characteristic of the leukotrienes is their ability to cause prolonged, smooth contraction of smooth muscle. This activity is described further in Chapter 19.

Migration of Leukocytes

Emigration of leukocytes is an active process that takes place independently of the increased vascular permeability of acute inflammation. The leukocytes bind to the vascular endothelium, insert their pseudopods through the interendothelial junctions, and migrate between these cells and the basement membrane (Fig. 5–3). Subsequently, the cell moves through the basement membrane into the tissue spaces under the influence of chemotactic factors.

Chemotactic Factors

Probably the most significant chemotactic factor (Table 5–4) produced in acute inflammation is a peptide derived from breakdown of the fifth component of complement, known as C5a. This small polypeptide not only attracts neutrophils to sites of complement activation, but also appears to trigger adherence to endothelial cells. C5a is relatively unstable and readily loses its terminal arginine to form C5a des arg. C5a des arg has lost its anaphylatoxic properties, but remains potently chemotactic and is probably of more importance than native C5a. You can find out more about C5a in Chapter 14.

When Hageman factor is activated by vascular damage, both kallikrein and plasminogen activator are generated and are chemotactic for neutrophils. Other neutrophil chemotactic factors include collagen, chemotactic lymphokines, chemotactic factors from macrophages, fibroblasts, and mast cells, as well as factors released by neutrophils themselves.

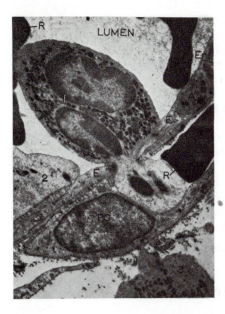

FIGURE 5–3. An inflamed venule of a rat: Cell I is a neutrophil emigrating from a capillary. (R = Red blood cells; E = endothelium, PC = periendothelial cell; Cell 2 and Cell 3 are neutrophils.) (From Marchesi, V. T., and Florey, H. W., Quart. J. Exp. Physiol., *45:* 343, 1960. With permission.)

For example, leukoegressin is a chemotactic peptide derived from cleavage of IgG by neutrophil proteolytic enzymes.

Bacterial products are also chemotactic and thus attract neutrophils to sites of bacterial invasion. The most potent chemotactic factor known, in molecular terms, is leukotriene B_4 derived from arachidonic acid through the activities of lipoxygenase. Its activity is detectable at a concentration of $10^{-8}M$.

Once neutrophils have reached the site of tissue damage, they tend to become unresponsive to chemotactic agents, so enabling them to move away. At the same time, they proceed to ingest and destroy foreign material, as described in Chapter 4.

How to Demonstrate and Measure Chemotaxis

There are two established quantitative techniques for measuring chemotaxis. In one technique, the micropore filter method, cells are placed on top of a filter and the chemotactic substance is placed on the other side. During a period of incubation, the cells on top migrate through the channels of the filter and, if given sufficient time, will even-

---

TABLE 5–4 Chemotactic Factors for Neutrophils

C5a
Bacterial products
Fibrin degradation products
Collagen
Kallikrein
Leukotrienes
Lymphokines
Plasminogen activator

tually reach the bottom chamber. The technique may be rendered quantitative either by counting the number of migrating cells or by measuring the distance they have migrated into the filter (Fig. 5–4).

An alternative technique is the under agarose method. In this method, holes are punched in a sheet of agarose in a petri dish. Cells placed in a central well are allowed to migrate under the agar toward a well containing medium alone (i.e., a negative control) or a chemoattractant. After incubation, the agar can be removed, and the cells adhering to the plastic or glass surface fixed and stained. The distance travelled can be estimated, and the specific cell types involved can be examined easily. Although the agarose method is very simple, it is about 50 to 100 times less sensitive than the micropore filter method.

Ward, P. A., and E. G. Maderazo, E. G. *Micropore filter method. Leukocyte chemotaxis. Manual of Clinical Immunology.* 2nd ed. American Society for Microbiology. Washington, D.C., 1980.

Nelson, R. D., Quie, P. G., and Simmons, R. L. *Chemotaxis under agarose: A new and simple method for measuring chemotaxis and spontaneous migration of human polymorphonuclear leukocytes and monocytes.* J. Immunol., 115,1650–1655, 1975.

Immunologically Mediated Inflammation

Acute inflammation, as described above, is commonly associated with tissue damage due to trauma or microbial invasion and is thus the most usual type of acute response. Inflammation is also, however, a protective response, and it may, under some circum-

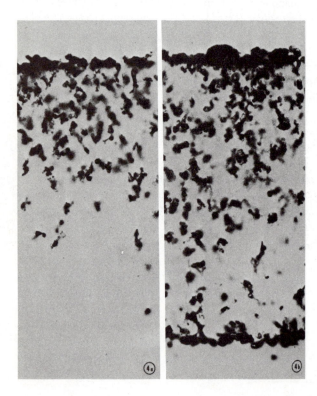

FIGURE 5–4. Sagittal section of a millipore filter after incubation of neutrophils: **A** using serum in the bottom chamber; **B** using chemotactic factor generated by LPS and serum. The top of the figure represents the surface to which the neutrophils were applied. (From Snyderman, R., et al. J. Exp. Med., *128:* 274, 1968. With permission.)

stances, be promoted by immunological processes. Immunologically mediated inflammation is known as **hypersensitivity** and is classified into four major types (Fig. 5–5). These are described in detail in Chapters 20 to 23, but are introduced here for convenience.

Type I or **immediate hypersensitivity** is an acute reaction mediated by antibody (IgE and some minor IgG subclasses) attached to mast cells or basophils. If antigen enters tissues and binds to this cell-fixed antibody, then the mast cells or basophils will respond

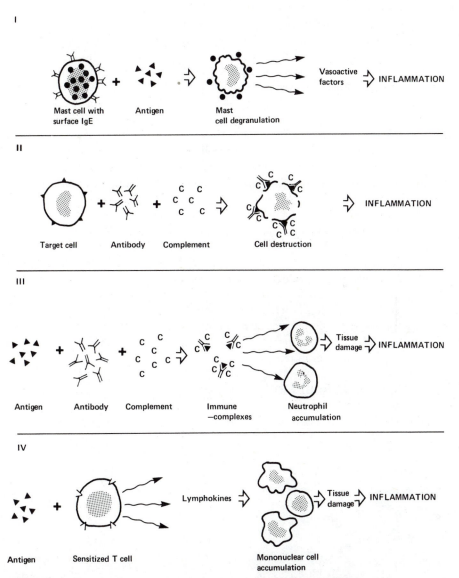

FIGURE 5–5. The four types of immunologically mediated inflammation (hypersensitivity) as classified by Gell and Coombs. (From Tizard, I. Veterinary Immunology. 2nd ed. W. B. Saunders, Philadelphia, 1982. With permission.)

by releasing their content of vasoactive factors. As a result, the tissues will be rapidly flooded by high levels of histamine, serotonin, kinins, and leukotrienes. These factors will, of course, cause a very severe local acute inflammatory response. The agents released by mast cells are normally neutralized by enzymes found within eosinophils. Because most cells also release eosinophil chemotactic factors, massive accumulations of eosinophils at the site of inflammation are characteristic of this type of hypersensitivity (Fig. 5–6).

Type II or **cytotoxic hypersensitivity** is an inflammatory response that occurs when cells are destroyed through the action of antibodies and complement or by cytotoxic cells. Cells that may cause cytotoxicity include activated T cells, NK cells, macrophages, neutrophils, and K cells acting through ADCC. (You can find out more about complement in Chap. 14 and about cytotoxic cells in Chap. 12.)

Type III or **immune-complex hypersensitivity** occurs because antibody bound to antigen will activate complement even if deposited in tissues (Chap. 14). Activation of complement by these immune complexes will result in the production of C5a and C567, and as a result, neutrophils will be attracted to sites of immune-complex formation. Unfortunately, under these circumstances, neutrophils may also release their lysosomal enzymes into tissues and thus cause severe damage. Neutrophil-activated plasmin will activate more complement, attract more neutrophils, and provoke platelet aggregation and the release of platelet-derived vasoactive factors. The C3a and C5a anaphylatoxins will also contribute to a severe acute inflammatory response.

Type IV or **delayed hypersensitivity** involves the participation of cell-mediated immune reactions in acute inflammation. If antigen is injected into an animal possessing appropriately sensitized T lymphocytes, then a local inflammatory reaction may result. This form of reaction is known as delayed hypersensitivity, since it generally takes at least 24 hours after administration of antigen for the response to reach maximal intensity (Fig. 5–7). The inflammation results from the release of vasoactive factors from mast cells and basophils under the influence of factors released from the sensitized lymphocytes (lymphokines) and is characterized by infiltration of the site with mononuclear cells (Fig. 5–8). This form of reaction occurs in response to many bacterial antigens as well as in response to virus-infected cells and in graft rejection.

The Control of Acute Inflammation

Since acute inflammation has the potential to cause severe tissue damage, it must be rigidly controlled. Human plasma contains several factors that can effect this control. They

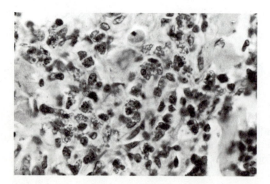

FIGURE 5–6. A photomicrograph of a lesion in horse skin brought about by allergy to worm larvae. The skin is infiltrated by large numbers of eosinophils reflecting the occurrence of a Type I hypersensitivity.

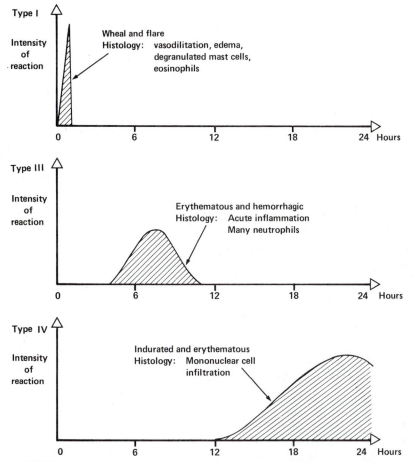

FIGURE 5–7. A schematic diagram showing the time course, character, and histology of inflammatory skin reactions resulting from the intradermal injection of antigen and mediated through Type I, III, and IV hypersensitivity reactions. (From Tizard, I. Veterinary Immunology. 2nd ed. W. B. Saunders, Philadelphia, 1982. With permission.)

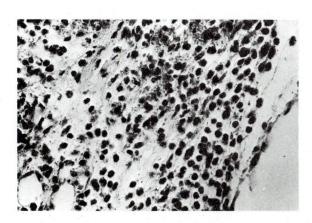

FIGURE 5–8. The characteristic mononuclear cell infiltration of a delayed hypersensitivity reaction. In this case, the response of a sensitized mouse to an extract of the protozoan *Toxoplasma gondii.* (Courtesy of Dr. C. H. Lai.)

may either inhibit the enzymes that generate inflammatory mediators, or, alternatively, they may directly inactivate the mediators.

Inhibitors of enzymes that will affect acute inflammation include several antiproteases such as α_1-antitrypsin and α_2-macroglobulin. These block the proteases released from neutrophil lysosomes, as well as thrombin, plasmin, and C1 esterase. Direct inhibitors of mediators include a plasma carboxypeptidase that removes the C-terminal arginyl residue from C5a, C3a, and bradykinin. There is, in addition, a complete series of inhibitors of the complement cascade.

Probably the major route by which mediators are destroyed is the action of eosinophils, which possess a complete battery of enzymes specifically capable of destroying the major inflammatory mediators (Chap. 20).

Chronic Inflammation

Several hours after neutrophils have arrived at the inflammatory focus, the macrophages begin to arrive. These macrophages are attracted by many of the factors that attract neutrophils, as well as by collagen-breakdown products and by lymphokines released from antigen-sensitized lymphocytes (Fig. 5–9).

The macrophages will not only eliminate invading bacteria, but also serve to get rid of tissue and neutrophil debris and any fibrin deposits that may be present. Macrophages, which are found in an inflammatory focus, also tend to be "activated." As a result, they release plasminogen activator which, by generating plasmin, causes degradation of fibrin. By releasing fibronectin, activated macrophages also attract fibroblasts to the site of inflammation, and some of the peptides derived by breakdown of fibrin have a similar effect. These fibroblasts proliferate, under the influence of macrophages, and commence to synthesize the collagen required to repair any damage. The collagen is deposited in the lesion

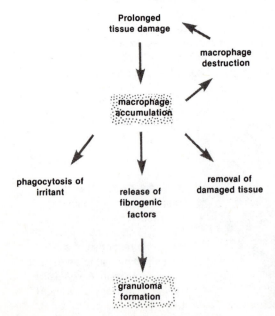

FIGURE 5–9. A schematic view of the process of chronic inflammation. Prolonged tissue damage leads to macrophage accumulation and granuloma formation over a relatively long period of time.

and then gradually remodeled over several weeks or months as the area gradually returns to normal.

The fate of the healing process following acute inflammation depends, to a large extent, on the success (or otherwise) of the acute inflammatory response. If the cause of the inflammation is rapidly and completely removed, then healing will follow uneventfully. Under some circumstances, however, the offending material may persist. The usual reason it persists is that it is insusceptible to destruction by neutrophil and macrophage enzymes. Thus, prolonged chronic inflammation is mediated by substances such as asbestos particles, *Mycobacterium tuberculosis* (which is covered by a waxy coat), and schistosome eggs (which are covered by an inert cuticle). Under these circumstances, there is a continuing chemotactic stimulus for macrophages and fibroblasts and excessive laying down of collagen fibers around the irritant focus. The net result of this is the formation of a **granuloma** (Fig. 5–10).

If these foreign bodies are nonantigenic, for example silica, talc, and mineral oil, few neutrophils or lymphocytes will be found in the lesion, but epithelioid and giant cells are formed in an attempt to destroy the material (Fig. 4–14). If the foreign body is toxic for macrophages, as in asbestosis, there may be a significant release of macrophage enzymes leading to tissue damage, and eventually to excessive fibrosis and scarring.

If the foreign material is immunogenic, then the initial inflammatory response may be similar to that seen in a delayed hypersensitivity reaction. As a result of the release of lymphokines from lymphocytes and continuous immune stimulation, this type of granuloma will contain lymphocytes, as well as macrophages and fibroblasts and probably also some neutrophils, basophils, and eosinophils. The macrophages may form giant cells. Other lymphokines, such as interleukin 1 (Chap. 11), may promote collagen formation by fibroblasts. The types of antigen that provoke this form of hypersensitivity granuloma include intracellular bacteria, such as *M. tuberculosis, M. leprae, B. abortus,* and the salmonellae, parasites such as schistosomes and filaria, and some metals that can act as haptens, such as zirconium and beryllium.

These chronic granulomatous responses, due either to immunological or foreign-body reactions are of importance since they may progress and enlarge to such an extent that they may extend into and destroy normal tissues. Thus in silicosis and berylliosis, for example, severe sickness and death may result from the replacement of normal lung tissues by granulomata.

Acute-Phase Proteins

When macrophages participate in inflammatory responses they release a small protein called interleukin 1. (This was once called leukocyte pyrogen or leukocyte activating factor). Interleukin 1 has several very important biological activities. First, it has an immunoregulatory function that is discussed further in Chapter 11; second, interleukin 1 acts on the hypothalamus to cause a fever; third it acts on the liver to stimulate the synthesis and release of certain newly formed proteins into the bloodstream. These proteins are usually associated with the presence of injury, infection, and inflammation. They are called **acute-phase proteins** (Table 5–5). (Inflammatory macrophages may also release prostaglandins that can also provoke hepatocytes to synthesize acute-phase proteins).

The most studied of the acute-phase protein is known as C reactive protein. The

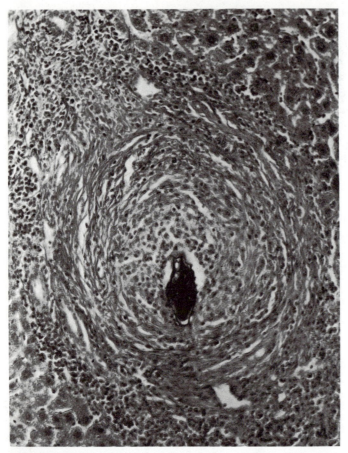

FIGURE 5–10. A section of liver from a patient infested by the parasite *Schistosoma mansoni.* An egg from the parasite is seen within the center of a granuloma that contains large numbers of eosinophil granulocytes. (Hematoxylin and eosin; original magnification ×100. (From Bellanti, J. A. Immunology II. W. B. Saunders, Philadelphia, 1969. With permission.)

concentration of this protein in blood increases up to a thousandfold in animals with extensive tissue damage. It returns to normal levels once the damage is resolved. The function of CRP is largely unknown. It is immunosuppressive and may prevent the production of autoantibodies to proteins released by damaged cells. CRP binds to damaged tissues and cell membranes where it activates the complement system. The benefits of this are unclear but it might accelerate healing by enhancing the inflammatory response. CRP has many properties in common with antibody molecules and is discussed further on page 93.

A second protein whose blood level rises several hundredfold in acute inflammation is serum amyloid A (SAA). SAA is the major protein of reactive amyloid, a pathological protein, described in Chapter 18. SAA is potently immunosuppressive, and it may act as a feedback inhibitor of interleukin 1 production.

TABLE 5-5 The Major Acute-Phase Proteins

Protein	Amount of Increase	Probable Function
C reactive protein (CRP)	Several hundredfold	Immunosuppressive, activates complement
Serum amyloid A (SAA)	Several hundredfold	Immunosuppressive
Haptoglobin	Two to fourfold	Binds hemoglobin, reduces serum iron levels
Alpha 1 acid glycoprotein	Two to fourfold	Potentiates clotting
Alpha 1 antitrypsin and alpha 1 antichymotrypsin	Two to fourfold	Inhibit serum proteases—limits tissue damage
Fibrinogen	Two to fourfold	Fibrin precursor
Ceruloplasmin	About 50%	Copper binding, scavenges free radicals
C3-Third component of complement	About 50%	Protective—part of the complement pathway

Ceruloplasmin, a copper binding protein that has the ability to "scavenge" oxygen-derived free radicals and, thus, inhibits some of the products of the respiratory burst, is another acute-phase protein. It is suggested that ceruloplasmin serves to protect tissues against superoxide-induced tissue injury. Alpha 1 antitrypsin and alpha 1 antichymotrypsin, both of which inhibit leukocyte proteases and, like ceruloplasmin, protect tissues against injury, are also elevated in inflammatory states.

As discussed in Chapter 17, many invading bacteria require iron for maximal proliferation and pathogenicity. Haptoglobin is an acute-phase protein that, by binding free hemoglobin, remove iron from circulation. As a result, serum iron levels drop significantly in acute inflammatory states and effectively reduce the ability of serum to support bacterial growth.

Sources of Additional Information

Becker, E. L., and Henson, P. M. *In vitro* studies of immunologically induced secretion of mediators from cells and related phenomena. Adv. Immunol., *17:* 93–193, 1973.

Bornstein, D. L. Leukocyte pyrogen: a major mediator of the acute phase reaction. Ann. N.Y. Acad. Sci., *389:* 323–337, 1982.

Borsos, D. L. Granulomatous inflammation. Progr. Allergy., *24:* 184–267, 1978.

Hurley, J. V. The sequence of early events in inflammation. In Vane, J. R., and Ferreira, S. M., eds. Handbook of Experimental Pharmacology. Springer Verlag, New York, 1978, pp. 26–67.

Jacob, M. S., et al. Complement-induced granulocyte aggregation: an unsuspected mechanism of disease. N. Engl. J. Med., *302:* 789–794, 1980.

Lewis, F. A., and Austin, K. F. Mediation of local homeostasis and inflammation by leukotrenes and other mast cell-dependent compounds. Nature, *293:* 103–108, 1981.

Movat, H. Z. Pathways of allergic inflammation: the sequelae of antigen antibody complex formation. Fed. Proc., *35:* 2435–2440, 1976.

McCarthy, K., and Henson, P. M. Induction of lysosomal enzyme secretion by alveolar macrophages in resonse to the purified fragments: C5a and C5a des-arg. J. Immunol., *123:* 2511–2517, 1979.

Oppenheim, J. J., Rosenstreich, D. L., and Potter, M. Cellular Functions in Immunity and Inflammation. Elsevier/North Holland, New York, 1981.

Spector, W. G., and Willoughby, D. A. The inflammatory response. Bacteriol. Rev., *27:* 117–154, 1963.

Weissmann, G., Smolen, J. E., and Korchatz, H. M. Release of inflammatory mediators from stimulated neutrophils. N. Engl. J. Med., *303:* 27–34, 1980.

6

The Nature of Antibodies

It was not long after Pasteur had launched the science of immunology that the protective component of many immune responses was found to reside in serum and given the name antibody. It was considerably later that Heidleberger (in 1930) showed that antibodies were proteins by demonstrating that pneumococcal polysaccharide antigen precipitated protein antibodies from antiserum.

The Properties of Antibodies

Antibodies can, in fact, be detected in many body fluids, for example, tears, respiratory-tract secretions, saliva, intestinal contents, urine, and milk. They are present in highest concentrations and most easily obtained in large quantities for analysis from blood serum. Antibodies, like other proteins, may be characterized by such features as their solubility in strong salt solutions, their electrostatic charge and isoelectric point, their molecular weight, and their antigenicity.

Solubility in Salt Solutions

Many years ago, when protein chemistry was in its infancy, it was found that some serum proteins could be precipitated out of solution if mixed with an equal volume of a saturated solution of ammonium sulfate. These proteins were called **globulins** to differentiate them from the proteins that remained in solution, which were called **albumins.**

Since antibody activity is precipitated by treatment of serum with ammonium sulfate in this way, antibodies are classified as globulins. The specific proteins that have antibody activity are called **immunoglobulins** and abbreviated Ig.

Electrostatic Charge

Proteins consist of chains of assorted amino acids. Some of these amino acids are basic and some are acidic. The overall electrostatic charge on any protein will, therefore, depend upon its amino-acid composition. Since the charge on an amino acid depends upon the pH of the solution in which they are dissolved, their overall charge is pH-dependent and is minimal at the isoelectric point of the protein. Because of this, a mixture of different proteins may be fractionated by subjecting it to an electrical potential at a standard pH. This technique is known as electrophoresis. The positively charged proteins are attracted toward the cathode. The neutral molecules will remain stationary, while the negatively charged molecules are attracted to the anode. Each protein will move at a rate dependent on its net charge.

When whole serum is electrophoresed, it consistently separates into four major fractions (Fig. 6–1). The most negatively charged fraction consists of a single, homogeneous protein known as serum albumin, since it is not precipitated by ammonium sulfate. The other three major fractions are all globulins and are classified into α, β, and γ globulins according to their electrophoretic mobility. Antibody activity is mainly found in the most cathodal fraction, the γ globulins. However, some immunoglobulins are also found among the β globulins.

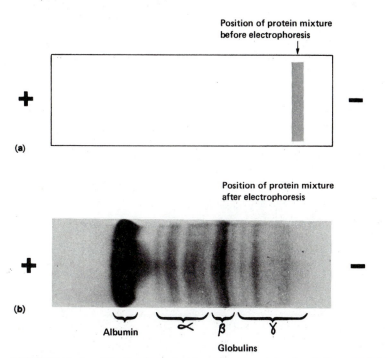

Position of protein mixture
before electrophoresis

+   **–**

(a)

Position of protein mixture
after electrophoresis

+   **–**

(b)

Albumin   ∝   β   γ

Globulins

FIGURE 6–1.   Electrophoresis of serum on a strip of cellulose acetate. (Courtesy of Dr. S. H. An. From Tizard I. Veterinary Immunology. 2nd ed. W. B. Saunders, Philadelphia, 1982. With permission.)

How to Electrophorese Serum

Serum is usually electrophoresed on a solid support that will permit fluid to flow without permitting extensive diffusion of proteins. Typical supports include paper, agar, starch gels, and cellulose acetate. The electrophoresis support is arranged in such a way that it is saturated with buffer, and each end is electrically connected to a power supply. This connection may be made simply by connecting the support to a buffer bath with wicks.

    A small volume of serum is placed on the support and a potential voltage applied. The voltage and the duration of the process are adjusted according to the size of the strip. When the electrophoresis is completed, the current is disconnected, and the strip is removed and stained with a protein stain such as amino black, acidic fuchsin, or ponceau S. After washing to remove unbound dye, each component in the mixture will be revealed as a stained band (Fig. 6–1).

Molecular Weight

Proteins may be characterized by their molecular weight, which can be measured by several techniques. (Figs. 6–2 and 6–3). When serum immunoglobulins are examined by ultra-

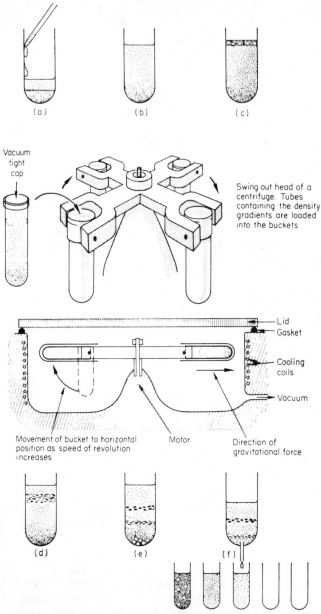

FIGURE 6-2. The technique of density-gradient ultracentrifugation: (a) A plastic centrifuge tube is filled with layers of sucrose solution of gradually decreasing concentration. (b) After standing for 12 hours, the layers have diffused into one another to form an even density gradient. (c) The serum to be separated is carefully layered on top. The tube is then placed in the head of an ultracentrifuge and spun at about 60,000 rev/min (175,000 g) for 6 hours. At this speed, air resistance is considerable so the bowl of the centrifuge is evacuated. The centrifuge tubes are sealed so that the contents do not boil (because of the very high vacuum) and disturb the gradient. The bowl is also refrigerated so that the specimen can be maintained at an even temperature. In practice, in order to withstand the enormous gravitation forces that are generated, it is necessary

Saline being added to carry the
serum through the column

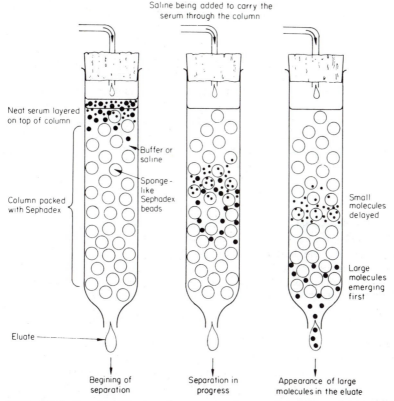

Neat serum layered
on top of column

Buffer or
saline

Sponge-
like
Sephadex
beads

Column packed
with Sephadex

Small
molecules
delayed

Large
molecules
emerging
first

Eluate

Begining of
separation

Separation in
progress

Appearance of large
molecules in the eluate

FIGURE 6–3. Gel-filtration chromatography may be employed to separate serum proteins on the basis of their size. (From Herbert, W. J. Veterinary Immunology. Blackwell Scientific Publications, Oxford, 1974. With permission.)

centrifugation, it is found that most have a sedimentation constant of 7S but some may have sedimentation constants of 8, 11, or 19S.

When the molecular weights of immunoglobulins are estimated, they are found, as might be expected from the sedimentation constants, to be heterogeneous. The 7S molecules have a molecular weight of 180,000 Mr, the 8S molecules are about 200,000 Mr, the 11S molecules are about 360,000 Mr, and the 19S molecules are about 900,000 Mr. The 19S molecules can be split by chemical treatment into five 7S units and are, clearly, pentamers

---

to use a much stronger design of head than that shown. (d) and (e) As centrifugation proceeds, the proteins in the serum sediment through the gradient until they reach a layer of density similar to their own. The heaviest proteins fall right to the bottom. (f) To collect the separated materials after centrifugation, the bottom of the tube is pierced with a needle, and the contents are allowed to flow out into a series of small test-tubes. (From Herbert, W. J. Veterinary Immunology. Blackwell Scientific Publications, Oxford, 1974. With permission.)

of a basic unit. Similarly, the 11S molecules can be split into two 7S subunits and are, therefore, dimers.

The Measurement of Molecular Weight by Ultracentrifugation

The rate at which a molecule will sink through a solution depends upon a number of variables. These include not only its molecular weight, but also its shape, the density of the suspending fluid, the viscosity of the suspending fluid, and the forces to which it is subjected. It is, therefore, possible to determine the sedimentation rate of a protein in solution and, by controlling the other variables, estimate its molecular weight.

The equation that governs this calculation is:

$$M = \frac{RTS}{D(1 - V\rho)}$$

where M is the molecular weight, R is the gas constant, T is the temperature in absolute degrees, D is the diffusion coefficient of the protein, V is the volume of 1g of the protein in solution, and ρ is the density of the suspending fluid.

S is the sedimentation coefficient. (This is usually expressed as the S_{20w} or standard sedimentation coefficient, which is the sedimentation coefficient of a particle or molecule at 20°C at infinite dilution in water.) The S value is usually measured in Svedberg units. It is measured by the formula $S = \frac{dx}{dt}/\omega^2X$ where $\frac{dx}{dt}$ is the rate of sedimentation, at a distance X from the center of the axis of a centrifuge rotor with an angular velocity of ω radians/sec.

Assuming that the molecules being examined are spherical, one can subject protein solutions to ultracentrifugation and thus calculate both their S_{20w} values and their molecular weights (Fig. 6-2).

The Measurement of Molecular Weight by Gel Filtration

The size of molecules may be estimated by measuring the rate at which they can pass through a glass tubular column filled with beads consisting of a cross-linked dextran gel (Fig. 6-3). (Dextran molecules can be cross-linked in such a way that they form a mesh of constant size.) This technique is called "gel filtration." When a protein solution is poured over these beads, very large molecules cannot penetrate the dextran mesh and will therefore be rapidly flushed through the column. In contrast, small molecules penetrate and are retained within the beads; their passage through the column is thus slowed down. The rate of passage of a molecule through the column is, therefore, related directly to its size. Its approximate molecular weight may be calculated by reference to a standard curve.

Antigenic Structure

Immunoglobulins, being proteins, function as potent antigens when injected into an animal of a different species. Human immunoglobulins, for example, will promote a strong antibody response when injected into a rabbit. By analysis of anti-immunoglobulin serum it is possible to show that there are five major immunoglobulin classes. Each is antigenically unique and each possesses its own characteristic antigenic determinants.

TABLE 6-1   The Major Immunoglobulin Classes of Man

	IgG	IgM	IgA	IgE	IgD
Most usual sedimentation coefficient	7S	19S	11S	8S	7S
Molecular weight	160,000	900,000	360,000	200,000	160,000
% carbohydrate	3	12	7	12	12
Electrophoretic mobility	γ	β	β-γ	β-γ	γ
Heavy chain	γ	μ	α	ϵ	δ
Subclasses	$\gamma_1, \gamma_2, \gamma_3, \gamma_4$	none	α_1, α_2	none	none
Light chains	κ or λ	κ or λ	κ or λ	κ or λ	κ or λ
Molecular formula	$\gamma_2\kappa_2$	$(\mu_2\kappa_2)_5$	$(\alpha_2\kappa_2)_n$	$\epsilon_2\kappa_2$	$\delta_2\chi_2$
	$\gamma_2\lambda_2$	$(\mu_2\chi_2)_5$	$(\alpha_2\gamma_2)_n$	$\epsilon_2\kappa_2$	$\delta_2\chi_2$
			(n = 1, 2, 3)		
Serum concentration mg/100 ml	800–1600	50–200	150–400	0.002–0.05	1.5–40
Half-life (days)	21	5	6	2	3

The major immunoglobulin in serum, called immunoglobulin G (usually abbreviated IgG) is a 7S molecule, with a molecular weight of 180,000 and characteristic γ antigenic determinants. The second major immunoglobulin is called immunoglobulin M (IgM). IgM is a 19S molecule with a molecular weight of 900,000 and μ antigenic determinants. The third immunoglobulin class is immunoglobulin A (IgA). IgA is commonly found in body secretions such as saliva, milk, or intestinal fluid. It is an 11S molecule with a molecular weight of 360,000 and α antigenic determinants. Immunoglobulin D (IgD), found in very low concentrations in plasma, is a 7S molecule, molecular weight 180,000 and δ determinants. Immunoglobulin E (IgE) is an 8S molecule with a molecular weight of 200,000 and ϵ antigenic determinants that mediates some allergic reactions (Table 6-1).

The Structure of Immunoglobulins

Immunoglobulin G

IgG is the major immunoglobulin class in mammalian serum. Its structure can serve as a model for the other immunoglobulins. IgG is a glycoprotein with a molecular weight of 180,000 and a sedimentation coefficient of 7S. On electron microscopy, it can be seen to be Y-shaped (Fig. 6-4). If the molecule is treated with a compound such as 2-mercapto-ethanol, which breaks interchain disulfide bonds, the molecule falls apart into four separate polypeptide chains. Two of these chains are identical, each being about 60,000 Mr and are called "heavy" chains. The other two chains are also identical, but are about 30,000 Mr and are thus termed "light" chains (Fig. 6-5).

If pure IgG is digested with the proteolytic enzyme papain, it splits into three approximately equal-sized fragments (Fig. 6-6). Two of these fragments retain the ability to bind antigen and are, therefore, called the antigen-binding fragments (Fab fragments). The third fragment obtained by papain treatment is sometimes crystallizable. This crystallizable fragment is called the Fc fragment.

If IgG is treated with the proteolytic enzyme pepsin, the molecule is cleaved in a

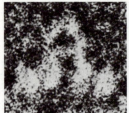
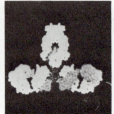
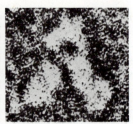

FIGURE 6-4. A comparison of a computer-generated space-filling model of the hinged Dob protein (see Fig. 6-17) to electron micrographs of rabbit IgG (original magnification ×2,042,500). (From Roux K. H., and Metzger, D. W. J. Exp. Med., *129:* 2548, 1982 With permission.)

somewhat different manner. The Fc fragment is split into very small peptides and thus completely destroyed. The two Fab fragments, however, remain joined together to produce a fragment called F(ab)′2 (Fig. 6-6). This fragment possesses two antigen binding sites. If F(ab)′2 is treated so that its disulfide bonds are reduced, it breaks into two Fab fragments, each of which has only one antigen binding site. Further disruption of the interchain disulfide bonds in the Fab fragments indicates that these each contain a light chain and half of a heavy chain (this is called the Fd fragment).

All of these observations may be synthesized into a workable model of IgG structure. The Y-shaped molecule possesses two binding sites for antigen, which are located on the "arms" of the Y (the Fab regions). The "tail" of the Y forms the Fc region. The heavy chains extend the full length of the molecule. The light chains are found in the N-terminal half of the molecule in the Fab regions.

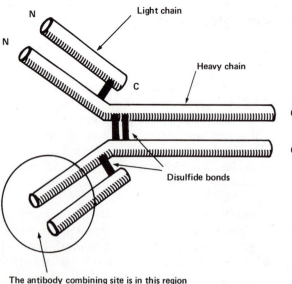

The antibody combining site is in this region

FIGURE 6-5. A simple model of an IgG molecule: N is the amino terminal of each peptide chain; C is the carboxyl terminal of each chain. (From Tizard I. Veterinary Immunology. 2nd ed. W. B. Saunders, Philadelphia, 1982. With permission.)

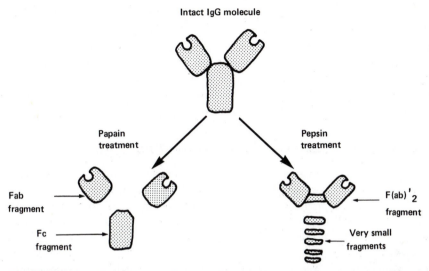

FIGURE 6-6. The effects of digestion by the proteolytic enzymes papain and pepsin on IgG. (From Tizard, I. Veterinary Immunology. 2nd ed. W. B. Saunders, Philadelphia, 1982. With permission.)

Subclasses of IgG

Even within the major immunoglobulin classes, there exist variants known as subclasses and subtypes. These may be identified on the basis of differences in antigenic structure, electrophoretic mobility, or differences in biological activities (Table 6–2). For example, the light chains of immunoglobulin molecules are of two subtypes termed kappa (κ) and lambda (λ), which have very different amino-acid sequences. In humans, about 65 percent of immunoglobulin molecules have κ chains, while 35 percent have λ chains; the subtype ratio differs in other species. κ and λ chains are antigenically different and can be readily identified by means of specific antibody.

The heavy chains of human IgG are divided into four different subclasses designated

TABLE 6–2   The Subclasses of Human IgG

	IgG1	IgG2	IgG3	IgG4
% of total IgG in serum	65	24	7	4
Heavy chain	γ_1	γ_2	γ_3	γ_4
Interheavy chain disulfide bonds	2	4	13	2
Complement fixation	++++	++	++++	(+)
Half-life (days)	23	23	8	23
Binding to Fc receptors on:				
neutrophils	+	+	+	+
macrophages	+	−	+	−
K cells	+	−	+	−
Placental passage	+	−	+	+
Sensitize guinea-pig skin	+	−	+	+

$\gamma1$, $\gamma2$, $\gamma3$ and $\gamma4$. All normal individuals possess all four subclasses. IgG molecules with $\gamma1$ heavy chains are known as IgG1, those with $\gamma2$ heavy chains are IgG2, etc. Not only are these heavy chains antigenically different, but they are also chemically and biologically distinct (Table 6–2). Thus, IgG3 has the shortest half-life, the lowest synthetic and highest catabolic rate, and an unusually high number of interchain disulfide bonds. Autoantibodies to clotting factors commonly tend to be IgG4 while autoantibodies to DNA tend to be IgG1 and IgG3. The reasons for these differences are unknown.

The Primary Structure of Immunoglobulins

The immunoglobulins found in any serum sample are a complex mixture of molecules with antibody activity against a wide spectrum of antigenic determinants. They thus represent a sample of the antibodies produced by that individual in response to a multitude of different antigenic stimuli. Because of their structural heterogeneity, it is not possible to use serum antibodies to analyze immunoglobulin structure in more than the general terms described above.

Immunoglobulins are secreted, however, by plasma cells and occasionally a single plasma cell may become neoplastic. As a result, a clone of cancerous plasma cells may arise and produce a single, absolutely homogeneous (monoclonal), immunoglobulin product. As the tumor grows, vast quantities of this homogeneous immunoglobulin appear in serum and must be removed. Since a plasma-cell tumor is known as a **myeloma,** the immunoglobulin product is called a myeloma protein (see p. 195). Myeloma proteins may be purified and their structure analyzed in detail.

One of the first tasks undertaken when myeloma proteins were recognized as perfectly homogeneous immunoglobulins was to determine the sequence of amino acids in light and heavy chains.

Light Chain Sequences   When light chains are sequenced, they are found to contain about 214 amino acids. If several light chains from different myelomas are studied almost identical amino-acid sequences are found in the C-terminal half of each light chain. (The C-terminus is the end of the chain with a free carboxyl group.) In contrast, the sequences in the N-terminal half (the end with a free amino group) are different in each light chain examined (Fig. 6–7). For this reason, these two halves of each light chain are referred to as constant (C_L) or variable (V_L) regions.

Heavy Chain Sequences   The heavy chains of IgG each consist of about 445 amino acids. Sequencing shows that the 115 N-terminal residues are different in each myeloma protein examined and thus constitute a variable (V_H) region, while the remaining 330 residues toward the C-terminus are relatively invariant and, therefore, form a constant (C_H) region.

Variable Regions   When the amino-acid sequences of a very large number of V regions from both light and heavy chains are examined carefully, two features become apparent. First, the sequence variation is largely restricted to certain areas within the entire variable region. Between these areas are relatively constant segments. (Figs. 6–7 and 6–8). These constant segments are called framework regions while between them are located hypervariable regions.

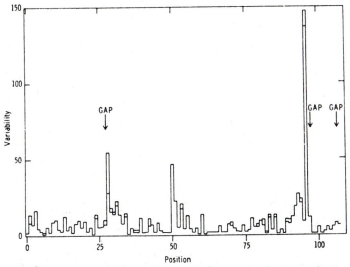

FIGURE 6-7. The variability at each different amino-acid position for the variable region of immunoglobulin light chains. (The variability is calculated as the number of different amino acids at a given position divided by the frequency of the most common amino acid at that position. An absolutely invariant residue has a value of 1.) Note the three hypervariable regions. GAP indicates positions at which insertions have been found. (From Wu, T. T., and Kabat, E. A. J. Exp. Med., *132:* 237, 1970. With permission.)

Light chains of both the κ and λ types each possess three hypervariable regions, whereas there are four hypervariable regions in heavy-chains (Fig. 6-8). Each hypervariable region is relatively short, consisting of from six to ten amino-acid residues.

When the sequences of framework regions are examined, it is clear that they, too, are not absolutely constant, but also show some variability. Examination of this framework variability reveals that variable regions can be classified into subgroups. Thus, in humans, there are three subgroups of V_κ regions, five subgroups of V_λ regions, and three subgroups of V_H regions. In the mouse, there are several hundred V_κ region subgroups but only two V_λ region subgroups. The number of different V_H region subgroups in the mouse is also relatively large but probably less than the number of V_κ region subgroups. Because each of the variable-region subgroups described above is distinctly different from the other, it is believed that each V-region subgroup is coded for by a separate V-region gene (see Chap. 8).

Constant Regions When the amino-acid sequences of the constant regions of immunoglobulin light and heavy chains were examined, several interesting features were revealed. First it became clear that each chain consisted of a set of repeated linear segments. Thus, there is remarkable similarity between the 110 amino-acid residues of the C_L region and three distinct segments, also of approximately 110 residues, making up the C_H region (Fig. 6-9). These repeating constant region segments are known as **homology regions.** It is believed that they have developed as a result of the repeated duplication of a single, primordial gene coding for a basic chain of 110 amino acids. Presumably, this gene first duplicated at an early evolutionary stage to form a linked constant and variable region and,

```
                         10                        20                        30

Tie  (γ1)  GLU VAL GLN LEU VAL GLU SER GLY GLY GLY LEU VAL GLN PRO GLY GLY SER LEU ARG LEU SER CYS ALA ALA SER GLY PHE THR PHE SER
Was  (γ1)  _____ LEU _____ SER _____
Jon  (γ3)  ASP _____ LYS _____
Zap  (α1)  _____ ALA _____ GLY _____
Tur  (α1)  _____ LEU _____
Nie  (γ1)  PCA _____ GLN _____ VAL _____ ARG _____
Gal  (μ)   _____ ASP _____ ARG _____ (ASX VAL LEU

LAY        ALA _____ LEU _____
POM        _____ LEU _____


                         40                        50                        60

Tie        THR SER ALA VAL TYR [    ] TRP VAL ARG GLN ALA PRO GLY LYS GLY LEU GLU TRP VAL GLY TRP ARG TYR GLU GLY SER SER LEU THR
Was        ___ ASP ___ MET ___ [    ] _____ ALA ___ LYS ___ GLN GLU ALA ___ ASN SER
Jon        ___ ALA TRP MET LYS [    ] _____ VAL _____ VAL ___ GLN VAL VAL GLU LYS
Zap        ___ THR SER ARG PHE [    ] _____ GLU PHE ___ VAL GLN _____ ALA ILE SER
Tur        ARG VAL LEU SER SER [    ] _____ SER GLY ___ LEU ASN ALA _____ ASN LEU
Nie        ARG TYR THR ILE HIS [    ] _____ ALA VAL MET SER TYR ASX GLY ASX ASX LYS
Gal        ASX ASX PHE)MET THR [    ] _____ ALA ASN ILE LYS GLX ASX GLY ___ GLX GLX

LAY        ALA _____ MET SER [    ] _____ ALA ___ LYS _____ ASN GLY ASN ASP LYS
POM        SER _____ MET SER [    ] _____ ALA ___ LYS _____ ASX GLY ASN ASP LYS


                         70                        80                        90

Tie        HIS TYR ALA VAL SER VAL GLN GLY ARG PHE THR ILE SER ARG ASN ASP SER LYS ASN THR LEU TYR LEU GLN MET LEU SER LEU GLU PRO
Was        ___ PHE ___ ASP THR ___ ASN _____ ASN ARG _____ ALA
Jon        ALA PHE ___ ASN _____ ASN _____ ILE ___ VAL THR ___
Zap        _____ ASP _____ ALA _____ ASN THR GLY ___ ALA
Tur        ___ PHE _____ ALA _____ GLN ALA
Nie        _____ ASP _____ ASN _____ ASN ___ ASN _____ ARG ___
Gal        ASX ___ VAL ASP _____ LYS _____ ASP ASN ALA _____ SER _____ ASN _____ ARG VAL

LAY        _____ ASP _____ ASN _____ ASN GLY ___ GLN ALA
POM        _____ ASP _____ ASN _____ LEU ___ ASN _____ GLN AL/


                         100                       110                       120

Tie        GLX ASX THR ALA VAL TYR TYR CYS ALA ARG VAL THR PRO ALA ALA ALA SER LEU THR PHE SER ALA VAL TRP GLY GLN GLY THR LEU VAL
Was        _____ PHE ARG GLN PRO PHE VAL GLN [    ] ___ PHE ASP ___ PHE _____
Jon        _____ VAL VAL SER THR [    ] SER MET ASP_____ PRO ___
Zap        _____ THR ARG ___ GLY GLY TYR [    ] ____ ASP _____
Tur        _____ LEU SER VAL THR ___ VAL [    ] ALA PHE ASP _____ LYS ___
Nie        _____ ILE ARG ASP THR ___ MET [    ] ___ PHE ___ HIS _____
Gal        _____ GLY TRP GLY [    ] GLY GLY ASP TYR _____

LAY        ___ VAL SER ___ ILE _____ ASP ALA GLY PRO TYR VAL ___ PRO _____ PHE ___ HIS _____
POM        _____ LEU _____ ASP ALA GLY PRO TYR VAL ___ PRO _____ PHE ___ HIS TYR _____
```

FIGURE 6–8. Seven complete V_H amino-acid sequences. Identity with the first protein (Tie) is indicated by a line. Residues that differ from Tie are noted. It is easy to see that some regions exhibit tremendous variability—for example, residues 31 to 36, 51 to 67, 86 to 90, and 101 to 114. These are known as hypervariable regions. (From Capra, J. D., and Kehoe, J. M. Proc. Natl. Acad. Sci., *71:* 4032–4036, 1974. With permission.)

SEQUENCE HOMOLOGY IN EU CONSTANT REGIONS

```
                                    110                              120
EU C_L  (RESIDUES 109-214)  THR VAL ALA ALA  PRO SER VAL PHE  ILE  PHE PRO PRO SER
EU C_H1 (RESIDUES 119-220)  SER THR LYS GLY  PRO SER VAL PHE  PRO  LEU ALA PRO SER
EU C_H2 (RESIDUES 234-341)  LEU LEU GLY GLY  PRO SER VAL PHE  LEU  PHE PRO PRO LYS
EU C_H3 (RESIDUES 342-446)  GLN PRO ARG GLU  PRO GLN VAL TYR  THR  LEU PRO PRO SER

                                              130
ASP GLU GLN  -   -  LEU LYS SER GLY THR ALA SER VAL VAL CYS LEU LEU ASN ASN PHE
SER LYS SER  -   -  THR SER GLY GLY THR ALA ALA LEU GLY CYS LEU VAL LYS ASP TYR
PRO LYS ASP THR LEU MET ILE SER ARG THR PRO GLU VAL THR CYS VAL VAL VAL ASP
ARG GLU GLU  -   -  MET THR LYS ASN GLN VAL SER LEU THR CYS LEU VAL LYS GLY PHE

140                              150
TYR PRO ARG GLU ALA LYS VAL  -   -  GLN TRP LYS VAL ASP ASN ALA LEU GLN SER GLY
PHE PRO GLU PRO VAL THR VAL  -   -  SER TRP ASN SER  -  GLY ALA LEU THR SER GLY
SER HIS GLU ASP PRO GLN VAL LYS PHE ASN TRP TYR VAL ASP GLY  -  VAL GLN VAL HIS
TYR PRO SER ASP ILE ALA VAL  -   -  GLU TRP GLU SER ASN ASP  -  GLY GLU PRO GLU

160                              170
ASN SER GLN GLU SER VAL THR GLU GLN ASP SER LYS ASP SER THR TYR SER LEU SER SER
 -  VAL HIS THR PHE PRO ALA VAL LEU GLN SER  -  SER GLY LEU TYR SER LEU SER SER
ASN ALA LYS THR LYS PRO ARG GLU GLN GLN TYR  -  ASP SER THR TYR ARG VAL VAL SER
ASN TYR LYS THR THR PRO PRO VAL LEU ASP SER  -  ASP GLY SER PHE PHE LEU TYR SER

180                              190
THR LEU THR LEU SER LYS ALA ASP TYR GLU LYS HIS LYS VAL TYR ALA CYS GLU VAL THR
VAL VAL THR VAL PRO SER SER SER LEU GLY THR GLN  -  THR TYR ILE CYS ASN VAL ASN
VAL LEU THR VAL LEU HIS GLN ASN TRP LEU ASP GLY LYS GLU TYR LYS CYS LYS VAL SER
LYS LEU THR VAL ASP LYS SER ARG TRP GLN GLU GLY ASN VAL PHE SER CYS SER VAL MET

200                              210
HIS GLN GLY LEU SER SER PRO VAL THR  -  LYS SER PHE  -   -  ASN ARG GLY GLU CYS
HIS LYS PRO SER ASN THR LYS VAL  -  ASP LYS ARG VAL  -   -  GLU PRO LYS SER CYS
ASN LYS ALA LEU PRO ALA PRO ILE  -  GLU LYS THR ILE SER LYS ALA LYS GLY
HIS GLU ALA LEU HIS ASN HIS TYR THR GLN LYS SER LEU SER LEU SER PRO GLY
```

FIGURE 6–9. The complete sequence of the constant region of myeloma protein Eu is arranged in four blocks, each corresponding to a homology region. The shaded areas indicate sequence homology. Note particularly the cysteines at positions 134 and 194. It is these that link to form the intrachain loops (See Fig. 6–10.) (From Edelman, G. M. et al. Proc. Natl. Acad. Sci., *63:* 83, 1969. With permission.)

thus, a primitive light chain. The constant region was subsequently duplicated at least twice to form a heavy chain. Three constant homology regions make up a γ heavy chain. They are labelled from the N-terminal end, C_{H1}, C_{H2}, and C_{H3} (Fig. 6–10). A similar arrangement is found in α chains. In μ and ϵ chains an additional homology region known as C_{H4} is present (Fig. 6–16).

Homology regions are paired to form specialized regions within the immunoglobulin molecule known as **domains.** The structure of these provides a mechanism by which immunoglobulin molecules can exert additional biological activities. Thus, collectively, V_H and V_L form a domain that serves to bind antigen, and C_{H1} and C_L together act to stabilize the antigen-binding site. The paired C_{H2} regions of IgG form a domain that contains site for activation of the complement cascade (see Chap. 14). This domain also influences the catabolic rate of IgG, while the adherence of IgG to phagocytic cell Fc receptors is mediated through a site on the C_{H3} domain formed by paired C_{H3} regions although its conformation is influenced by the proximity of the C_{H2} domain. Structures within the heavy chain also regulate placental transfer of IgG and antibody-mediated cellular cytotoxicity (Chap. 11) although these are probably due to the combined activities of several domains.

Other Functions of Immunoglobulin Homology Regions Immunoglobulin homology regions appear to be able to function as very useful protein "building blocks." As a result, similar structures are widely employed in nonimmunoglobulin molecules (Fig. 6–11).

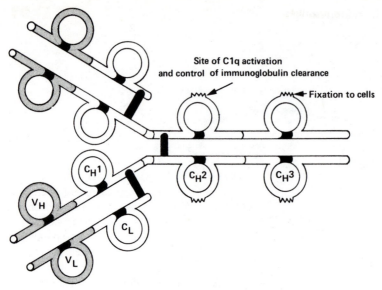

FIGURE 6–10. A schematic diagram showing the homology regions of IgG. (From Tizard, I. Veterinary Immunology. 2nd ed. W. B. Saunders, Philadelphia, 1982. With permission.)

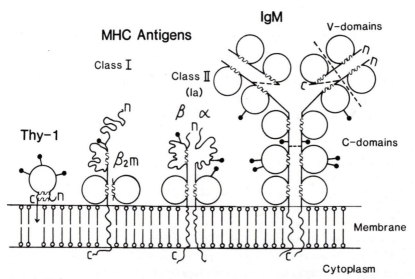

FIGURE 6–11. Immunoglobulin-related molecules found at lymphoid cell surfaces. Ig domains and their homologous regions in the other molecules are represented by circles. Intrachain disulphide bonds are shown by the $\frac{S}{S}$ symbols and interchain bonds in IgM by dashed lines. N-linked carbohydrate structures are shown by ˥, and n and c identify the N-terminus and C-terminus of the polypeptides with the exception of β_2-microglobulin (β_2-m). The polymorphic determinants of the major histocompatibility (MHC) antigens are found mainly in the heavy chains of Class I antigens and the β chains of Class II antigens. (From Williams, A. F. Bioscience Reports, *2:* 281, 1982. With permission.)

β-2 Microglobulin (β₂M) A small protein (11,800 Mr), β_2M is found on the membranes of all nucleated cells, in serum, seminal fluid, and colostrum. On cell membranes, it forms part of the Class I histocompatibility antigens (see Chap. 3), the receptor for phytohemagglutinin (see Chap. 10), and the thymus leukemia (TL) antigen (see Chap. 10). β_2M has an amino-acid sequence and structure very similar to that found in C_H homology regions. As a result, it can fix complement and bind to macrophage Fc receptors. The function of β_2M is unclear, although it does seem to enhance the immunogenicity of proteins with which it is associated.

C-Reactive Protein C-reactive protein (CRP), so-called for its ability to precipitate the C polysaccharide of *Strep pneumoniae*, has a molecular weight of 135,000. It is absent from normal serum, but appears in the blood of individuals suffering from acute inflammation or severe tissue damage. C-reactive protein has a structure similar to a C_{H3} immunoglobulin homology region. It can, therefore, activate the complement cascade and will promote phagocytosis, but its basic biological function is unclear.

Thy-1 Antigen A characteristic feature of lymphocytes that mature within the thymus is that they develop a cell-surface-protein antigen known as Thy 1 (Chap. 10). Thy 1 possesses a sequence homology very similar to that of an immunoglobulin constant homology region.

Immunoglobulin-like regions have also been reported in the brain peptide, β endorphin, in the heavy chain of some Class I histocompatibility antigens, and in the α chain of the HLA-DR molecules (Fig. 6–11). The occurrence of these homologies is unlikely to be of major immunological significance, but probably reflects the general usefulness of the basic structure and the evolution of these proteins from a common precursor molecule.

The Hinge Region On electron microscopy of IgG, it can be readily observed that the Fab regions are mobile and can swing freely around the center of the molecule as if they are hinged (Fig. 6–12). This hinge consists of a group of about 15 amino acids located between the C_{H1} and C_{H2} regions. The exact sequence of amino acids in the hinge is very variable. There is no homology between the hinge and other heavy-chain regions, and the sequence is unique for each immunoglobulin class and subclass.

A remarkable feature of the hinge region is the presence in it of a large number of hydrophilic and proline residues (Table 6–3). The hydrophilic residues tend to open up this region and thus make it accessible to proteolytic cleavage. As a result, it is in this region that pepsin and papain act. This region also contains all the interchain disulfide bonds (although IgD has a hinge region without cysteine residues, and hence no interchain links).

Proline, because of its configuration, produces a 90° "bend" in a polypeptide chain. Since amino acids can rotate freely around peptide bonds, the effect of closely spaced prolines is to produce a "universal joint" around which the immunoglobulin chains can swing freely (Fig. 6–13).

Immunoglobulin M

IgM (Fig. 6–14) is found in the second highest concentration after IgG in most mammals, with the exception of humans, where the IgA concentration is slightly greater that that of IgM (Table 6–4). Structurally, IgM is formed by five basic 180,000 Mr subunits. As a

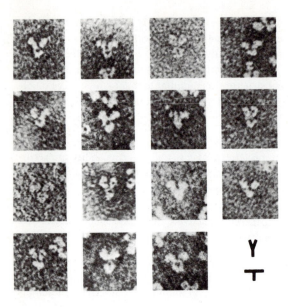

FIGURE 6–12. A series of electron micrographs of IgG showing the variable orientation of the Fab regions, as a result of the flexibility of the hinge region, and an interpretative diagram illustrating the two extremes of the basic "Y" configuration observed. (From Roux, K. H., and Metzger, D. W. J. Exp. Med., *129:* 2548, 1982. With permission.)

result, its molecular weight is 900,000. Each of the basic subunits consists of two κ or two λ light chains and two μ (mu) heavy chains. Since each subunit possesses two antigen-binding sites it might be anticipated that the valency of IgM for antigen would be 10. In practice, this valency is more commonly found to be 5 as a result of steric hindrance between antigen molecules. IgM has carbohydrate residues attached to the C_{H3} domain and an additional, fourth constant homology region (C_{H4}). The site for complement activation by IgM is located on this C_{H4} region.

The IgM monomers are linked together by disulfide bonds in a circular fashion to form a star. A small cystein-rich polypeptide called the J chain (15,000 Mr), coded for by a separate gene, binds two of the units to complete the circle. Since IgM molecules are normally secreted intact by plasma cells, the J chain must be considered to be an integral part of the molecule.

IgM is the major immunoglobulin class produced in a primary immune response. It is also produced during a secondary response, but this is commonly masked by the production of very large quantities of IgG. In humans, for example, about 32 mg/kg of IgG is produced daily as opposed to 2.2 mg/kg of IgM. Although produced in relatively small

TABLE 6–3   Amino-Acid Sequences Within the Hinge Regions of Human IgG Subclasses

	225						230				
Human γ 1	Lys	Thr	His	Thr	Cys	Pro	Pro	Cys	Pro	Ala	Pro	Gly
Human γ 2	Cys	Cys	Val	Glu	Cys	Pro	Pro	Cys	Pro	Ala		
Human γ 3	Thr	Pro	Pro	Pro	Cys	Pro	Arg	Cys	Pro	Ala	Pro	Glu
Human γ 4	Tyr	Gly	Pro	Pro	Cys	Pro	Arg	Cys	Pro	Ala	Ser	Glu

Note the large number of proline residues that confer flexibility and the cysteine residues that are involved in interchain-disulfide-bridge formation.

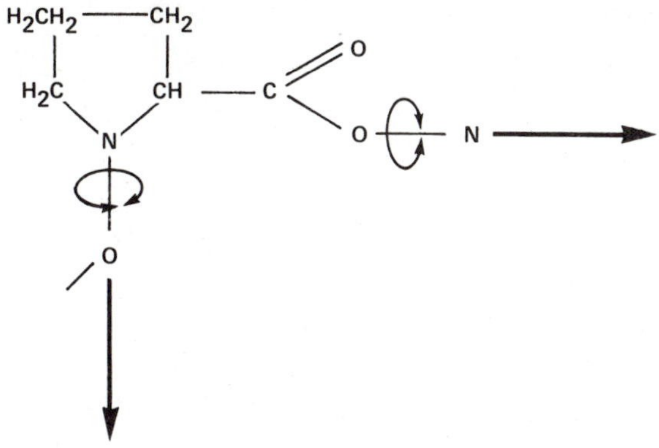

H₂CH₂————CH₂
H₂C   CH ——— C
       N   O
                       O   N ⟶

FIGURE 6–13. The structure of the amino acid proline demonstrating how, when inserted in an amino-acid chain, it produces a right-angle bend. Because peptide bonds are free to rotate, three prolines in series effectively function as a "universal joint." (From Tizard, I. Veterinary Immunology. 2nd ed. W. B. Saunders, Philadelphia, 1982. With permission.)

quantities, when considered on a molar basis, IgM is more efficient than IgG at activating the complement cascade, at opsonization, at virus neutralization and at agglutination.

Because of their very large size, IgM antibodies are essentially confined to the blood vascular system and are therefore of little importance in conferring protection in tissue fluids or body secretions.

IgM molecules, possibly in the monomeric form, function as antigen receptors on B cells (Chap. 10). This membrane-bound IgM differs from the secreted form in that the C-terminus of the C_{H4} region is longer and contains hydrophobic residues that enable it to interact with cell-membrane lipids (see Chap. 8).

Immunoglobulin A

Monomeric IgA has a molecular weight of 150,000 (6.8S), but it is normally found as a dimer. Each molecule has a typical four-chain structure consisting of paired κ or λ chains

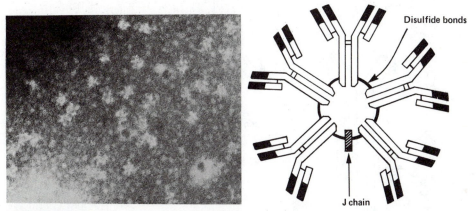

FIGURE 6–14. The structure of IgM and an electron micrograph of this immunoglobulin from bovine serum. Approximate magnification × 240,000. (Courtesy of Drs. K. Nielsen and B. Stemshom. From Tizard, I. Veterinary Immunology. 2nd ed. W. B. Saunders, Philadelphia, 1982. With permission.)

**TABLE 6–4 Immunoglobulin Levels
in Human Serum**

Class and Subclass	mg/100 ml
IgG1	800
IgG2	400
IgG3	100
IgG4	40
IgM	100
IgA1	350
IgA2	40
IgD	3
IgE	.01

and two α (alpha) heavy chains (Fig. 6–15). In dimeric IgA, the molecules are joined by a J chain linked to the Fc regions. Higher polymers of IgA are occasionally found free in serum.

In many species of mammal, including man, subclasses of IgA are recognized. In humans, differences in heavy-chain structure give rise to IgA1 and IgA2. There are two

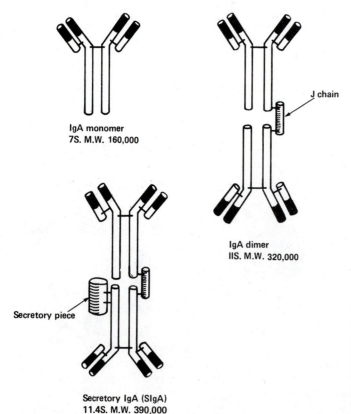

IgA monomer
7S. M.W. 160,000

J chain

IgA dimer
IIS. M.W. 320,000

Secretory piece

Secretory IgA (SIgA)
11.4S. M.W. 390,000

FIGURE 6–15. The structure of the major forms of IgA. (From Tizard, I. Veterinary Immunology., 2nd ed. W. B. Saunders, Philadelphia, 1982. With permission.)

variants of IgA2. One variant lacks disulfide bonds between the heavy and light chains, and the molecule is, therefore, held together only by noncovalent forces. Interchain bonds are present in the other IgA2 variant and in all IgA1 molecules. IgA is synthesized largely by plasma cells located on body surfaces. The IgA produced by the cells in the intestinal wall may either pass directly into the intestinal lumen or, alternatively, diffuse into the bloodstream. IgA within the bloodstream binds to receptors on hepatocytes as it passes through the liver and is carried through them into the bile. As the IgA is transported through intestinal epithelial cells or through hepatocytes, it binds to a glycoprotein of 71,000 daltons known as secretory component (or secretory piece). Secretory component binds covalently to IgA dimers to form a complex molecule called secretory IgA (SIgA). Secretory IgA is the predominant immunoglobulin in intestinal secretions, and it is the secretory component that serves to protect IgA from digestion by gastrointestinal proteolytic enzymes. The production of secretory component is independent of the production of IgA. Secretory IgA is of critical importance in protecting body surfaces against invading micro-organisms, since it is the major immunoglobulin in the intestinal, respiratory, and urogenital tracts, in milk and in tears.

Immunoglobulin E

IgE (Fig. 6–16) is composed of paired κ or λ light chains and two ϵ (epsilon) heavy chains. Each heavy chain contains an additional constant homology region and, as a result, has a molecular weight of 190,000 and a sedimentation coefficient of 8S.

IgE is found in very low concentrations in the serum of unparasitized individuals (20–500 ng/ml) but is nevertheless of major importance, since it mediates Type I hypersensitivity reactions (i.e., allergies and anaphylaxis; see Chap. 20) and is largely responsible for immunity to invading parasites.

IgE is unique in that its Fc region binds strongly to a receptor on mast cells and basophils, and, together with antigen, mediates the release of inflammatory agents from these cells. IgE has the shortest half-life of all immunoglobulins (2–3 days) and is readily denatured by mild heat treatment.

Immunoglobulin D

Immunoglobulin D molecules consist of two δ (delta) heavy chains and two κ or λ light chains. Its molecular weight is about 170,000 Mr and its sedimentation coefficient is 7S.

IgD is found in very low concentrations in plasma and is very difficult to study because it is extraordinarily susceptible to proteolysis. Since proteolytic enzymes are generated when blood clots, IgD is usually absent from serum. Like IgE, IgD is readily denatured by mild heat treatment. The reason for this fragility is that IgD has no interchain disulfide bonds between its heavy chains and a very exposed hinge region.

IgD antibodies with activity against thyroid tissue, insulin, penicillin, nuclear antigens, and against diphtheria toxoid have been described. Nevertheless, extensive IgD production is not a common feature of conventional immune responses. IgD is primarily a cell-membrane immunoglobulin found on the surface of B lymphocytes in association with IgM (Chap. 10). This lymphocyte-bound IgD has a very hydrophobic C_{H3} region, which is associated with the cell-membrane lipids. It may exist in the form of half molecules. IgD serves, in this location, as a specific antigen receptor.

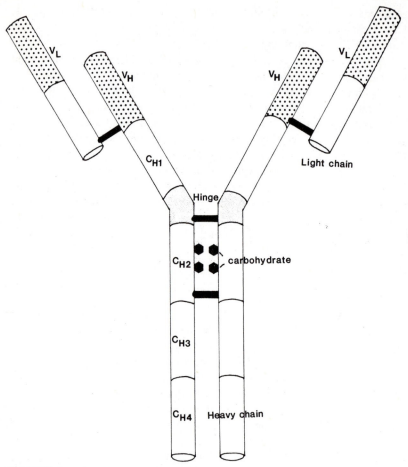

FIGURE 6-16. The structure of IgE.

The Three-Dimensional Structure of Immunoglobulins

While the primary structure of a protein is based upon the sequence of amino-acid residues in a polypeptide chain, the reader should be well aware that these chains are not composed of straight, sticklike molecules. The shape of a polypeptide chain may be very complex, because each amino acid in a chain forms an angle with its neighbor, influenced by the charged and hydrophobic interactions between nearby residues. The final structure that develops is generally the most thermodynamically stable configuration.

As might be anticipated, the overall three-dimensional structure of immunoglobulin molecules is relatively constant. This applies not only to the constant parts of the molecule, but also to the variable regions. The occurrence of hypervariable regions within the variable regions, however ensures that there are profound differences in molecular shape in the region of the antigen-binding site.

Overall, a typical monomeric immunoglobulin G molecule consists of three globular regions (Fig. 6–17) (two Fab regions and Fc) linked by a flexible hinge region. Closer examination of each of these globular regions shows that they can be divided into domains corresponding to paired homology regions. Thus, the Fab globular regions each consist of two interacting domains (V_H–V_L and C_{H1}–C_L), while the Fc globular region contains either two or three domains depending upon the immunoglobulin class (i.e., C_{H2}–C_{H2}, C_{H3}–C_{H3}, and in IgE or IgM, C_{H4}–C_{H4}). The polypeptide chains within each domain are closely intertwined. In the Fab globular region, however, there is a deep cleft between the two variable-region chains. The peptides of the hypervariable regions line this cleft; as a

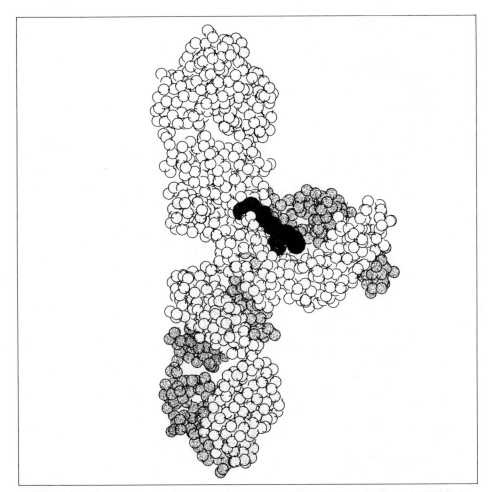

FIGURE 6–17. The three-dimensional structure of the myeloma immunoglobulin Dob. One complete heavy chain is white, the other is dark gray; the two light chains are lightly shaded. The large, black spheres represent the individual hexose units of the complex carbohydrate. The reader may find it useful to compare this diagram with Figures 6-4 and 6-11. (From Silverton, E. W. Proc. Natl. Acad. Sci., *74:* 5140–5144, 1977. With permission.)

result, the surface of the cleft shows great variability in its shape and constitutes the antigen-binding site.

Because immunoglobulins are bilaterally identical, the cleft on each Fab globular region will be identical and, as a result, the molecule will be bivalent and able to cross-link two identical antigenic determinants. Between the two C_{H2} regions in the IgG molecule, there exists a large, solvent-filled space in which are located carbohydrate residues. This space appears to be required in order to maintain the correct configuration of the Fc region and to allow it to mediate its biological activities. It can be seen very clearly in Figure 6–4.

Immunoglobulins as Antigens

Because immunoglobulin molecules are proteins, they can serve as very effective antigens when used to immunize mammals of a different species. When the resulting anti-immunoglobulin (or antiglobulin, for short) antibodies are carefully analyzed, three major categories of antigenic determinants may be recognized (Fig. 6–18).

First, as described earlier, the dominant antigenic determinants are those found on the immunoglobulins of all animals of a species. These include the determinants specific for each immunoglobulin class such as γ for IgG, μ for IgM and α for IgA, etc. In addition there are subclass-specific determinants found, for example, on γ_1 and γ_2 heavy chains, and the light-chain subtype-specific determinants κ and λ. The collective term for class and subclass- and subtype-specific antigenic determinants such as these is **isotype.**

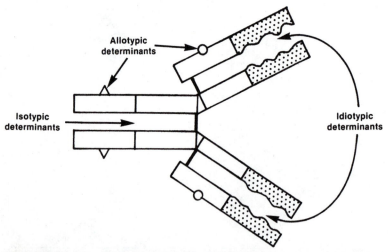

FIGURE 6–18. The antigenic structure of an immunoglobulin molecule: Isotypic determinants are found on the heavy chains of all molecules of a specific isotype. On the heavy chains, these determine the immunoglobulin class or subclass. On the light chains, these determine the subtype. Allotypic determinants are inherited variations that may be located in any region of the molecule. Idiotypic determinants are associated with the hypervariable regions.

Allotypes

The second major group of antigenic determinants are those found on the immuno-globulins of some, but not all, animals of a species. Antibodies to these **allotypes** may be produced by injecting the immunoglobulins of one animal into another of the same species. Any "foreign" determinants will provoke antibody formation. The presence of allotypic determinants on an immunoglobulin is genetically determined. Homozygous individuals have the same determinants on all immunoglobulins of a specific class. Heterozygous individuals have approximately half of their immunoglobulins of one allotype and half with the allotype coded by the alternative allele. The phenomenon occurs because, although they possess two chromosomes, antibody-producing cells in a heterozygous individual use only one chromosome at a time and, therefore, will each make only one allotype from each allelic group. This phenomenon is called **allelic exclusion.**

How Allotypes Were First Identified

In the disease known as rheumatoid arthritis (Chap. 21), an autoantibody is produced that is known as **rheumatoid factor.** Rheumatoid factor is directed against an immunoglobulin bound to antigen and is thus an antiglobulin. Grubb and his colleagues in 1956 found that erythrocytes coated with nonagglutinating antibodies, were agglu-tinated by rheumatoid factors. Some human sera, called Gm(a+) could inhibit the agglutination caused by the rheumatoid factors, while other sera (Gm(a−)) could not. Further studies showed that Gm(a) determinant (now called G1m(1)) was present only on the heavy chain of IgG1 and was inherited as a domi-nant mendelian trait. Presumably, the rheumatoid factors were directed against this determinant, and the addition of Gm(a+) immunoglobulins in sera to the mixture caused competitive inhibition. It is now possible to induce anti-Gm antibodies by immu-nization of Gm-negative individuals.

Grubb, R. Agglutination of erythrocytes coated with "incomplete" anti-Rh by certain rheumatoid arthritis sera and some other sera. Acta. Pathol. et Microbiol. Scand., 39:195–197, 1956.

Allotypes of Humans   In man, five sets of allotypic markers have been found (Table 6–5): Gm, Km, Mm, Am, and Hv. The Gm determinants are found on γ heavy chains and are thus restricted to IgG molecules. There are about 25 different Gm determinants,

TABLE 6–5   Human Immunoglobulin Allotypes

Location	Allotype
κ light chains	Km 1, 2, 3
Heavy-chain variable regions	Hv 1
γ 1 heavy chain	G1m 1, 2, 3, 4, 17
γ 2 heavy chain	G2m 23
γ 3 heavy chain	G3m 5, 6, 11, 13, 14, 15, 16, 21, b, c
γ 4 heavy chain	G4m 4a, 4b
μ heavy chain	Mm 1
α 2 heavy chain	A2m 1, 2

each denoted by two numbers. The first number denotes the immunoglobulin subclass on which they are found; the second number denotes the allotype. These determinants are restricted to certain IgG subclasses and homology regions. Thus, G1m (4) and G1m (17) are restricted to the C_{H1} region of IgG1 molecules, G3m (5) and G3m (21) are found on the C_{H2} region of IgG3 molecules and so on. A single γ heavy chain may possess several Gm determinants and these may be inherited in association. Thus G1m (1) is commonly associated with G1m (17) on the same IgG1 molecule.

The allotypic determinant Mm (1) has been identified on μ chains while A2m (1) and A2m (2) are found on $α_2$ chains (the heavy chains of the IgA2 subclass).

The Hv (1) determinant is found on the V_H region. As a result it is found on IgG, IgM and IgA.

The Km antigenic determinants, by contrast, are found on κ light-chain constant regions. As a result, they are present on all the immunoglobulin classes and subclasses. There are three alternative Km determinants. Km 1, which is associated with a valine at position 153 and a leucine at position 191, Km 1,2, which is due to an alanine at position 153 and a leucine at position 191, and Km 3, which has an alanine at position 153 and a valine at position 191. These three behave like alleles of a single gene.

Rabbit Allotypes   Rabbit allotypes (Table 6–6) are inherited through at least eleven gene loci. Eight of these loci code for determinants in the constant regions of light and heavy chains; thus, e and d are in the C_H region, b is in $C_κ$ while c is in $C_λ$, and f is found in $C_α$.

Allotypes a, x, and y are associated with determinants in the V_H region. By using specific antisera, these allotypes can be found on IgG, IgM, IgA, and IgE. This implies that a single V-region gene carrying these allotypes must be able to interact with a series of different heavy-chain constant-region genes. Since crossovers have been observed to occur between the V_H allotype a and the allotypes e and d on the C_H region, this also implies that the V_H and C_H genes must be relatively far apart (see also Chap. 8).

Mouse Allotypes   Allotypic determinants have been found in mouse IgG1, IgG2, IgM, IgA, and IgD and on light chains. Those found on heavy chains are denoted by the prefix

TABLE 6–6   Rabbit Immunoglobulin Allotypes

Location	Locus	Alleles
κ light chain	b	b 4, b 5, b 6, b 9
λ light chain	c	c 7, c 21
VH regions	a	a 1, a 2, a 3
	x	x 32
	y	y 33
γ heavy chain	d	d 11, d 12
	e	e 14, e 15
α heavy chain	f	f 71, f 72, f 73
	g	g 74, g 75
μ heavy chain	ms	ms 1, ms 2, ms 3, ms 4, ms 5, ms 6
	n	n 81, n 82

Igh followed by a number, thus, Igh-1, Igh-2, etc. The Igh allotypic loci are coded for by genes clustered on chromosome 12.

Allotypes in Other Species Allotypes have been demonstrated in most other mammalian species. Cattle have four allotypes, three on C_γ and one on C_L. Pigs have four allotypes, dogs have an IgM allotype, and chickens have four γ allotypes.

Idiotypes

The third group of antigenic determinants on immunoglobulins exist as a result of the unique structures generated by the hypervariable regions on light and heavy chains. These determinants are known as **idiotopes.** The collection of idiotopes on an immunoglobulin is known as its **idiotype.**

It is not easy to make specific anti-idiotype serum, since, if purified serum immunoglobulins are used as antigens, the immunodominant determinants are isotypic or allotypic. If, however, the immunizing immunoglobulin is a homogeneous preparation, for example, a myeloma protein, then the relative dose of an individual V-region determinant is much higher, and anti-idiotype antibodies may be generated. Alternatively, it has been found that some rabbit antipneumococcal polysaccharide antibodies tend to be very homogeneous, and they, too, may be used as antigens for the production of anti-idiotype serum.

If these immunoglobulins are used as antigens and the antiglobulins provoked are carefully absorbed, the antibodies remaining may have a specificity for antigenic determinants located in the hypervariable regions of the V regions. These are **anti-idiotype antibodies.** As is found with the rabbit V_H allotypes, the same idiotype may be associated with several different antibody classes reflecting the fact that one V-region gene may be paired with several alternative C-region genes. Thus, for example, when a cell switches from IgM to IgG production, its V regions may remain unchanged, while its C regions switch.

Sources of Additional Information

Capra, J. D., and Kehoe, J. M. Variable region sequence of five human immunoglobulin heavy chains of the V_{HIII} subgroup, definitive identification of four heavy chain hypervariable regions. Proc. Natl. Acad. Sci. USA., *71:* 845–848, 1974.

Davies, D. R., Padlan, E. A., and Segal, D. M. Three dimensional structures of immunoglobulins. Ann. Rev. Biochem., *44:* 639–667, 1975.

Edelman, G. M. The structure and function of antibodies. Sci. Am., *223*(2): 34–42, 1970.

Lin, L-C., and Putnam, F. W. Primary structure of the Fc region of human immunoglobulin D: implications for evolutionary origin and biological function. Proc. Natl. Acad. Sci. USA., *78:* 504–508, 1981.

Milstein, C. Monoclonal antibodies. Sci. Am., *243:* 66–74, 1980.

Natvig, J. B., and Kunkel, H. G. Human immunoglobulin, classes, subclasses, genetic variants and idiotypes. Adv. Immunol., *16:* 1–59, 1978.

Nisonoff, A., Hopper, J. R., and Spring, S. B. The Antibody Molecule. Academic Press, New York, 1975.

Oi, V., et al. Lymphocyte membrane IgG and secreted IgG are structurally and allotypically distinct. J. Exp. Med., *151:* 1260–1274, 1980.

Osler, A. G. On the precedence of 19S antibodies in the early immune response. Immunochemistry, *15:* 714–720, 1978.

Uzgiris, E. E., and Kornberg, R. D. Two-dimensional crystallization technique for imaging mac-romolecules, with application to antigen-antibody-complement complexes. Nature, *301:* 125–129, 1983.

Wu, T. T., and Kabat, E. A. An analysis of the sequences of the variable regions of Bence-Jones proteins and myeloma light chains and their implications for antibody complementarity. J. Exp. Med., *132:* 211–250, 1970.

7

The Combination of Antigen with Antibody

The Chemical Basis of Antigen-Antibody Bonding

When an antigenic determinant and its specific antibody combine, they interact through the chemical groups found on the surface of the antigenic determinant and on the surface of the hypervariable regions of the immunoglobulin molecule.

In classical chemical reactions, molecules are assembled through the establishment of firm, covalent bonds. These bonds, however, can only be broken by the input of a significant amount of energy—energy that is not readily available in body systems. By contrast, the formation of noncovalent bonds provides a rapid and reversible way of forming complexes and therefore permits reuse of molecules in a way that covalent bonding would not allow. Noncovalent bonds, however, act over very short intermolecular distances and, as a result, form only when two molecules approach very closely (Table 7–1).

The binding of antigen to antibody is exclusively noncovalent. As a result, the strongest binding occurs when the two components are very closely approximated and, ideally, when the shape of the antigenic determinants and the shape of the antigen-binding site conform to each other. This requirement for a very close conformational fit has been likened to the specificity of a key for its lock.

The major bonds formed between antigen and antibody are hydrophobic in nature. Many of the nonpolar side chains of proteins are hydrophobic. When antigen and antibody molecules come together, these side chains interact and exclude water molecules from the area of interaction. Since this exclusion frees some water molecules from constraints imposed by the proteins, it results in a favorable gain in entropy, and the complex is, therefore, energetically stable.

A second type of noncovalent interaction is that mediated through hydrogen bonds (Fig. 7–1). When a hydrogen atom covalently bound to one electronegative atom (as in an $-OH$ group for example) gets close to another electronegative atom (for example, an $0 = C-$ group), then the hydrogen is shared between the electronegative atoms. This situation is energetically favorable, and is known as a hydrogen bond. The major hydrogen bonds formed in antigen–antibody interaction are $O-H-O$, $N-H-N$, and $O-H-N$. In addition, since hydrogen bonds normally pre-exist between proteins and water molecules when in aqueous solution, the complexing of antigen to antibody by hydrogen bonds normally requires relatively little net energy change.

TABLE 7–1 Major Forces through which Antigenic Determinants and Antibodies Interact

Bonding Force	Relationship between Force and Distance*	Stabilization Energy† (kcal mole^{-1})
Electrostatic	$1/d^2$	5–10
Hydrogen bonding	$1/d^2$	2–5
Hydrophobic interactions	$1/d^7$	1–5
Van der Waals	$1/d^7$	0.5

*This is the distance between molecules.

†The stabilization energy of a bond is a reflection of the ease with which it is broken. It may be compared with that of covalent bonds, which is in the region of 40–140 kcal mole^{-1}.

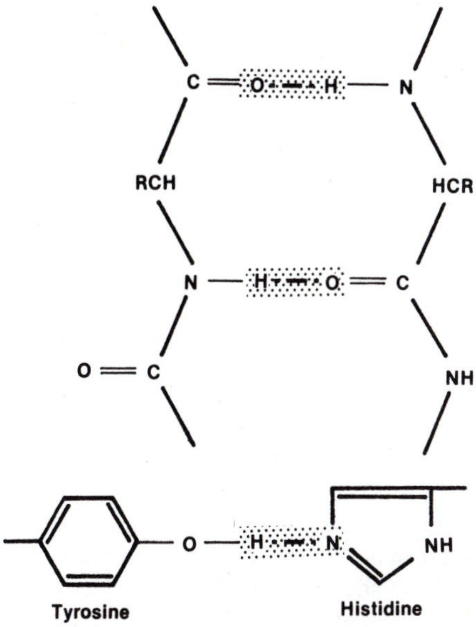

FIGURE 7–1. Hydrogen bonds such as these link polypeptide chains and are, therefore, of importance in the combination of antigen and antibody.

We might anticipate that electrostatic bonds formed between oppositely charged amino acids may contribute to antigen–antibody binding. The charge on many protein groups however, is commonly neutralized by electrolytes in solution, and, as a result, the relative importance of electrostatic bonds is unclear.

When two atoms approach very closely, a nonspecific attractive force called a Van der Waals force becomes operative. This force, while very weak, may become collectively important. It occurs as a result of a minor asymmetry in the charge of an atom due to the position of its electrons.

The Strength of Binding between Antigen and Antibody

The binding of antibody to its antigen is mediated, as described above, by several types of noncovalent bonds. Each of these is relatively weak in itself, but collectively they may have a significant binding strength. All of these bonds, however, act only across a very short distance and weaken very rapidly as that distance increases. Thus electrostatic-bond and hydrogen-bond strengths fall off in inverse proportion to the square of the distance between the interacting molecules, and the Van der Waals forces and hydrophobic forces decline in inverse proportion to the seventh power of that distance. Clearly, therefore, the strongest binding between antigen and antibody will occur only if their shapes match perfectly. Notwithstanding this fact, antigens can bind to antibodies when they fit less than perfectly, although, clearly, the number of bonds established and the strength of binding will be less.

Measurement of Binding Strength

Because the combination of antigen and antibody is a reversible reaction

$$Ag + Ab \rightleftharpoons Ag\,Ab,$$

the strength of binding of the reactants can be defined through an affinity constant (K) by the mass action equation:

$$K = \frac{[AbAg]}{[Ab][Ag]},$$

where [Ab] is the concentration of antibody-binding sites. [Ag] is the concentration of free antigenic determinants and [AbAg] the concentration of immune complexes *at equilibrium*.

How to Measure Antibody Affinity

Antibody affinity may be measured by means of a method known as equilibrium dialysis. This technique involves placing a mixture of univalent hapten (H), for example, dinitrochlorobenzene, and antibody (Ab) in a dialysis sac (Fig. 7–2). The antibody cannot pass through the dialysis membrane, but the hapten does so freely. When equilibrium is reached, any hapten bound to the antibody [AbH] is retained within the sac. On the other hand, the unbound hapten, being free to diffuse through the membrane, will be at an equal concentration both inside and outside the sac. If the total amount of hapten inside and outside the sac is measured, the amount of hapten bound to the antibody is easily measured by subtraction, and the process can be repeated using different hapten concentrations. (1) At equilibrium, therefore,

$$K = \frac{[Ab\,H]}{[Ab][H]}. \tag{1}$$

This can be simplified to:

$$K = \frac{b}{A_F \cdot c}$$

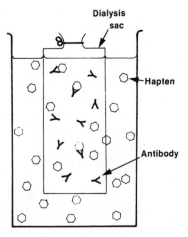

FIGURE 7–2. Equilibrium dialysis: Antibody is confined within the dialysis sac while the hapten is free to diffuse through the membrane. When equilibrium is reached, the concentration of free hapten will be identical both inside and outside the sac. However, additional hapten will be bound to antibody inside the sac. By measuring the concentration of hapten inside and outside the sac at different hapten concentrations, the amount of bound hapten and hence the affinity of the antibody may be calculated.

where b is the concentration of bound hapten, A_F is the concentration of uncomplexed antibody-binding sites, and c is the concentration of free hapten *at equilibrium.* However A_F can also be expressed as

$$(nA_T - b) \tag{2}$$

where n is the number of binding sites on an antibody molecule (its valency) and A_T is the total concentration of antibody in the system. Thus equation 2 can be expressed as:

$$K = \frac{b}{(nA_T - b)c} . \tag{3}$$

If we divide this by A_T, we get:

$$K = \frac{b/A_T}{cnA_T/A_T - cb/A_T} . \tag{4}$$

Now b/A_T is the ratio of the moles of hapten bound per mole of antibody in the inner chamber, and we can call this ratio r. Equation 4 may therefore be simplified:

$$K = \frac{r}{cn - cr} \tag{5}$$

which can be rearranged to:

$$r/c = -Kr + Kn \tag{6}$$

In this system, both r and c are variables, while K and n are constants. Equation (6) can therefore be considered to be a form of the straight-line equation ($y = ax + b$), where a is the slope and b the intercept of the abscissa. Thus, if r/c is plotted against r, the slope will be $-K$, the intercept on the abscissa will be Kn, and the intercept on the ordinate will be n, the valency of the antibody (Fig. 7–3). (This is known as a Scatchard plot).

When equilibrium dialysis is performed, it is usual to place a constant concentration of antibody (A_T) in the dialysis sac and permit it to react with a series of different hapten concentrations. The hapten concentration outside the sac is c, and r is the concentration of bound hapten in the dialysis sac divided by the total antibody concentration.

At the free antigenic determinant concentration $[Ag_c]$, where only half the antibody binding sites are filled, then the concentration of antigen bound to antibody will be equal to the concentration of free antibody, that is, $[AbAg] = [Ab]$. As a result, the equation may be simplified to:

$$K = \frac{1}{[Ag_c]}$$

In other words, K will be equal to the reciprocal of the concentration of free antigenic determinants *when half the antibody-binding sites are occupied.*

If an antibody has a very high *affinity* for its antigen, then very little antigen will be required in order to half-saturate the antibody-binding sites. For example, antibody affinity constants can reach values as high as 10^{11} liters per mole. (This means that as small an

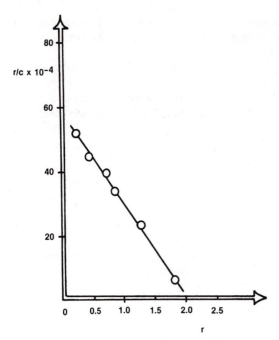

FIGURE 7–3. A plot of r/c against r (A Scatchard plot) for an absolutely pure immunoglobulin—for example, a hybridoma product. The intercept on the ordinate is 2.0 and indicates the valency of the immunoglobulin. The affinity of this antibody can be read from the abscissa with r = 1 and is approximately 3 $\times$ 10^5 liters/mole.

amount as 10^{-11} moles per liter of free antigenic determinant [hapten] is required to occupy half the binding sites on a mole of this antibody). Normally, antibody affinities fall within the range of 10^5 to 10^{10} liters per mole.

Another way of expressing the affinity of an antibody for its antigen is by the change in free energy (ΔF), which occurs when the two components interact. Because ΔF depends upon the concentration of the reactants, it is more usual to use the standard free energy ($\Delta F°$). This is the loss or gain of free energy in calories that occurs when 1 mole of Ab and 1 mole of hapten combine. $\Delta F°$ is independent of the concentration of the reactants and is related to the affinity constant by this equation:

$$\Delta F° = -RT \ln K$$

where lnK is the natural log of the affinity constant, $-R$ is the gas constant (1.987 cal/mole-deg), and T the absolute temperature.

$\Delta F°$ for antibody hapten reactions ranges from about $-6,000$ to $-11,000$ calories per mole of hapten bound. This energy change is due to the formation of noncovalent bonds. Thus, the formation of hydrogen bonds is exothermal, releasing about 1000 cal/bond. The formation of hydrophobic bonds is athermal with little free energy change.

Terminology

Avidity tends to mean different things to different people. Some authors use it to describe the increased affinity that occurs as a result of multiple antigen-binding sites on an immunoglobulin. Others use it to describe the strength of binding of a serum with a complex antigen, while still others use it to indicate the *rate* of reaction between antigen and antibody. The term is probably best avoided!

Affinity Labelling

If a hapten is designed so that it is chemically reactive and will bind covalently to nearby amino acids, then it can be used to label and so identify the amino acids that contribute to the antibody-binding site. For example, one can use a hapten with an azide side chain. Once it has bound to antibody, the resulting immune complexes are irradiated with ultraviolet light. The azide is thus converted to a reactive nitrene radical, which then binds covalently to nearby amino acids. When the complex is analyzed, the hapten can be shown to be attached to amino-acid residues located in the hypervariable regions of both light and heavy chains, although the label usually binds preferentially to heavy chains.

Antibody Heterogeneity

If a sample of pure monoclonal antibody is reacted with a simple hapten and r/c plotted against r, the points obtained will fall in a straight line (Fig. 7–3) as described previously.

If, however, a serum sample is reacted with the hapten, the line is not straight but curved (Fig. 7–4). The reason is that even a single antigenic determinant provokes the production of many different idiotypes in a serum, each having a different affinity for the antigenic determinant. Since affinity is calculated as the equilibrium constant when half the antibody-binding sites are occupied, it is usual to read the slope at a point where $r =$

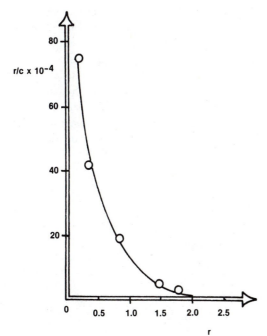

FIGURE 7–4. A Scatchard plot for an IgG fraction from serum. The intercept on the ordinate is 2.0 indicating the average valency of the mixture of immunoglobulins. The line is curved, since a great mixture of different antibody molecules is present. This may be compared to Figure 7-3, in which a pure immunoglobulin is examined. The average affinity of the mixture can be read from the abscissa when r = 1 and is approximately 1.5 $\times$ 10^5 liters/mole.

1 and thus measure the *average* affinity of the antibody populations when half the sites are occupied.

Affinity Maturation

If the affinity of antibodies produced at different times following administration of antigen is measured, it is found that the average affinity of IgG antibodies gradually increases as an immune response progresses. It is also found that the affinity of antibodies tends to rise as the dose of immunizing antigen is lowered.

Bennacerraf and Siskind suggested that these two phenomena were linked. They suggested that a high initial dose of antigen is capable of provoking many different clones of antibody-producing cells with high, medium, or low affinity for antigen. As a result, the average affinity of the antibodies produced is relatively low. As an immune response progresses, however, the amount of available antigen is gradually reduced. When less antigen is available, it tends to stimulate only those cells with a high affinity for the antigen. Therefore, the antibody produced late in an immune response will have a relatively high average affinity.

It is curious that this change in affinity only occurs in the IgG response. It may well be that the increase in affinity is also mediated through genetic mechanisms—for example, a form of directed somatic mutation in the hypervariable regions. This suggestion will be discussed further in Chapter 8.

The Biological Significance of Antibody Affinity

The affinity of a population of antibodies markedly affects their immunological properties. Perhaps the most important of these is antibody specificity. In general, high-affinity antibodies tend to be less specific for antigen than low-affinity antibodies. This is because high-affinity antibodies will combine strongly not only with their homologous antigen, but also with related haptens, for which their affinity may be much lower. By contrast, low-affinity antibodies, which can just be detected reacting with their homologous antigen, are unlikely to react *detectably* with any other antigen and thus give the appearance of high specificity (Table 7–2).

The strength of binding between antigen and antibody also influences the biological properties of the antibody. Thus, high-affinity antibodies are superior to low-affinity antibodies at virus and toxin neutralization. The firm binding of antibody to these antigens apparently reduces the possibility of dissociation and so prevents the release of free virus

TABLE 7–2   The Relationship between the Average Affinity of an Antibody Population and its Apparent Specificity

	Reaction with Related Antigens			
	A1	A2	A3	A4
High affinity anti-A1	+ + + +	+ + +	+ +	+
Medium affinity anti-A1	+ +	+	−	−
Low affinity anti-A1	+	−	−	−

The low-affinity serum appears to be most specific.

or toxin from the complex. High-affinity antibody is also more effective at removing foreign antigen from the bloodstream and is more effective at complement activation and erythrocyte destruction through hemolysis.

The Detection of Antigen–Antibody Combination

Antibody molecules combine reversibly with antigenic determinants to form immune complexes. The detection of these reactions forms the basis of the immunological subdiscipline of **serology.**

There are three general groups of techniques used to detect antigen–antibody combination. The most sensitive approach (in terms of the amount of antigen or antibody detectable) is to directly measure the immune complexes formed in an in vitro system. These techniques are known as primary binding tests.

The most widely employed approach, however, is to detect and measure the consequences of antigen–antibody interaction. These consequences include precipitation of soluble antigens, clumping (agglutination) of particulate antigens, neutralization of bacteria, viruses, or toxins, and activation of the complement system. These tests are known as secondary binding tests. They are commonly less sensitive than primary binding tests, but do not usually require sophisticated techniques.

The third type of test, the tertiary binding test is used to measure the consequences of immune responses in vivo. Thus, the determination of the protective effects of antibody falls into this category. This type of test is clearly much more complex than the primary or secondary binding tests, but the results reflect the practical significance of the immune response.

Primary Binding Tests

In general, primary binding tests are performed by allowing the reactants to combine and then measuring the amount of immune complex formed. It is usually necessary to use radioisotopes, fluorescent dyes, or enzyme-labelling in order to identify one of the reactants. After allowing the complexes to form, they are separated from the uncombined antigen or antibody, and the amount of label in these immune complexes is then estimated. Some specific examples of primary binding tests are described below.

Radioimmunoassays for Antibody   One widely employed primary binding test for antigen is called the radio allergosorbent test (RAST). In this technique, antigen-impregnated cellulose disks are immersed in test serum so that antibody binds to them. After washing to remove unbound antibody, the disk is immersed in a radiolabelled antiglobulin solution. The antiglobulin will bind to the disk only if antibodies have first bound to the antigen. By counting the radioactivity of the disk after washing, it is possible to measure the level of specific antibody in the serum. If antiglobulins specific for a single immunoglobulin class or subclass are used, it is possible to measure the level of antibodies of that class or subclass in a serum. The RAST is most commonly used to measure levels of specific IgE in allergic individuals.

Radioimmunoassays for Antigen   Competitive radioimmunoassays are widely employed to detect extremely small quantities of antigen. For example, they were first developed to measure insulin in plasma, the concentration of which is far below the limits of conventional chemical assays. These radioimmunoassays are usually based on the principle that unlabelled antigen can displace radiolabelled antigen from immune complexes, and that the amount of labelled antigen released in this way is directly related to the amount of unlabelled antigen added to the system (Fig. 7–5).

The most commonly used competitive radioimmunoassay utilizes antigen labelled with an isotope such as ^3H, ^{14}C or ^{125}I. When labeled antigen is mixed with its specific antibody, they combine to form immune complexes that may be precipitated with ammonium sulfate, or with an antiglobulin serum. Under standard conditions, the radioactivity remaining in the supernatant fluid is relatively constant and provides an estimate of the proportion of antigen bound by antibody. If unlabelled antigen is added to the standardized mixture of labelled antigen and antibody, it will compete with the labelled antigen for the binding sites on the antibody. As a result, some labelled antigen will be prevented from binding to antibody, and hence the amount of radioactivity in the supernatant will be increased. If a standard curve is first constructed by using known amounts of unlabelled antigen added to a standard system, then the amount of antigen in a test sample may be measured by reference to this standard curve.

Tests Involving Enzyme-Labelled Reagents   The most important of the techniques involving enzyme-labelled reagents are the enzyme-linked-immunosorbent assays (ELISAs). As with other primary binding tests, they may be used to detect and measure either antibody or antigen.

In the indirect ELISA for antibody, use is made of the ability of polystyrene surfaces

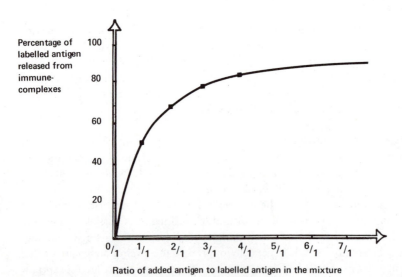

FIGURE 7–5.   The principle of competitive radioimmunoassay: The preparation of isotope-labelled antigen released from immune complexes into supernatant fluid is related to the amount of unlabelled antigen added to the mixture. (From Tizard, I. Veterinary Immunology. 2nd ed. W. B. Saunders, Philadelphia, 1982. With permission.)

to adsorb protein antigens. Polystyrene tubes are first coated with antigen by incubating the antigen solution in the tubes overnight (Fig. 7–6). (Specific details of each ELISA vary but the general principles are described here.) After unbound antigen is removed by washing, test serum is added to the tubes so that any antibodies in the serum will bind to the antigen on the tube wall. After incubation and washing to remove unbound antibody, the presence of bound antibodies is detected by addition of an enzyme-linked antiglobulin. This antiglobulin binds to the antibody and, following incubation and washing, may be detected and measured by addition of the enzyme substrate. The enzyme and substrate are selected so that a colored product develops in the tube. The intensity of the color change is, therefore, proportional to the amount of enzyme-linked antiglobulin that is bound, which in turn is proportional to the amount of antibody present in the serum under test. The color that develops may be estimated visually or, preferably, read in a spectrophotometer.

A modification of this technique can be used to detect antigen. In this case, the tubes are first coated with specific antibody. The antigen solution to be tested is then added, and, after allowing it to bind, the tubes are washed and specific antibody is added. The amount of second antibody bound is measured using an enzyme-labelled antiglobulin and substrate, as described for the indirect technique. In this test, the intensity of the color reaction is related directly to the amount of bound antigen.

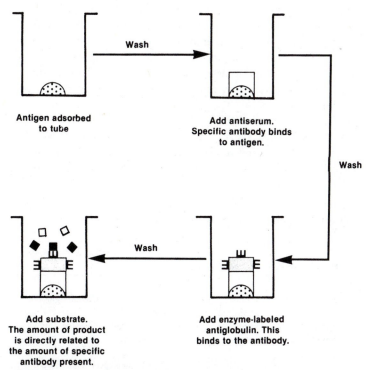

Antigen adsorbed to tube

Add antiserum. Specific antibody binds to antigen.

Wash

Wash

Add substrate. The amount of product is directly related to the amount of specific antibody present.

Wash

Add enzyme-labeled antiglobulin. This binds to the antibody.

FIGURE 7–6. A schematic diagram showing the procedure for the indirect ELISA technique. (From Tizard, I. Veterinary Immunology. 2nd ed. W. B. Saunders, Philadelphia, 1982. With permission.)

The enzymes used to label antiglobulins in the ELISA techniques are chosen primarily on the bases of cost and their ability to be easily assayed. They include alkaline phosphatase, lysozyme, horseradish peroxidase, and β-galactosidase. Because of its relative simplicity, the indirect ELISA shows promise of becoming a useful aid in the immunodiagnosis of many bacterial, viral, and parasitic infections.

Tests Involving Immunofluorescence   Fluorescent dyes are also very commonly employed as labels in primary binding tests. The most important of these is fluorescein isothiocyanate (FITC). FITC is a yellow compound that is readily conjugated to immunoglobulins without affecting their reactivity. When irradiated with invisible ultraviolet or blue light (290 and 495 μm), it re-emits a visible green light (525 μm) and is thus readily detected using an ultraviolet light source. FITC-labelled immunoglobulins may be employed in a number of techniques, the most important of which are the direct and indirect fluorescent antibody tests (Table 7–3).

Direct Fluorescent Antibody Test   The direct fluorescent antibody test (Fig. 7–7) is usually used to identify the presence of antigen. Antibody directed against a specific antigen, such as a bacterium or virus, may be labelled with FITC. A tissue section or smear containing this organism is incubated with the labelled antiserum and then washed to remove unbound antibody. If examined by dark-field illumination under a microscope with an ultraviolet light source, any antigenic structures that have bound the labelled antibody may be seen to fluoresce brightly (Fig. 7–8). This direct test can be used in many different situations. It can be used, for example, when examining the sputum of humans suspected of shedding *Mycobacterium tuberculosis,* or in other cases where bacteria are present in very low numbers. It may also be employed to detect viruses growing in tissue culture or in tissues from infected individuals. It is thus possible, for example, to detect rabies virus in the brains of infected animals.

Indirect Fluorescent Antibody Test (IFA)   The indirect fluorescent antibody test (Fig. 7–7) may be used for the detection and measurement of antibodies in serum or for the demonstration and identification of antigens in tissues or cell cultures. When testing for

TABLE 7–3   Comparison of Techniques Involved in Direct and Indirect Fluorescent Antibody Tests

Test	Direct Fluorescent Antibody Test	Indirect Fluorescent Antibody Test
Requirements	Antigen? Fluorescent-labelled anitbody	Antigen Fluorescent-labelled antiglobulin Antibody?
Method	1. Put FITC-labelled antibody onto suspected antigen preparation	Put suspected antiserum onto known antigen preparation
	2.	Wash, then cover with FITC-labelled antiglobulin
	3. Wash and examine	Wash and examine
Detects	Fluorescence indicates presence of antigen	Fluorescence indicates presence of antibodies in serum

DIRECT FLUORESCENT
ANTIBODY TEST

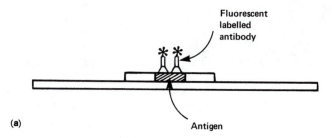

(a)

INDIRECT FLUORESCENT
ANTIBODY TEST

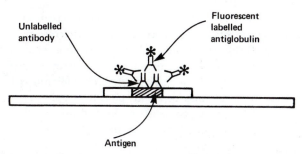

(b)

FIGURE 7–7. **a)** The direct fluorescent antibody test is employed to detect antigen by means of FITC-labelled antibody directed against that antigen. The labelled antibody will only bind to specific antigen, and therefore fluorescence seen under the ultraviolet microscope indicates that antigen is present in the material under examination. **b)** The indirect fluorescent antibody test is employed to detect and measure either antigen or specific antibody. Antigen present in a frozen section, smear, or culture will bind antibody from serum. After washing, this antibody may be detected by using a FITC-labelled antiglobulin serum. (From Tizard, I. Veterinary Immunology. 2nd ed. W. B. Saunders, Philadelphia, 1982. With permission.)

antibody, antigen is employed as a tissue smear, section, or cell culture on a glass slide. Antigen is first incubated in a serum suspected of containing antibodies to that antigen, and the serum is then washed off, leaving antibodies bound to the antigen. These bound antibodies may be visualized by incubating the slide in FITC-labelled antiglobulin serum. When this serum is removed by washing and the slide is examined, fluorescent areas on

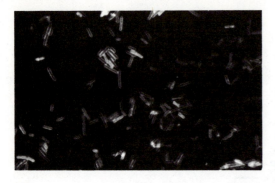

FIGURE 7–8. Direct immunofluorescence of a smear of *Clostridium chauveoi.* (Courtesy of Dr. C. L. Gyles. From Tizard, I. Veterinary Immunology. 2nd ed. W. B. Saunders, Philadelphia, 1982. With permission.)

the slide indicate that antibody was present in the test serum. The quantity of antibody in the test serum may be estimated by examining increasing dilutions of serum on a number of different antigen preparations.

The indirect fluorescent antibody test has a number of advantages over the direct techniques. Since each antibody molecule binding to antigen will itself bind several labelled antiglobulin molecules, fluorescence will be considerably brighter than in the direct test. Similarly, by using antiglobulin sera specific for each immunoglobulin class, the class of specific antibody present in the serum may also be determined.

Other Labels Used in Primary Binding Tests   Several other labels have been employed as alternatives to radioisotopes, enzymes, or fluorescent dyes in primary binding tests. For example, reagents linked to the iron-containing protein ferritin may be used to identify the location of antigens in tissues examined by electron microscopy. The ferritin molecule is a protein of 700,000 daltons containing 23 percent iron as ferric hydroxide or phosphate. The iron is concentrated within the molecule and, on electron microscopy, can be detected as a characteristic electron-dense spot. Therefore, if ferritin is linked to an immunoglobulin, the location of antigen may be readily observed on electron micrographs. A similar technique employs the enzyme peroxidase conjugated to immunoglobulin, and the presence of the enzyme is then identified by histochemical techniques.

The Physical Consequences of Antigen-Antibody Combination

Secondary Binding Tests

The reaction between antigen and antibody is commonly followed by a second stage of reaction, which is determined by the physical state of the reactants. Thus, if antibodies combine with soluble antigens in solution under appropriate conditions, the resulting complexes may precipitate out of solution. If, however, the antigens are particulate (for example, bacteria or erythrocytes), then they will agglutinate (clump).

Precipitation

If a suitable amount of a clear solution of soluble antigen is mixed with its homologous antiserum and incubated at 37°C, the mixture becomes cloudy within a few minutes, then flocculent, and finally a precipitate settles to the bottom of the tube within an hour or so. If increasing amounts of soluble antigen are mixed with a constant amount of antibody, the results obtained are determined by the relative proportions of the reactants. No obvious precipitate is formed at low antigen concentrations. As the amount of antigen increases, larger quantities of precipitate result until the amount is maximal. With the addition of more antigen, however, the amount of precipitate begins to diminish, until eventually none is observed in tubes containing a large excess of antigen (Fig. 7–9).

In the first stage of these reactions, only a little antigen is complexed to antibody, and, since antibody is in excess, free antibody may be found in the supernatant, and little precipitate is deposited. In the tubes where maximal **precipitation** occurs, both antigen and antibody are completely complexed, and neither can be detected in the supernatant. This is known as the equivalence zone, and the ratio of antibody to antigen is here said to be in optimal proportions. When antigen is added to excess, then little precipitate is formed, although soluble immune complexes are present, and free antigen may be found in the supernatant.

These results may be explained by the fact that antibodies are usually bivalent and therefore are able to cross-link only two antigenic determinants at a time, but protein antigens are multivalent, since they possess a relatively large number of determinants. In the mixtures containing excess antibody, each antigen molecule is effectively covered with antibody, which prevents cross-linkage and thus precipitation. When the reactants are in optimal proportions, the ratio of antigen to antibody is such that extensive cross-linking occurs. As the antigen–antibody complex grows in size, it becomes insoluble and eventually precipitates (Fig. 7–10). In mixtures where antigen is in excess, each antibody molecule is bound to a pair of antigen molecules. Further cross-linkage is impossible in this case, and, since these complexes are small and soluble, no precipitation occurs. The cells of the mononuclear-phagocytic system are most efficient at binding and removing from the bloodstream

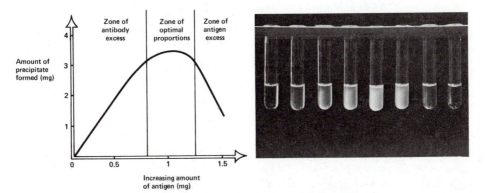

FIGURE 7–9. A photograph showing the effect of mixing increasing amounts of bovine serum albumin with a constant amount of rabbit antiserum to that antigen. The tube with the greatest amount of precipitate is the one in which the ratio of antigen to antibody is considered to be in optimal proportions. A quantitative precipitation curve of this test graphically shows the effect of adding increasing amounts of antigen to a constant amount of antibody. (From Tizard, I. Veterinary Immunology. 2nd ed. W. B. Saunders, Philadelphia, 1982. With permission.)

Antibody is bivalent

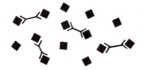

Antigen is multivalent

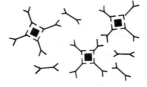

Antigen mixed with excess antibody

Antibody mixed with excess antigen

Antigen and antibody mixed in optimal proportions

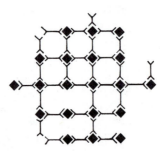

FIGURE 7–10.
The mechanism of precipitation: In antibody excess and in antigen excess, only small soluble immune complexes are produced. At optimal proportions, however, large insoluble complexes are generated. (From Tizard, I. Veterinary Immunology. 2nd ed. W. B. Saunders, Philadelphia, 1982. With permission.)

complexes formed at optimal proportions and in antibody excess. Immune complexes formed in antigen excess are poorly removed by phagocytic cells in vivo but are deposited within vessel walls and in glomeruli, where they contribute to an acute inflammatory response classified as a Type III hypersensitivity reaction (Chap. 22).

If antigen and antibody solutions are layered, one on top of the other, without mixing, the components will diffuse into each other. Where the ratio of the reagents is in optimal proportions, a band of precipitate forms. A technique such as this, sometimes called a ring test, has been used in forensic medicine to identify the origin of a piece of tissue. Antiserum against serum of the species under test is allowed to react in a capillary tube with an extract of tissue from the unknown animal. A line of precipitate at the interface of the two fluids constitutes a positive reaction. Unfortunately, this technique requires a certain steadiness of hand, and the result is easily obscured if the two solutions are inadvertently mixed. The reaction, however, can be stabilized by conducting the test in gels such as agar.

Nephelometry A rapid quantitative method of measuring antigen by means of precipitation is the technique of nephelometry, which relies on the ability of a suspension of particles, such as immune complexes, to scatter a narrow beam of light. Thus, a standard solution of antibody (usually in excess) and a solution of antigen are mixed and incubated for a standard time so that immune complexes form. When a beam of light from a helium-neon laser is passed through this suspension in a cuvette, the degree of light scatter can be measured. By means of a standard curve drawn up previously using antigen solutions of known concentration, the amount of antigen in the unknown solution can be rapidly measured.

Immunodiffusion A simple method of detecting the precipitation reaction is to cut two round wells, 5 mm in diameter and about 1 cm apart, in a layer of agar in a petri dish. If one well is filled with antigen and the other with antiserum, the reactants will diffuse out radially. A circular concentration gradient therefore is established for each reactant, and these eventually overlap. Optimal proportions for the occurrence of precipitation will occur in one zone of the superimposed gradients, and an opaque white line of precipitate will appear in this region (Fig. 7–11). This technique is known as the double-diffusion test and, since it was first described by the Swedish immunologist Dr. O. Ouchterloney, is sometimes known as the Ouchterloney technique.

If several different antigen-antibody mixtures are used (for example, antibodies against whole serum), each component is unlikely to reach optimal proportions in exactly the same position in the agar. Consequently, a separate line of precipitation is produced for each interacting set of antigens and antibodies present. Immunodiffusion techniques may also be used to determine the relationship between antigens. If two antigen wells and one antibody well are set up as in Figures 7–11 and 7–12, then lines of precipitate will form between each antigen well and the antibody well. If these two lines are completely confluent, then the two antigens are considered to be identical. If the lines cross over, then the two antigens are different, whereas if the lines merge with spur formation, then a partial identity exists, each antigen possessing antigenic determinants in common. The line that continues as a spur possesses antigenic determinants not present in the other.

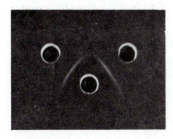

FIGURE 7–11. Precipitation in agar gel: Antigen and antibody diffusing from their respective wells precipitate in a region where optimal proportions are achieved. In this example, the two top wells each contain identical antigens. The antibody is in the bottom well. The precipitation lines fuse as a result of the identity of the antigens. (From Tizard, I. Veterinary Immunology. 2nd ed. W. B. Saunders, Philadelphia, 1982. With permission.)

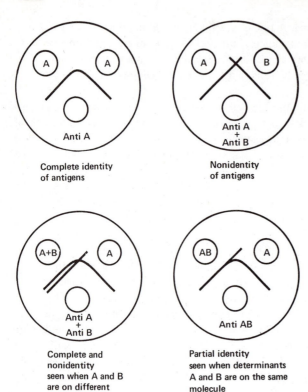

Complete identity
of antigens

Nonidentity
of antigens

Complete and
nonidentity
seen when A and B
are on different
molecules

Partial identity
seen when determinants
A and B are on the same
molecule

FIGURE 7-12. The use of the gel-diffusion technique to determine the relationship between two antigens. (From Tizard, I. Veterinary Immunology. 2nd ed. W. B. Saunders, Philadelphia, 1982. With permission.)

Radial Immunodiffusion   If antigen is allowed to diffuse from a well into agar in which specific antiserum is already incorporated, then a ring of precipitate indicating the zone of optimal proportions will form around the well. The area within this ring is directly proportional to the amount of antigen added to the well. If the technique is first standardized using known amounts of antigen, then a standard curve may be constructed, and unknown solutions of antigen, accurately assayed. This is also called the Mancini technique (Fig. 7–13).

If, instead of being permitted to diffuse into agar-containing antiserum as in the radial immunodiffusion technique, the antigen is driven into the antiserum agar by electrophoresis, then the ring of precipitation around each well becomes deformed into a "rocket" shape. The length of the "rockets" is proportional to the amount of antigen placed in each well. This technique, known as electroimmunodiffusion, "rocket" electrophoresis, or electroimmunoassay, may also therefore be employed to quantitate antigen (Fig. 7–14).

Immunoelectrophoresis and Related Techniques   While double-diffusion techniques give a separate precipitation line for each antigen–antibody system in a mixture, it is often difficult to resolve all the components in a very complex mixture in this way. One technique that may be used to improve the resolution of the system is to separate the antigen mixture by electrophoresis prior to undertaking immunodiffusion. This technique is known as immunoelectrophoresis and is usually employed to identify proteins in body fluids.

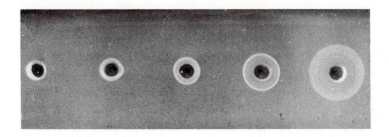

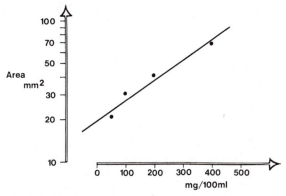

FIGURE 7–13. Radial immunodiffusion: In this case, antiserum to IgA is incorporated in the agar and is used to measure serum IgA levels. (From Tizard, I. Veterinary Immunology, 2nd ed. W. B. Saunders, Philadelphia, 1982. With permission.)

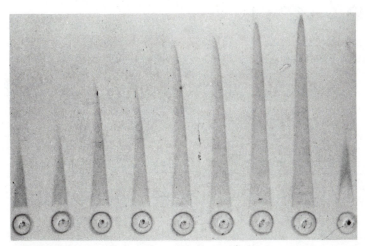

FIGURE 7–14. Electroimmunodiffusion: In this example, the level of the iron-binding protein lactoferrin from milk is being estimated. The height of each ''rocket'' is proportional to the amount of antigen placed in each well. (Courtesy of Dr. R. Harmon. From Tizard, I. Veterinary Immunology. 2nd ed. W. B. Saunders, Philadelphia, 1982. With permission.)

Immunoelectrophoresis involves the electrophoresis of the antigen mixture in agar gel in one direction. A trough is then cut in the agar just to one side of and parallel to this line of separated proteins. Antiserum is placed in this trough and allowed to diffuse laterally. When the diffusing antibodies encounter antigen, curved lines of precipitate are formed. One arc of precipitation forms for each of the constituents in the antigen mixture (Fig. 7–15). This technique can be used to resolve the proteins of normal serum into between 25 and 40 distinct precipitation bands. The exact number depends upon the strength and specificity of the antiserum employed (Fig. 7–16). By means of this technique, it is possible to identify the absence of a normal serum protein such as occurs in individuals with a congenital deficiency of some complement components. It is also possible to detect the presence of excessive amounts of a particular component, as is found in individuals with plasma-cell tumors (myelomas).

Two-Dimensional Immunoelectrophoresis   Two-dimensional immunoelectrophoresis is a combination of simple electrophoresis and electroimmunodiffusion. The first stage inovlves the electrophoresis of a serum mixture such as serum in one direction. Following this first stage, the current is reset at a right angle to the first electrophoretic run and the serum re-electrophoresed into agar containing polyspecific antiserum (Fig. 7–17). As a result, a series of large precipitate arcs are formed in the agar. These arcs may be quantitated by measuring their surface area. Individual components can be identified either by means of specific antisera or by looking for a line of identity with a known antigen.

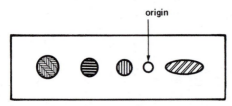

Stage 1.   Serum placed in a well on an agar plate is electrophoresed

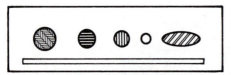

Stage 2.   Antiserum is placed in a trough cut parallel to the electrophoretic run

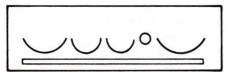

Arcs of precipitate form as each serum protein meets its specific antibody

FIGURE 7–15.   The principles of immunoelectrophoresis. (From Tizard, I. Veterinary Immunology. 2nd ed. W. B. Saunders, Philadelphia, 1982. With permission.)

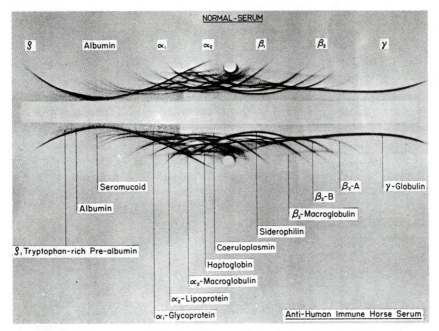

NORMAL-SERUM

β | Albumin | α_1 | α_2 | β_1 | β_2 | γ

Seromucoid
Albumin
β_2-A | γ-Globulin
β_2-B
β_2-Macroglobulin
Siderophilin
β_1 Tryptophan-rich Pre-albumin
Coeruloplasmin
Haptoglobin
α_2-Macroglobulin
α_2-Lipoprotein
α_1-Glycoprotein | Anti-Human Immune Horse Serum

FIGURE 7-16. Immunoelectrophoretic pattern obtained by first electrophoresing human serum, and then developing with antihuman immune horse serum. (From Carpenter, P. L. Immunology and Serology, 3rd ed. W. B. Saunders, Philadelphia, 1975. With permission.)

Counterimmunoelectrophoresis When electrophoresed in agar gel, some antibodies move cathodally because of a flow of buffer through the agar toward the cathode. This phenomenon is called electroendosmosis. If an antigen is strongly negatively charged so that it moves toward the anode in spite of this flow, then it is possible by a suitable arrangement of wells in an agar plate to drive antigen and antibody together by electrophoresis. A precipitate may be produced in this way within a few minutes. This technique

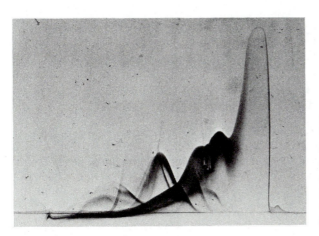

FIGURE 7-17.
Two-dimensional immunoelectrophoresis of normal catfish serum. The anode is on the right. The point of application is on the left. (Courtesy of Dr. D. H. Lewis.)

is known as counterimmunoelectrophoresis and may be used for the rapid identification of bacteria and mycoplasma and for the diagnosis of some viral diseases.

Titration of Antibodies

Although the detection of the presence of antibodies or antigen is sufficient for many tests, it is usually desirable to arrive at some estimate of the amount of reactants present. In the case of tests designed to detect the presence of specific antibody, this quantitation is often accomplished by titration. Titration is a procedure in which the serum under test is made up in a series of increasing dilutions (Fig. 7–18). Each dilution is then tested for activity in the test system. The reciprocal of the highest dilution giving a positive reaction is known as the **titer,** or **titre** (depending on geographical location) and provides a measure of the amount of antibody in that serum.

Agglutination

In the same way that bivalent antibodies may link soluble antigens to form an insoluble complex that then precipitates, antibody may crosslink particulate antigens, resulting in their clumping or **agglutination** (Fig. 7–19). Agglutination may be produced, therefore, by mixing a suspension of antigenic particles, such as bacteria, with antiserum. Antibody combines rapidly with the particles, the primary interaction, but agglutination is a much

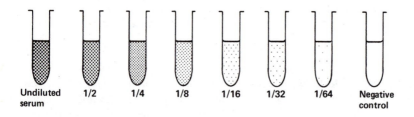

| Undiluted serum | 1/2 | 1/4 | 1/8 | 1/16 | 1/32 | 1/64 | Negative control |

A constant amount of antigen is added to each tube

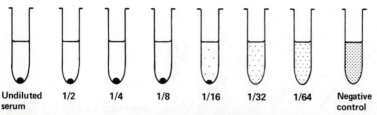

| Undiluted serum | 1/2 | 1/4 | 1/8 | 1/16 | 1/32 | 1/64 | Negative control |

FIGURE 7–18. The principle of antibody titration: Serum is first serially diluted in a series of tubes. A constant amount of antigen is then added to each tube and the mixture incubated. By the end of the incubation period in this example, agglutination has occurred in all tubes up to a serum dilution of 1/16. The titer of the serum is therefore 1/16. (From Tizard, I. Veterinary Immunology. 2nd ed. W. B. Saunders, Philadelphia, 1982. With permission.)

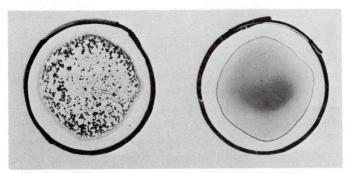

FIGURE 7–19. Bacterial agglutination (on the left) compared to a nonagglutinated bacterial suspension on the right.

slower process, since adherence between particles occurs only when they touch each other. Normally, these suspensions are stable, their constituent particles prevented from clumping by a net negative charge, or zeta potential, on their surface. However, immunoglobulins are relatively positively charged and, on coating particles, they therefore reduce this zeta potential. In addition, immunoglobulins can bridge charged particles by extending out beyond the effective range of this potential. As a result, the particles can approach closely, bind together, and agglutinate.

　　Antibodies differ in their capacity to promote agglutination. IgM antibodies are considerably more efficient than IgG or IgA antibodies in producing this form of reaction (Table 7–4).

　　If excess antibody is added to a suspension of antigenic particles, then, just as in the precipitation reaction, it is possible for each particle to be so coated by antibody that agglutination is inhibited. This lack of reactivity seen at high antibody concentrations is termed a **prozone.** Another cause of prozone formation is the presence in a serum of antibodies that do not cause agglutination even when bound to the particles. These nonagglutinating antibodies are also known as **incomplete antibodies.** The reasons for their lack of agglutinating activity are not completely clear; one possible reason is that the antigenic determinants with which they react lie deep within the surface coat of the particle—so deep, in fact, that cross-linking cannot occur. An alternative suggestion is that they are capable of

TABLE 7–4　Role of Specific Immunoglobulins in Diagnostic Tests

Property*	IgG	IgM	IgA
Agglutination	+	+++	+
Complement-fixation (heterologous guinea pig complement)	+	+++	−
Precipitation	+++	+	±
Neutralization	+	++	+
Time of appearance after exposure to antigen	3–7 days	2–5 days	3–7 days
Time to reach peak titer	7–21 days	5–14 days	7–21 days

*The properties listed may vary somewhat between species.

only restricted movement in their hinge region (Chap. 6) causing them to be functionally "monovalent."

Antiglobulin Tests   If it is necessary to test for the presence of incomplete antibodies on the surface of particles such as bacteria or erythrocytes, then a direct **antiglobulin test** may be used (Fig. 7–20). The washed particles are mixed with an antiglobulin serum, and, if incomplete antibodies are present, agglutination will occur.

In order to test for the presence of incomplete antibodies in a serum, an indirect antiglobulin test is used. In this technique, the serum under test is first incubated with antigen particles, which adsorb the incomplete antibodies. After washing to remove unbound antibody, the coated particles are mixed with an antiglobulin serum. On reacting with bound antibody, the antiglobulin will cross-link the particles and cause agglutination.

Passive Agglutination   Since agglutination is a much more sensitive technique than precipitation, it is sometimes considered desirable to convert a precipitating system to an agglutinating one. One way this may be done is by chemically linking soluble antigen to inert particles such as erythrocytes, bacteria, or latex, so that specific antibody will cause these sensitized particles to agglutinate. Erythrocytes appear to be among the best particles for this purpose, and tests that employ coated erythrocytes are termed passive hemagglutination tests. Some antigens, such as the bacterial lipopolysaccharides, adsorb naturally to erythrocytes, and it is possible to use this phenomenon to advantage in diagnostic tests.

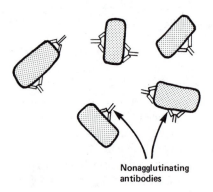

Nonagglutinating
antibodies

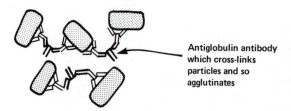

Antiglobulin antibody
which cross-links
particles and so
agglutinates

FIGURE 7–20. The principle of the direct antiglobulin test. The presence of an antiglobulin antibody is required to agglutinate erythrocytes coated with nonagglutinating antibody. (From Tizard, I. Veterinary Immunology. 2nd ed. W. B. Saunders, Philadelphia, 1982. With permission.)

Unfortunately, these lipopolysaccharides are also adsorbed to erythrocytes in vivo so that the erythrocytes are destroyed by the antibacterial immune responses; as a consequence, anemia is a feature of many diseases caused by Gram-negative organisms.

The Biological Consequences of Antigen-Antibody Interaction

The combination of antigen and antibody, while it may block the toxic sites on toxins or prevent viruses binding to cells, will not, by itself, cause antigen elimination or destruction. It is only through reactions mediated by the constant regions of antigen-bound antibody that the major protective effector mechanisms are triggered. Given the variety of structures in each homology region of all the immunoglobulin classes and subclasses, it is clear that these can constitute a system which provides a choice of the biological consequences of immune complex formation. Antibody molecules may therefore be considered to function as transducers which convert the initial antigen–antibody interaction into a protective response. After combining with antigen, antibody acquires the ability to activate the complement cascade, to bind effectively to phagocytic cells or to provoke the degranulation of mast cells and basophils. (Activation of the complement cascade and the serologic tests that utilize this phenomenon are discussed in Chap. 14.) The most significant of these effects is the triggering of the antibody response itself, which occurs when antigen binds to cell-membrane immunoglobulins on B lymphocytes (Chap. 11).

It is still not entirely clear how many of these reactions are initiated. One suggestion is that a conformational change occurs in the Fc region as a result of antigen combining with the Fab region, and the result is the generation of new, biologically active sites. Alternatively, and probably more likely, the active sites pre-exist hidden in the uncomplexed antibody molecule. When antigen binds to the antibody, the resulting conformational changes result in exposure of these hidden sites (Fig. 7–21). A third suggestion is that these

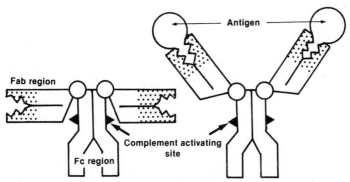

FIGURE 7–21. The complement activating site is located on the C_{H2} area of the Fc region. Free immunoglobulin does not, therefore, activate the classical complement pathway because the site is normally masked. Combination of antigen with the immunoglobulin results in exposure of the activating site and therefore permits activation of C1q.

reactions are dose-dependent and aggregation results in the accumulation of sufficient active sites to trigger the reactions.

Many cells possess specific surface receptors for immunoglobulin Fc regions. These Fc receptors permit the attachment of immunoglobulins or immune complexes to a cell surface (Table 7–5).

Fc receptors on lymphocytes for Cγ chains consist of a single polypeptide chain of 28,000 to 30,000 Mr and a single Fc γ binding site. They also contain free fatty acids and phospholipids. Some lymphocytes (the B lymphocytes) may have Fc receptors for all the major immunoglobulin classes, while others, especially those T lymphocytes that suppress the immune response (suppressor cells) have Fc γ receptors and those T lymphocytes that enhance the immune response (helper cells) possess Fc μ receptors.

Macrophages and neutrophils also possess Fc receptors. Immune complexes binding to these receptors initiate changes in cellular activity that lead to phagocytosis of the complexes. The mechanisms involved are unclear. The Fc receptor permits firm attachment of the complexes to the cells and probably provokes local cell-membrane synthesis. This may lead to complete enclosure of the complexes within a cell or, alternatively, if the amount of cell-bound complex is small, serve to move the cell toward the complexes in a form of chemotaxis. Both macrophage and lymphocyte Fc receptors may be shed from those cells into the extracellular fluid. These free receptors may bind to other nearby cells and so permit them to bind immune complexes also. In this way, they may act as mitogens and as suppressive factors. You can read more about this process in Chapters 10 and 13.

A second type of response seen following antigen–antibody–cell-membrane interaction is degranulation. This occurs in mast cells, platelets and occasionally, in neutrophils. For example, if antigen binds and links two mast-cell-fixed IgE moleclues, then intracellular enzymes are activated and cause the cell to release the contents of its granules into the extracellular fluid (Chap. 20). Platelets that bind immune complexes release not only vasoactive factors but also procoagulants and adenosine diphosphate, which potentiates the reaction. On occasion, neutrophils respond to immune complexes by releasing the contents of their lysosomes into extracellular fluid.

TABLE 7–5 Fc Receptors on Cells of the Immune System

Cell	FcR for			
	γ	μ	α	ϵ
B* lymphocyte	+	+	+	+
T$_H$* lymphocyte	−	+	−	−
T$_S$* lymphocyte	+	−	−	−
NK cell*	+	−	−	−
Mast cell†	+	−	−	+
Basophil	+	−	−	+
Neutrophil	+	−	−	−
Eosinophil	+	+	−	+
Macrophage	+	(+)	−	+
Platelets	+	−	−	−

*See Chapter 10.

†See Chapter 20.

A third form of response to antigen–antibody–cell-membrane interaction is the generation of cell-mediated cytotoxic activity (Chap. 11). Cells that can participate in this process (known as antibody-dependent cellular cytotoxicity [ADCC]) and destroy foreign (allogeneic) cells on contact, include macrophages, neutrophils and some lymphocyte subpopulations. All these cells exert their cytotoxicity regardless of whether they first bind to antibody-coated target cells or if they bind antibody first and then bind to antigens on target-cell surfaces. A similar toxic effect may be mediated by eosinophils that bind to helminths, destroying them through IgG or IgE bound to the helminth surface (Chap. 17). Fc receptors are found, not only on the cells of the immune system, but throughout the body. Thus they have been found in splenic red pulp, hepatic lobules, renal glomeruli, alveolar walls, intestinal villi, synovia, subcutis, and the sinuses of lymph nodes. Their role in these locations is unclear.

Most serum immunoglobulins cannot bind to cell Fc receptors unless they are first complexed with antigen. Nevertheless, some antibodies, known as cytophilic or cytotropic antibodies, may bind to Fc receptors even when uncomplexed. Examples of cytophilic antibodies include IgE antibodies, which are cytophilic for mast cells, and sheep IgG2, which is cytophilic for neutrophils and appears to act as a cell-bound opsonin, since it enhances the phagocytic ability of these cells.

(You can read more about Fc receptors and their activities on p. 166.)

Sources of Additional Information

Delaat, A. N. C. Primer of Serology. Harper and Row, New York, 1976.

Frieden, E. Non-covalent interactions. J. Chem. Educ., *52:* 754–761, 1975.

Friedman, H., Linna, T. J., and Prier, J. E., eds. Immunoserology in the Diagnosis of Infectious Diseases. University Park Press, Baltimore, 1979.

Haber, E., and Krause, R. M., eds. Antibodies in Human Diagnosis and Therapy. Raven Press, New York, 1977.

Hill, H. R., and Matsen, J. M. Enzyme-linked immunosorbent assay and radioimmunoassay in the serologic diagnosis of infectious diseases. J. Inf. Dis., *147:* 258–263, 1983.

Journal of Immunological Methods. Elsevier North Holland (Biomedical Press), Amsterdam.

Metzger, H. Effects of antigen binding on the properties of antibody. Adv. Immunol., *18:* 169–207, 1974.

Richards, F., et al. On the specificity of antibodies. Science, *189:* 130–137, 1978.

Rose, N. R., and Friedman, H., eds. Manual of Clinical Immunology, ed. 2. American Society for Microbiology, Washington, D.C., 1980.

Siskind, G. W., and Benacerraf, B. Cell selection by antigen in the immune response. Adv. Immunol., *10:* 1–50, 1969.

Spiegelberg, H. L. Biological activities of immunoglobulins of different classes and subclasses. Adv. Immunol. *19:* 259–294, 1974.

Weir, D. M., ed. Handbook of Experimental Immunology, ed. 3. Blackwell Scientific Publishers, Oxford, 1978.

Wictor, T. T., Flamand, A., and Koprowski, H. Use of monoclonal antibodies in diagnosis of rabies virus infection and differentiation of rabies and rabies-related viruses. J. Virol. Methods., *1:* 33–46, 1980.

Yalow, R. S. Radioimmunoassay: A probe for fine structure of biologic systems. Science, *200:* 1236–1245, 1978.

8

The Generation of Antibody Diversity

The early studies of Landsteiner on the specificity of the immune responses to haptens (Chap. 2) added a new degree of complexity to our understanding of the immune system. Landsteiner's investigations suggested that almost any organic molecule, could, when used as a hapten, provoke an absolutely specific immune response. Since the number of potential haptens was phenomenally large, the number of different antibodies that could be produced by an animal must be equally enormous. Any theory of antibody production was, therefore, required to account for this phenomenal variability of antibody molecules.

The earliest theories assumed that the variability of antibodies was so great that antibodies directed against all possible antigenic determinants could not exist preformed but must be synthesized on demand following exposure to antigen. These theories, therefore, suggested that antigen would function as a template around which its specific antibody would be constructed. Once built, the newly formed antibody, it was postulated, would be stabilized by interchain bonding and then released into the bloodstream.

Theories of this type (known as instructive theories since the antigen "instructed" the antibody), although attractive, were never supported by experimental evidence. For example, it could never be shown that antigen was present when antibodies were being synthesized. More important, instructive theories could never be reconciled with the realities of protein synthesis and the central dogma of molecular biology, namely, that information flows only from DNA through RNA to protein, not the reverse.

An alternative group of theories was developed that held that the information needed to make all possible antibodies was already stored in an animal's genome. In this case, all that is required for an antibody to be produced is that the necessary gene be "selected" by exposure to specific antigen. Consequently, the specific immunoglobulin could be synthesized through use of appropriate messenger RNA. This type of selective theory is not only compatible with our knowledge of molecular biological mechanisms, but also with our knowledge of the factors that govern protein configuration.

The shape of a protein molecule is in no way governed by a physical template. The shape of a protein depends upon the configuration of its constituent peptide chains, and this configuration is, in turn, governed by the amino-acid sequence within the chains. Each amino acid in a peptide chain exerts an influence on its neighbouring amino acids, which determines their positions relative to each other. It also affects, but to a lesser extent, the position of more remote amino acids. The final configuration of a peptide chain, therefore, represents the total effect of all amino acids in the chain. Thus, the shape of a protein is only determined by its amino-acid sequence, and that sequence is determined by the nucleotide sequence in the DNA coding for that specific molecule.

Some Basic Molecular Genetics

It has been known for many years that DNA, consisting of a chain of nucleotides, codes for messenger RNA by transcription employing the enzyme RNA polymerase (Fig. 8–1).

The bases in the messenger RNA chain are then read sequentially by transfer RNA (tRNA) and translated into a polypeptide chain within the ribosomes of the cell.

For many years, it was believed that there was a direct correspondence between the DNA, the mRNA and the final polypeptide chain product and that a single DNA chain was eventually translated into a colinear polypeptide chain. However, once it became possible to sequence mammalian DNA, it was found that genes were not, in

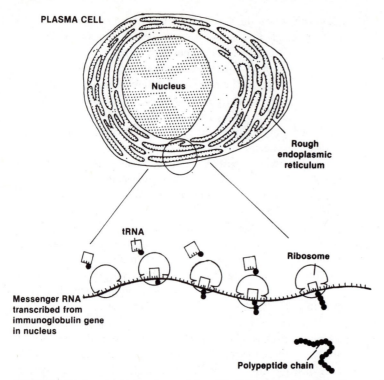

FIGURE 8–1. A schematic and simplified diagram depicting the synthesis of a protein, in this case, immunoglobulin from a plasma cell: The genes for this protein are translated from DNA in the nucleus into messenger RNA through a number of intermediate steps. This messenger RNA acting through transfer RNA transcribes this information into a polypeptide chain.

fact, uninterrupted sequences of nucleotides coding for single polypeptide chains. It became apparent that, within genes for individual proteins, there exist segments of DNA that do not code for peptides. These noncoding DNA segments may be deleted from the DNA before transcription or from the mRNA after transcription. If deleted from the DNA before transcription, these noncoding segments are simply called "spacers." If the complete DNA is transcribed into mRNA before deletion, then the noncoding sequences are called "introns," and the expressed sequences are called "exons" (Fig. 8–2).The production of immunoglobulins employs both deletion techniques so spacers, introns, and exons are found in immunoglobulin genes. The mRNA is *processed* so that the introns are removed and the exons joined together in the correct order through a process known as splicing. The mechanism of splicing is unclear, but it may reasonably be assumed that a splicing enzyme or enzymes acts at a defined position on the mRNA to split and splice it. Analysis of the base sequences at the borders of introns and exons shows that there is indeed a characteristic splicing sequence. Thus, as a rule, the base sequence of an intron begins with guanine-uridine and ends with adenine-guanine. It is possible that this, in conjunction with the correct conformation, permits splicing to occur in exactly the correct position. It is this phe-

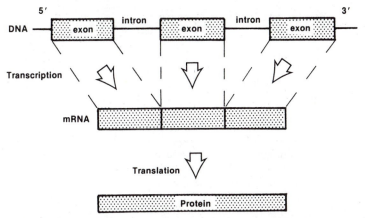

FIGURE 8–2. The DNA coding for most proteins consists of a series of expressed regions, known as exons, separated by intervening sequences, called introns. Only the exons are transcribed through a number of intermediate stages to form a continuous messenger RNA segment, which is then translated into a polypeptide chain.

nomenon of splicing that provides the first clue to the problem of immunoglobulin diversity.

Each nucleotide is linked to its neighbors through the 3′ site and the 5′ site on the ribose ring. The 3′ site binds to its neighbor's 5′ site. Because of this binding, each nucleic acid chain has polarity. One end has a free 3′ end, the other has a free 5′ end. When printing nucleotide sequences, it is usual to place the 5′ end on the left and the 3′ end on the right.

Immunoglobulin Diversity

In 1965, Dreyer and Bennett suggested that if the variable and constant regions of immunoglobulin light and heavy chains were coded for by different gene segments (as opposed to a single gene for an entire heavy or an entire light chain), then it could provide a situation in which a single constant region could be combined with any one of a large number of different variable regions. Subsequent studies of the genetics, the serology, and the structure of immunoglobulin molecules confirmed the correctness of this suggestion. (See, for example, the discussion on allotypes and idiotypes in Chap. 6).

This finding immediately simplified the major problem of all selective theories of antibody formation, namely, the very large quantity of information that had to be stored. Instead of having to retain information about all possible antibody molecules, it is only necessary to store the information (genes) about all the variable regions and to match these, when required, with a relatively small number of constant-region genes in order to produce a complete range of immunoglobulin molecules.

Subsequent studies have demonstrated that three unlinked gene families are in fact

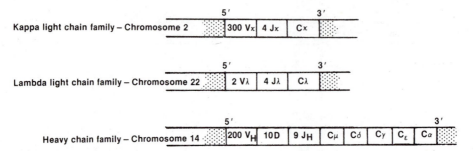

FIGURE 8–3. The three families of human immunoglobulin genes: Each is located on a separate chromosome. The gene for the J *chain* found in IgM and IgA and used to link immunoglobulin monomers together is located on chromosome 5.

employed to code for immunoglobulin molecules. Each of these families consists of a large number of gene segments coding for variable regions (V genes) associated with one or several genes for constant regions (C genes). One of these families, located on chromosome 14 in man and 12 in mice codes for immunoglobulin-heavy chains. One family on chromosome 2 in man and 6 in mice codes for κ light chains, while the third family on chromosome 22 in man and 16 in mice codes for λ light chains (Fig. 8–3).

Light-Chain Diversity

When carefully examined, the light-chain gene families in mice have consistently shown that a single copy of a C gene segment is required to code for the C_L region, while several different gene segments are required to code for the V_L regions. Thus Tonegawa and his colleagues showed, in the germ cells of mice, that V_λ and C_λ genes were separate. The V_λ gene segment codes for most of the V_λ region up to the amino acid located at position 95 from the N-terminus. The C_λ gene segment on the other hand, codes for the C-terminal end of the chain starting at position 110. The intervening 15 amino acids in the V_λ region are coded for by a short segment known as J_λ (J for joining or junctional). V and J segments are separated by a spacer of unknown length while J and C segments are separated by a spacer of 1150 base pairs. When B cells develop, and synthesize λ chains, the spacers are removed so that the 3' end of V_λ segment is joined to the 5' end of J segment and thus forms a continuous sequence.

In mice λ chains account for only 5% of total serum immunoglobulin. The λ light chain family consists of only two V_λ segments, four J_λ segments (one of which is defective) and six C_λ gene segments. On the other hand, the kappa light chain family contains about 90 to 300 V_K gene segments clustered in 30 to 100 groups each containing up to ten related gene segments. The κ light chain family also contains five related J_K gene segments and a single C_K segment. In man, the V_K gene pool contains 15 to 20 genes clustered in 3 or 4 subgroups.

In order for a complete light chain to be produced, a single V gene segment must be selected, the spacer deleted and its DNA spliced to the DNA for a J and C gene segments as the B cell develops. Just prior to light-chain production, the rearranged gene is transcribed. V–J segments remain separated from the C segment during transcription to mes-

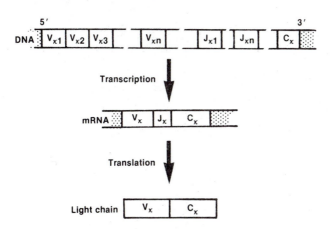

FIGURE 8-4. The production of a κ light chain: One V and one J region gene are selected for transcription before being linked to a C region in RNA, and translated into a complete light chain.

senger RNA. The V–J transcript is then spliced to the C transcript and the completed mRNA sequence is then translated to yield a complete light chain (Fig. 8–4).

The splicing process described above can generate V-region diversity in three ways. First, as occurs in the case of the V_K family, only one of a possible 90 to 300 V_K segments is selected for transcription as is only one of the four J_K segments. This random coupling of segments will provide a source of variability, since there are clearly some 1200 to 3000 different V_K–J_K combinations possible. Second, the splicing of V and J is imprecise and the joining ends of the V_K and J_K segments can vary from one recombination to another by as many as ten nucleotides. Third, sequence analysis of the V–J splice site indicates that one or more nucleotides are inserted into the junction. Their origin is unknown.

The V–J splicing site, occurring at around position 96–97 will clearly give rise to a highly variable region in the completed light chain and indeed, it corresponds to the site of the third hypervariable region and to a major idiotypic determinant (idiotope).

While V–J splicing accounts thus for the formation of the third hypervariable region on light chains, it must be clear to the reader that much variability is left unaccounted for. Indeed, what about the first two hypervariable regions? And how can we explain the variability of mouse λ light chains or human κ chains, where the size of the V gene pool is relatively small? Clearly, other mechanisms of generating antibody variability must be operating.

Heavy-Chain Variable-Region Diversity

The mechanisms that have been associated with heavy-chain diversity are similar in principle to those described previously for light chains (Fig. 8–5).

First, there are at least 20 groups of V_H genes, each of which can contain up to ten V_H gene segments. Consequently the V_H gene pool can contain up to 200 V_H different segments. Second, there are probably a number of J_H segments (4 in mice, 9 in humans) situated 3′ to the V_H segments. Third, there exists a set of short DNA segments located between the V_H and J_H segments. These short segments, known as D segments (D for diversity), contribute to the generation of hypervariability in the V_H–J_H splicing region. There appear to be about twelve distinct D segments ranging from 6 to 17 base pairs in

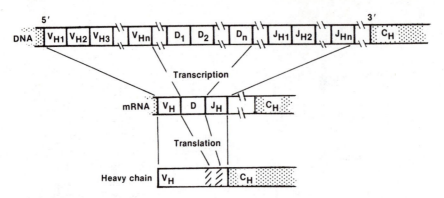

FIGURE 8–5. The arrangement of the genes that code for the variable region of immunoglobulin heavy chains: One V_M, one D, and one J_H gene are selected for translation into a heavy-chain V region. Their junctional diversity contributes to the hypervariability in this area.

length in mice. Thus, the entire V region of an immunoglobulin-heavy chain requires the splicing of V_H, D, and J_H segments. The assembly of the complete V_H gene from V_H, D, and J_H segments appears to be random. The use of a third segment selected from a pool in this way will clearly greatly increase the diversity that is generated due to combinational joining. Thus, if there are 200 V_H, 12 D, and 4 J_H segments, it is in theory possible to produce $200 \times 12 \times 4 = 9.6 \times 10^3$ different V–D–J combinations. In addition, the presence of two splice sites multiplies the potential for diversity arising as a result of imprecise joining of the DNA.

Although these mechanisms will provide a means whereby great diversity may be generated in the VDJ DNA, it should be borne in mind that not all combinations of segments will necessarily provide usable amino-acid sequences. The junctional rearrangement may be so severe that the entire chain may be so improperly arranged as to be useless. Abortive rearrangements of this type have been found to be a feature of myeloma cells. Indeed it may well be that many B cells, as a normal process, undergo abortive gene segment rearrangements and die without generating immunoglobulin. Perhaps abortive rearrangements are the rule while usable combinations may prove to be the exception.

The Mechanism of V–J and V–D–J Splicing

Molecular geneticists have developed a number of different models to account for gene segment rearrangements within chromosomes (Fig. 8–6). These models include:

1. Copy insertion: A gene segment may be duplicated and the copy inserted in the correct position beside the second gene segment.
2. Excision-insertion: The first gene segment may be excised before being inserted beside the second segment.
3. Looping out-deletion: The two gene segments may come together by looping out and then excising the spacer DNA.

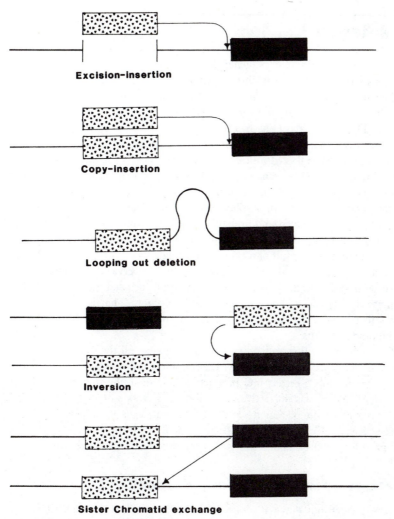

FIGURE 8–6. Different mechanisms by which gene segments can be joined. It is probable that unequal sister chromatid exchange is the major mechanism in splicing V gene segments to J gene segments.

4. Inversion: If the two gene segments are in the opposite orientation in the genome, then one may be excised and inverted before insertion.
5. Sister chromatid exchange: When the chromosome duplicates during mitosis, an unequal crossing over occurs between gene segments on sister chromatids so joining the gene segments.

    At the present time, looping out-deletion, sister chromatid exchange, inversion and deletion have all been implicated in variable region gene splicing.

Somatic Mutation

Although a tremendous variability can be generated by gene segment rearrangement and imprecise joining, as already pointed out, these mechanisms clearly cannot account for all the variability known to occur within the V regions. For example, there are two hypervariable regions in the V_L chain region and three in the V_H region that are quite separate from the V–J or V–D–J splice sites (Fig. 6–7).

If the amino-acid sequences of a large number of V regions are studied, however, it is possible to show a progressive departure from a basic sequence as the immune response progresses. These differences cannot be accounted for by gene segment rearrangement, but may, however, be due to somatic-point mutations.

For example, when nineteen antiphosphoryl choline myelomas were studied, it was clear that they were all closely related and probably all derived from a single V_H segment. Thus, ten were identical, while the remaining nine had numerous substitutions clearly derived by somatic mutation as a result of a change in a single base pair (Table 8–1). The mutations were tightly clustered at the sites of the first two hypervariable regions. This may be explained by postulating the existence of a very local, focussed mutagenic mechanism. A much more likely process, however, is somatic selection. That is, B cells whose immunoglobulin fails to bind antigen, are not selected for, do not, therefore, multiply and do not produce immunoglobulins.

When the phosphoryl choline antibodies were investigated, all the immunoglobulins that contain the basic sequence were of the IgM class, while the mutants were either IgG or IgA. Since IgM production precedes IgG production, it is tempting to suggest that the somatic mutation mechanism was not activated until after a responding cell has become committed to utilizing a specific V-region segment. The mutations will, therefore, occur during the course of B-cell differentiation. The occurrence of this form of somatic mutation may account, in part, for the process of affinity selection described in Chapter 6.

The Numbers of Different Antibody Molecules

It has already been pointed out that with 90 to 300 V_K exons and 4 J_K exons there are possibly as many as 280 to 1200 different V_K region sequences in mice. Similarly with 200

TABLE 8–1 Progressive Change in the Composition of the N-Terminal 36 Residues of Antibodies to Choline

		Proportion of Sequences Dissimilar to the Prototype Sequence
IgM	Light chains	1/12
	Heavy chains	0/12
IgG	Light chains	6/9
	Heavy chains	5/9
IgA	Light chains	2/9
	Heavy chains	5/9

SOURCE: Gearhart, P. J., et al. Nature *291*, 29, 1981. With permission.

V_H, 12 D, and 4 J_H exons there may be 9600 different V_H sequences. In addition, junctional site diversity will be increased by imprecise splicing although some of the combinations so formed may be of little functional use.

Since both light and heavy chains contribute to the antibody-binding site, the number of potential combinations and hence antigen binding specificities will be about 1×10^7, (1200 × 9600). This estimate does not, of course, take into account errors in splicing or somatic mutation. (These figures may be compared with a figure of 1×10^7 which has been estimated to be the number of antigenic determinants that the immune systems may recognize.)

Constant-Region Diversity

The constant regions of immunoglobulin-heavy chains vary according to the immunoglobulin class and subclass. Thus, while an immunoglobulin-heavy chain constant region attaches to only one V_H region, this constant region may belong to any one of the several immunoglobulin classes or subclasses. For each immunoglobulin class or subclass, there exists a set of four or five different C_H exons, each coding for a single homology region or a hinge region. Thus an IgM constant region is coded for by five $C\mu$ exons, an IgA constant region by four $C\alpha$ exons, etc. These C_H exons are arranged in a fixed pattern along the DNA chain (Fig. 8-7). During the course of an antibody response, the immunoglobulin classes are synthesized in a fixed sequence. Thus, a B cell first makes IgM and then both IgM and IgD. The IgM is first firmly bound to the cell membrane, then it is secreted. Finally, a B cell becomes committed to synthesizing immunoglobulins of one of the other major classes, IgG, IgA, and IgE. All these changes require that the cell transcribe the appropriate C_H genes and switch to the genes for another class as required.

Class Switching The exons required for all immunoglobulin heavy chains are arranged in linear fashion on chromosome 14 in man and chromosome 12 in mice (Fig. 8-

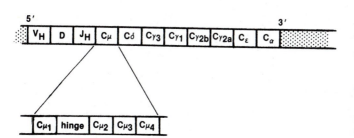

FIGURE 8-7. The arrangement of the genes coding for immunoglobulin heavy chains: Every immunoglobulin homology region within each class is coded for by a separate exon as shown here by the genes for a μ heavy chain. There is a fifth $C\mu$ exon 3' to $C\mu 4$ that is involved in cell-membrane binding (see Fig. 8-9).

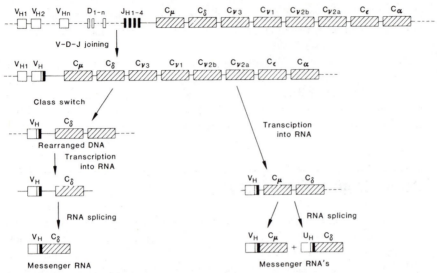

FIGURE 8–8. Heavy-chain gene assembly: The upper diagram shows the arrangement in germ-line cells of the gene segments for antibody heavy chains. The assembly of a complete variable-region gene (V_H) requires the joining of three gene segments, one of those designated V_{H1} through V_{Hn}, one D, and one J. After V–D–J joining, transcription of the rearranged DNA into RNA, followed by differential splicing of the transcript, allows the simultaneous production of messenger RNA's for two different classes of heavy chain (shown in the right-hand branch of the diagram). The messengers direct the synthesis of either an IgM or IgD heavy chain. The shift to the final class of heavy chain that will be produced by the cell involves a further gene rearrangement (left-hand branch). In this case, the cell will make an IgD heavy chain and the $C\mu$ gene segment has been deleted to bring the completed variable region gene nearer to the $C\delta$ gene segment. If the cell were going to make an IgA heavy chain, gene segments $C\mu$ through $C\epsilon$ would have to be deleted. The rearranged DNA is transcribed and the RNA copy spliced to form the final messenger. (From Marx, J. L. Science:, *212:* 1015–1018, 1981. Copyright 1981 by the American Association for the Advancement of Science.)

8). The selection of the required V–D–J segments is a very early event in the development of a B cell and this does not change after selection. On the other hand, the selection of genes for a specific immunoglobulin class is a relatively late event and may switch as the immune response progresses. Thus, V–D–J segments remain separated from the C region segments until after transcription into mRNA. Just prior to translation, the unwanted C region transcripts are excised and the required C region mRNA is spliced to the V–D–J transcript. Thus, if IgM is to be synthesized, the V-D-J transcript is spliced directly to the $C\mu$ transcript. On the other hand, if IgA is to be synthesized, the mRNA transcripts coding for $C\mu$ to $C\epsilon$ inclusive are excised and the V–D–J transcript spliced to the $C\alpha$ transcript.

IgM and Cell Membranes

The constant homology-region exons and the hinge-region exons of immunoglobulin-heavy chains are normally separated by introns. When the exons for IgM are investigated, there appears to be an additional exon 3′ to Cμ4, known as CμM. There is also a cleavage site within the Cμ4 exon. In order to produce membrane IgM, the Cμ4 exon is cleaved so that the 3′ segment of Cμ4 is deleted and the CμM exon is joined directly to Cμ4. CμM codes for a hydrophobic peptide that is capable of interacting with the lymphocyte membrane. In order to produce free IgM, however, the CμM exon is deleted from the mRNA and translation is stopped, after the intact Cμ4 is read.

IgM and IgD Production

During the course of B-cell maturation, the cells synthesize IgM and IgD simultaneously by transcribing the complete Cμ and Cδ exons into mRNA. This mRNA is then arranged in such a way that both VDJCμ is produced, coding for μ-heavy chains, and, VDJCδ is produced coding for δ-heavy chains (Fig. 8–9).

Heavy-Chain Switching

Heavy-chain class switching operates in a manner very different from V-gene segment splicing. It appears to be associated with each C$_H$ exon. On the 5′ side of each of these exons is a switching (S) region that can recognize and splice to the switching region of other heavy chain regions, e.g., 5′–VDJ–Sμ–Cμ–Sδ–Cδ–Sα–Cα–3′. Thus, in order for IgA to be produced, the Sα region binds to the Sμ region, looping out all the intervening exons and directly joining VDJ to Cα.

These switching regions are complex, apparently consisting of multiple sites and it may be that each S site may be designed for a different gene rearrangement. Thus, there may be a distinct site for joining Sμ to Sδ and, another for joining Sμ to Sα, etc.

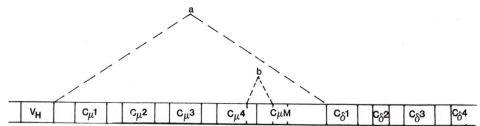

FIGURE 8–9. Diagram of chromosomal DNA coding for IgM and IgD in a B cell: The labelled rectangles are exons, and the intervening segments represent introns. In cells expressing both membrane IgM and membrane IgD, it is believed that the entire region is transcribed. Dotted line *a* joins the introns that are spliced to produce membrane IgD, with the elimination of all the Cμ exons. Dotted line *b* joins the introns that are spliced to produce the membrane form of IgM. Note that if the switch from membrane to secreted IgM occurs through termination of transcription after the μ segment, transcription of the δ gene will also be shut off. The switch from membrane to secreted δ chains is believed to occur as described for μ. (Some investigators call the 3′ segment of Cμ4, CμM and call the CμM depicted here Cμ5). (Reprinted by permission from *Nature*, Vol. 290, p. 543. Copyright © 1981 MacMillan Journals Limited.)

Sources of Additional Information

Baltimore, D. Somatic mutation gains its place among the generators of diversity. Cell, *26:* 295–296, 1981.

Brack, C., et al., A complete Ig gene is created by somatic recombination. Cell, *15:* 1–14, 1978.

Crews, S., et al. A single V$_H$ gene segment encodes the immune response to phosphorylcholine: Somatic mutation is correlated with the class of antibody. Cell, *25:* 59–66, 1981.

Dreyer, W. J., and Bennett, J. C. The molecular basis of antibody formation: A paradox. Proc. Natl. Acad. Sci., USA., *54:* 864–869, 1965.

Early, P., and Hood, L. Alletic exclusion and non-productive immunoglobulin gene rearrangements. Cell, *24:* 1–3, 1981.

Gershenfield, H. K., et al. Somatic diversification is required to generate the Vκ genes of MOPC 511 and MOPC 167 myeloma proteins. Proc. Natl. Acad. Sci., USA., *78:* 7674–7678, 1981.

Gottlieb, P. D. Immunoglobulin genes. Mol. Immunol., *17:* 1423–1435, 1980.

Hood, L. Two genes: one polypeptide chain—fact or fiction? Fed. Proc., *31:* 179–187, 1977.

Robertson, M. Chopping and changing in immunoglobulin genes. Nature, *287:* 390–392, 1980.

Sakano, H., et al. Domains and the hinge region of an immunoglobulin heavy chain are encoded in separate DNA segments. Nature, *277:* 627–633, 1979.

Seidman, J. G., et al. Antibody diversity. Science, *202:* 11–17, 1978.

Tonegawa, S. Somatic generation of antibody diversity. Nature, *302:* 575–581, 1983.

Valbuena, O., et al. Chromosomal location of mouse immunoglobulin genes. Proc. Natl. Acad. Sci. USA., *75:* 2883–2887, 1978.

9

Tissues of the Immune System

Although antigen is trapped and processed by the macrophages of the mononuclear-phagocytic system, the mounting of an immune response is a function of lymphocytes. These lymphocytes are the relatively featureless, small, round cells that constitute the predominant cell type of organs such as the spleen, lymph nodes, and thymus. Because their morphology has provided no clues as to their function, very little was known about the role of lymphocytes until relatively recently. They have now been shown, however, to be extraordinarily complex, and their major function appears to be the production of antibodies or specific effector cells in response to macrophage-bound antigen. These responses occur within lymphoid organs (Fig. 9–1), which, therefore, must provide an environment for efficient interaction between lymphocytes, macrophages, and antigen. In addition, control systems must be provided in order to regulate the immune responses, and this regulation can occur at two levels.

On the first level, the production of lymphocytes must be controlled so that their numbers are appropriate for the tasks involved. In addition, some form of "editing" of these cells must occur so that those produced are reactive only to foreign antigenic determinants and not to "self" antigens. On the second level, the magnitude of the response of each lymphocyte also must be regulated so that it is sufficient but not excessive for the body's requirements.

The tissue of the lymphoid system may, therefore, be classified on the basis of their roles in generating lymphocytes, in regulating the production of lymphocytes, and in providing a suitable environment for the interaction between processed antigen and antigen-sensitive cells (Fig. 9–2).

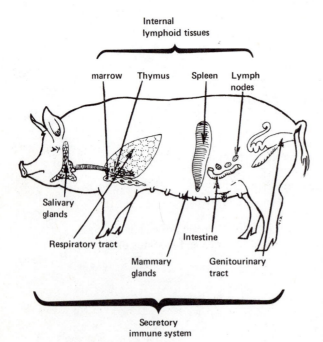

FIGURE 9–1. The major lymphoid tissues of an animal. (From Tizard, I. Veterinary Immunology. 2nd ed. W. B. Saunders, Philadelphia, 1982. With permission.)

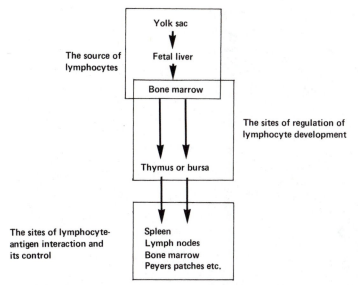

FIGURE 9–2. The role of the various lymphoid tissues. (From Tizard, I. Veterinary Immunology. 2nd ed. W. B. Saunders, Philadelphia, 1982. With permission.)

Sources of Lymphoid Cells

In the very young embryo, lymphoid stem cells are produced first by the omentum and later by the fetal liver and yolk sac. In the older fetus and adults, the bone marrow serves as the major source of lymphoid cells. This central role of the bone marrow is emphasized by the observation that, of all the tissues in the adult, it alone is able to prevent the death of animals that have been lethally irradiated. Therefore, it is presumably capable of providing all the cells necessary to restore the functions of the other lymphoid organs.

The bone marrow in adults serves three functions. Not only is it a hematopoietic organ serving as the source of all blood cells, including lymphocytes, but like the spleen, liver, and lymph nodes, it also contains many mononuclear phagocytes, and thus serves to remove particulate antigens from circulating blood. In addition, it functions as a major source of antibody. Because of these functions, the bone marrow consists of two compartments, a hematopoietic compartment and a vascular compartment. These two compartments alternate, like slices of cake, in wedge-shaped areas within long bones. The hematopoietic areas contain precursors of all the blood cells, as well as macrophages and lymphocytes, and are enclosed by a layer of adventitial cells (Fig. 9–3). The lymphocytes are either scattered among the other hematopoietic cells or else are found in discrete clusters. Macrophages are commonly associated with these clusters. In older individuals, these adventitial cells may become so loaded with fat that the hematopoietic tissue is masked, and the marrow may have a fatty yellow appearance. The vascular compartment consists of blood sinuses lined by endothelial cells and crossed by reticular cells and macrophages.

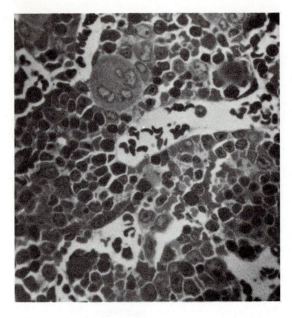

FIGURE 9–3. The hepatopoietic tissue in bone marrow is separated by radially oriented venous sinuses that communicate with a large central vein. The large multinucleated cell is a megakaryocyte, and other small cells are myeloid, lymphoid, and erythroid cell precursors. (Reprinted by permission of the publisher from J. J. Oppenheim, D. L. Rosenstreich, and M. Potter (eds.), Cellular Functions in Immunity and Inflammation. Copyright 1981 by Elsevier Science Publishing Co., Inc.)

Primary Lymphoid Organs

The organs whose function is to regulate the production and differentiation of lymphocytes are known as **primary lymphoid organs.** They include the thymus, found in both mammals and birds, and the bursa of Fabricius, found only in birds. These organs arise early in fetal life from outgrowths at the ectoendodermal junctions. The thymus arises from the endoderm of the third and fourth pharyngeal pouches, whereas the bursa develops from the cloacodermal junction. Because of this, each organ consists of a mass of epithelial cells. Lymphoid stem cells from the yolk sac, the fetal liver, and eventually the bone marrow, migrate to these organs via the bloodstream, and infiltrate the endothelial reticulum. It is in them that recognizable lymphocytes are first observed in the fetus (Table 9–1).

Thymus

The thymus is a pale, lobulated organ found in the anterior mediastinal space. The size of the thymus can vary considerably, its relative size being greatest in the newborn and its

TABLE 9–1 Comparison of Primary and Secondary Lymphoid Organs

	Primary Lymphoid Organ	Secondary Lymphoid Organ
Origin	Ectoendodermal junction	Mesoderm
Time of development	Early in embryonic life	Later in fetal life
Persistence	Involutes after puberty	Persists through adult life
Effect of removal	Loss of lymphocytes	No effect or only minor consequences
Response to antigen	Unresponsive	Fully reactive
Examples	Thymus; (bursa)	Spleen; lymph nodes

absolute size being greatest in puberty. After puberty, atrophy of the thymic parenchyma occurs, and the cortex is replaced by adipose tissue, but remnants of the thoracic thymus may persist in many animals until old age. In addition to this age-related involution, the thymus atrophies rapidly in response to stress, so that the thymus of individuals dying after prolonged sickness may be abnormally small.

Structure

The thymus (Fig. 9–4) consists of a series of lobules of loosely packed epithelial cells, and each lobule is covered by a connective tissue capsule. The outer part of each lobule, the cortex, is densely infiltrated with large numbers of rapidly dividing lymphocytes. In the inner part, the medulla, the epithelial cells are clearly visible since there are fewer lymphocytes. Within the medulla are round bodies known as thymic (Hassall's) corpuscles, whose function is not known. They contain the protein keratin and perhaps represent an abortive attempt at keratinization by the epithelial cells. Occasionally, the remains of a small blood vessel may be observed at their center. The blood supply to the thymus is derived from arteries that enter through connective-tissue septa and run as arterioles along the corticomedullary junction. The capillaries that arise from these arterioles enter the cortex and loop back to the medulla. These cortical capillaries are covered by a barrier composed of an endothelium, an abnormally thick basement membrane, and a continuous outer layer of epithelial cells. It appears that this barrier may effectively prevent circulating antigens from entering the thymic cortex, since blood vessels in the thymic cortex are impermeable to physiological tracers. No lymphatics enter the thymus.

Function

The function of the thymus was unknown until relatively recently, since its removal in adult animals has no immediately obvious effect. If, however, it is removed from newborn rodents, a number of important consequences result.

Neonatal Thymectomy

Thymectomy performed on mice within a day of birth results in these animals' becoming much more susceptible to infection and occasionally becoming runted. Closer

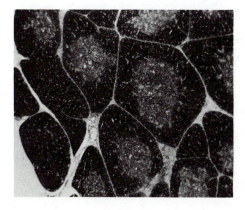

FIGURE 9–4. A section of thymus. Each lobule is divided into a cortex rich in lymphocytes, hence dark-staining, and a paler medulla consisting largely of epithelial cells (Original magnification ×45). (Specimen kindly provided by Dr. S. Yamashiro. From Tizard, I. Veterinary Immunology. 2nd ed. W. B. Saunders, Philadelphia, 1982. With permission.)

TABLE 9–2 Effects of Neonatal Thymectomy and Bursectomy on the Immune Responses and on Lymphoid Tissues

Function	Thymectomy	Bursectomy
Numbers of circulating lymphocytes	↓↓↓*	—
Presence of lymphocytes in thymus-dependent areas	↓↓↓	—
Graft rejection	↓↓↓	—
Presence of lymphocytes in thymus-independent areas and germinal centers	↓†	↓↓↓
Plasma cells	↓	↓↓↓
Serum immunoglobulins	↓	↓↓↓
Antibody formation	↓	↓↓↓

*Severely depressed.

†Slightly depressed.

examination of these neonatally thymectomized animals reveals that there is a drop in the number of their circulating lymphocytes and a marked depression in the ability of the animals to mount some type of immune response (Table 9–2). Their capacity to reject grafts is especially compromised, reflecting a total loss of the cell-mediated immune response. Antibody-mediated immunity is depressed also, but to a lesser extent.

Adult Thymectomy

Removal of the thymus from adult animals produces no immediately obvious results. If, however, animals are kept for several months after this operation, there is a progressive decline in the number of their circulating lymphocytes, and in their ability to mount cell-mediated immune responses (Table 9–3). We may interpret these results to suggest that, although the adult thymus is still functional, there exists a reservoir of thymus-derived lymphocytes that must be exhausted before the immunosuppressive effects of thymectomy become apparent.

The results of thymectomy indicate that the neonatal thymus acts as a source of many of the circulating blood lymphocytes. These are called **thymus-derived lymphocytes** or **T cells.** These thymus-derived lymphocytes actually originate in the bone marrow, but mature within the thymic cortex after being attracted by hormones secreted by thymic epithelial cells. These lymphocytes divide within the cortex at a rapid rate and this division is

TABLE 9–3 Loss of Thymic Function in Adult Thymectomized Animals

Time	Effect
1 hr	Disappearance of circulating thymic factor (Thymulin [FTS])
1 wk	Disappearance of Thy 1$^+$, E rosetting cells in blood
1 mo	Depression of responses to mitogens
	Depression of some suppressor cells
	Depletion of Thy 1$^+$ cells in spleen
1 yr	Depression of antibody formation
	Delay in skin allograft reaction
	Depression of GVH reaction

unaffected by the presence of antigen. Of the new cells produced, most appear to die there, while others (about 5% of the total in rodents and about 25% in calves) migrate to the thymic medulla and then emigrate to colonize the secondary lymphoid organs with T cells.

The thymus serves to provide an environment in which T cells can mature. The mature T cell released by the thymus must be able to participate in the immune responses yet be incapable of responding in an adverse manner to normal body constituents. The nature of the processing T cells within the thymus undergo appears to involve the development of these cells within a structure known as a nurse cell (Fig. 9–5). These nurse cells are very large and are capable of engulfing up to 50 thymic lymphocytes and then releasing them. Within this environment, the T-cell population acquires the capacity to recognize self-antigens based upon the recognition of histocompatibility antigens on the surface of thymic epithelial cells.

Thymic Hormones

The thymus also functions as an endocrine gland since thymic epithelial cells appear to release several hormone-like molecules. All these molecules are polypeptides and, at the present time, do not seem to be related (Table 9–4).

Thymosin The thymosins are a mixture of polypeptides with molecular weights between 1000 and 15000. They are classified according to their electrophoretic mobility into α, β, and γ thymosins. These peptides are able to induce the maturation and differentiation of pre-T cells. Thus, α_1 thymosin induces the appearance of the T-cell enzyme terminal deoxynucleotidyl transferase (TdT), Lyt antigens, and E receptors (see Chap. 10). α_2 thymosin induces the production of Lyt antigens and suppressor cells, whereas thymosins β_2 and β_4 induce TdT production in vitro and in vivo.

Thymopoietins Thymopoietins I and II are each polypeptides of 49 aminoacid residues. The biological activity is contained within a small pentapeptide (TP5) from thymo-

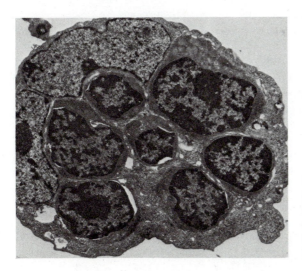

FIGURE 9–5. A photomicrograph of a thymic nurse cell. Within the cytoplasm of the cell can be seen seven lymphocytes. (Courtesy of Dr. H. Wekerle.)

TABLE 9-4   The Properties of the Major Thymic Hormones

Name	Physical Properties	Biological Activity
Thymic humoral factor	Peptide 3220 Mr.	Promotes T-cell differentiation.
Thymopoietin I and II	Proteins 5500 Mr.	Promotes T-cell differentiation. Enhances T-cell-mediated activities. Causes neuromuscular block.
Thymosin	Peptides 4982 Mr.	Regulate early thymocyte production. Induce deoxynucleotidyl transferase.
Thymulin (facteur thymique serique [FTS])	Nonapeptide 847 Mr.	Increases CAMP in T cells. Promotes T-cell maturation.
Thymostimulin	Peptides 12000 Mr.	Induces T-cell differentiation. Enhances tumor resistance. Present in serum

Note that the literature on thymic hormones contains descriptions of at least twelve other thymic-hormone-like agents.

poietin II. Thymopoietins induce the appearance of Thy-1 and TL antigens on cells from nude mice. They seem to exert an immunoregulatory activity since they can increase suppressor cell populations in some autoimmune disorders and restore immune competence in tumor-bearing and aged mice. They also have neuromuscular blocking activity.

Thymic Humoral Factor (THF)   THF is a peptide of 3220 daltons that can restore immune responsivness in neonatally thymectomized mice. It promotes T-cell differentiation and prevents the runting that tends to follow neonatal thymectomy. In man, THF has been used in an attempt to restore T-cell function in immunosuppressed patients.

Facteur Thymique Serique (FTS)   Also known as thymulin, or thymic serum factor, this nonapeptide is secreted by thymic epithelial cells and may be isolated from serum. FTS induces the appearance of T-cell markers on immature T cells and has variable effects on suppressor cell function depending on the dose employed. The level of FTS in serum declines in old or immunodeficient animals and following thymectomy.

Thymostimulin   This is a group of polypeptides smaller than 12000 daltons. They induce the appearance of the Thy-1 antigen and E receptors. Thymostimulin may also enhance resistance to some tumors in mice.

One of the difficulties encountered in determining the significance of factors isolated from thymus extracts is that they may not be specific for thymic cells. Thus cyclic AMP can induce T-cell differentiation and thymopoietin and THF appear to act by elevating lymphocyte cAMP levels. A peptide called ubiquitin has been isolated from a number of different organs including the thymus and has similar properties to the thymopoietins. Its biological significance is unclear.

Bursa of Fabricius

The bursa of Fabricius (Fig. 9-6) is a lymphoepithelial organ found in birds but not in mammals. It arises from the ectoendodermal junction as a round, saclike structure just

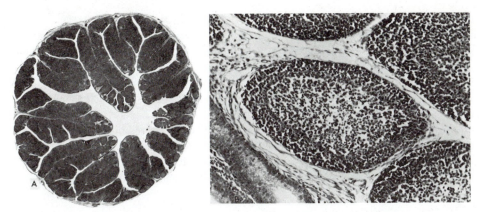

FIGURE 9–6. The bursa of Fabricius. (**A**) Low-power photomicrograph showing the complete bursa in a 14-day-old chick (original magnification ×5). (**B**) A single bursal follicle (original magnification ×360). (Specimen kindly provided by Dr. S. Yamashiro. From Tizard, I. Veterinary Immunology. 2nd ed. W. B. Saunders, Philadelphia, 1982. With permission.)

dorsal to the cloaca. The bursa reaches its maximal size about one to two weeks after the chick has hatched and then undergoes gradual involution.

Structure

Like the thymus, the bursa consists of lymphoid cells embedded in epithelial tissue. This epithelial tissue lines a hollow sac connected to the cloaca by a duct. Inside this sac, large folds of epithelium extend into the lumen, and, scattered through these folds, are follicles of lymphoid cells. Each lymphoid follicle is divided into a cortex and medulla. The cortex contains lymphocytes, plasma cells, and macrophages. At the corticomedullary junction there is a basement-membrane-and-capillary network, on the inside of which are epithelial cells. These medullary epithelial cells show frequent mitotic figures, and, toward the center of the medulla, appear to be replaced by lymphoblasts and lymphocytes, so that the center of the follicle may appear to consist solely of lymphocytes.

Function

The bursa may be removed either surgically or by infecting newborn chicks with a virus that causes bursal destruction (infectious bursal disease). Since the bursa involutes when chicks become sexually mature, premature bursal atrophy may also be provoked by administration of the hormone testosterone. When treated in these ways, birds show only a slight drop in the numbers of circulating lymphocytes, but they produce only very small quantities of antibody, and there is a loss of antibody-producing plasma cells. Since bursectomized birds can still reject foreign skin grafts, there appears to be little effect on the cell-mediated immune response. These birds are more susceptible than normal to bacterial infections.

These results have been interpreted to suggest that the bursa is a primary lymphoid organ, whose function is to serve as a maturation and differentiation site for the cells of the antibody-forming system. These cells are therefore called **B cells.** More recent studies, however, have suggested other interpretations. It can be shown, for example, that spleen cells from neonatally bursectomized birds, if transplanted into a normal bird, cause the recipient to lose its ability to make antibodies. It has been demonstrated that this phenomenon results from the development of a population of suppressor cells in the bursectomized bird. It is possible that the loss of antibody production in bursectomized birds is due, therefore, to the actions of these suppressor cells.

In addition, the bursa also functions as a secondary lymphoid organ—that is, it can trap antigen and undertake some antibody synthesis. Indeed, it also contains a small focus of T cells just dorsal to the bursal duct opening. It is probable, therefore, that the bursa has a number of different functions and can no longer be considered to be a pure primary lymphoid organ.

Bursal Equivalent of Mammals

Mammals do not possess a bursa of Fabricius; consequently, investigators have searched for an organ with equivalent function. In order to conform to the criteria of a primary lymphoid organ (see Table 9–1), the bursal equivalent might be expected to arise from an ectoendodermal junction and to atrophy at puberty, and the removal of such an organ from a newborn animal might be expected to prevent antibody production. No such organ has been identified. It now seems probable that bursal functions in the mammal are the joint responsibility of the intestinal lymphoid tissue, such as the Peyer's patches, and of the spleen, and the bone marrow.

Secondary Lymphoid Organs

In contrast to the thymus and bursa, the other lymphoid organs of the body arise from mesoderm late in fetal life and persist through adult life (see Table 9–1). They are responsive to antigenic stimulation and thus are poorly developed in germ-free animals. This is in marked contrast to the primary lymphoid organs, which do not normally respond to antigen and are thus of normal size in germ-free animals. Removal of individual secondary lymphoid organs does not significantly reduce an animal's immune capability. Examples of these secondary lymphoid organs include the spleen, the lymph nodes, and the lymphoid nodules of the gastrointestinal respiratory and urogenital tracts. These organs are rich in macrophages and dendritic cells that trap and process antigens and in T and B lymphocytes, which mediate the immune responses. The overall anatomical structure of these organs is, therefore, designed to facilitate antigen trapping and to provide maximal opportunities for processed antigen to be presented to antigen-sensitive cells.

Lymph Nodes

Structure

Lymph nodes are round or bean-shaped structures strategically placed on lymphatic channels in such a way that they can trap antigen being carried from the periphery of the body to the bloodstream. Thus, lymph nodes consist of a reticular network filled with lymphocytes, macrophages, and dendritic cells through which lymphatic sinuses penetrate (Fig.

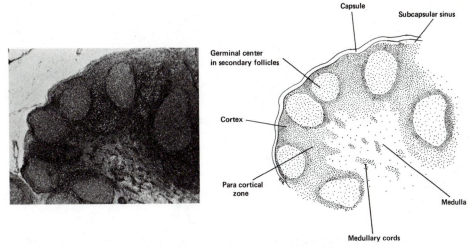

FIGURE 9–7. A portion of a lymph node (original magnification ×100). (Specimen kindly provided by Dr. S. Yamashiro. From Tizard, I. Veterinary Immunology. 2nd ed. W. B. Saunders, Philadelphia, 1982. With permission.)

9–7). A subcapsular sinus is found immediately under the connective-tissue capsule of the node; other sinuses pass through the body of the node but are particularly prominent in the medulla. Lymphatic vessels enter the node at various points around its circumference, and efferent lymphatics leave from a depression or hilus on one side. The blood vessels to and from a lymph node also enter and leave via the hilus.

The interior of a lymph node is divided into a peripheral cortex, a central medulla, and an ill-defined area between these two regions termed the paracortical zone. The cells in the cortex are predominantly B lymphocytes and are arranged in poorly defined nodules. Prior to exposure to antigen, these nodules are termed primary follicles. In lymph nodes that have been stimulated by antigen, the cells within primary follicles expand to form characteristic structures known as germinal centers. A follicle containing a germinal center is known as a secondary follicle. Some T cells are found in the cortex, in an area immediately surrounding each germinal center.

The cells in the paracortical zone are mainly T lymphocytes. In neonatally thymectomized or congenitally athymic animals, this area is deprived of cells and so can be considered a thymus-dependent area (Fig. 9–8). The cells of the medulla include B lymphocytes, macrophages, reticulum cells, and plasma cells. They are arranged in cellular cords between the lymphatic sinuses.

Lymphocyte Circulation

Lymph flows through the thoracic duct at about 500 ml per hour in man, and it contains about 1×10^8 lymphocytes per ml. If the thoracic duct is cannulated and the lymph removed, the number of lymphocytes in the bloodstream drops dramatically within a few hours. When the lymphoid tissues of a cannulated animal are examined, it can be shown that cells have also disappeared from lymph-node paracortical zones. The rapid depletion of lymphocytes by this technique makes it clear that thoracic duct cells must nor-

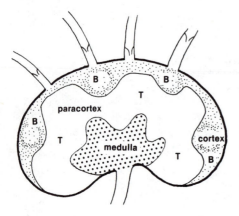

FIGURE 9–8. A diagram showing the major areas in which T and B cells are located within a lymph node. A significant number of T cells may also be found in the cortex. The medulla is rich in macrophages and plasma cells.

mally recirculate back to the lymphoid tissues through the bloodstream (Fig. 9–9). In fact, the lymphocytes that enter the vena cava from the thoracic duct spend only between two and twelve hours in the blood before returning to the lymphoid organs. They leave the bloodstream by way of the venules of the lymph-node paracortical zone. These venules (usually called, somewhat unnecessarily, postcapillary venules) possess an extremely tall endothelium. These high endothelial cells are unlike endothelial cells found elsewhere in the body, being somewhat monocytelike, having phagosomes, and being rich in nonspecific esterase. Circulating lymphocytes adhere to these endothelial cells and then migrate into the node by passing between the cells (Fig. 9–10). The binding of lymphocytes to this tall endothelium is energy-dependent, it requires calcium and an intact cytoskeleton, and the lymphocyte and the endothelial cell must be histocompatible. T cells percolate through the lymph node paracortex and then re-enter the lymphatic circulation via the efferent lymph. There is thus a continuing recirculation of these cells between lymph and blood. As a result of this circulation, the majority of lymphocytes found in peripheral blood are T cells (see Table 10–1).

A small proportion of the circulating T cells do not return to lymph nodes but enter

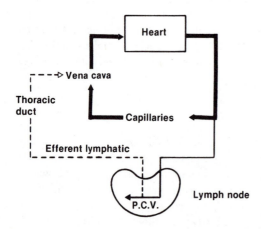

FIGURE 9–9. A schematic diagram depicting the circulation of lymphocytes. The majority of lymphocytes seen on a blood smear are recirculating cells. A small proportion, however, may be cells newly released by the bone marrow or the thymus (P.C.V. = postcapillary venule). (From Tizard, I. Veterinary Immunology. 2nd ed. W. B. Saunders, Philadelphia, 1982. With permission.)

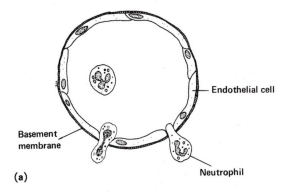

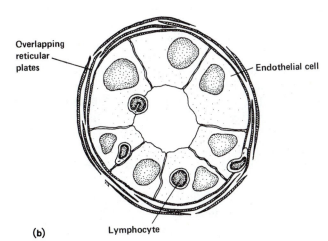

FIGURE 9-10. A diagram comparing the migration of neutrophils from a conventional capillary, as occurs in acute inflammation (**A**), with the migration of lymphocytes from a "postcapillary" venule within the paracortical zone of a lymph node (**B**). Neutrophils, when migrating from conventional capillaries, pass between endothelial cells and then directly through the basement membrane. In contrast, lymphocytes appear to migrate through the cytoplasm of the tall endothelial cells lining "postcapillary" venules and then infiltrate between overlapping reticular plates before gaining access to the node. (From Tizard, I. Veterinary Immunology. 2nd ed. W. B. Saunders, Philadelphia, 1982. With permission.)

the lymphoid tissues in the lung or intestine. These cells are specifically involved in the development of immune responses at body surfaces.

Response of Lymph Nodes to Antigen

Antigen deposited in tissues is carried by the flow of tissue fluid to local lymph nodes. Its fate within these nodes depends upon whether the animal has had previous exposure to the antigen. Lymph nodes possess two separate antigen-trapping systems. One system employs the macrophages present in the medulla. Since these cells can take up antigen in the absence of antibodies, this system can function relatively effectively on first exposure to antigen. The other system involves dendritic cells, which are found in the lymph-node cortex and in particular within secondary follicles. Dendritic cells possess a large array of cytoplasmic processes (see Fig. 4–16) and can thus form a web through which antigen must pass as it flows through the cortex. The efficiency of this web as an antigen-trapping device does depend, however, upon the presence of antibody, which is required for antigen to adhere to the dendritic cell processes.

If an animal possesses no antibodies to an injected antigen, then most of the antigen entering the node will be phagocytosed by macrophages situated in the medulla. The antigen-carrying macrophages then migrate to the cortical follicles, where antigen-sensitive cells are present. Once these cells respond, their antibody-producing progeny migrate to the medulla. Some of these antibody-producing cells are also released into the efferent lymph and, are thus carried to other lymph nodes downstream. Some time after antibody production is first observed in the medulla, germinal centers appear in the cortex, arising as a result of proliferation of cells within primary follicles. The dividing cells are usually relatively large and pale-staining, but compress the surrounding lymphocytes into a dense mantle around the germinal center (Fig. 9–11). Dendritic cells may form a cap on the peripheral side of the germinal center. Antigens that do not stimulate antibody production do not usually cause germinal center formation. The role of these germinal centers is to provide a focus for the production of the immunological memory cells that are required for a secondary response. It is also possible that they provide an environment in which B cells can undergo non-antigen-specific proliferation and thus increase the size of the available B-cell pool.

On second exposure to antigen, adherence to antibody-coated dendritic cells is the predominant means of antigen trapping. In a secondary response, the germinal centers tend to become less obvious as the activated memory cells migrate from the cortex to the medulla and out in the efferent lymph. Once this stage is completed, the germinal centers then show hyperplasia and limited antibody production. The migration of cells within the lymph node is necessary to ensure that antibody-producing cells are kept well away from antigen-sensitive cells. As will be discussed later (Chap. 13), this segregation prevents an immediate inhibition of the immune response through the negative feedback exerted by the antibody.

When responding to antigens that stimulate a cell-mediated rather than an antibody-mediated immune response, such as skin grafts, for example, the T-cell-rich paracortical areas respond by the production of large pyroninophilic cells (i.e., they stain with pyronin, which is a stain for RNA; thus, a cell with pyroninophilic cytoplasm is rich in ribosomes and is probably a protein-producing cell). These large pyroninophilic cells (known as lymphoblasts) give rise, in turn, to more small lymphocytes, which participate in the cell-mediated immune responsed (Chap. 12).

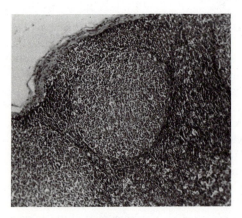

FIGURE 9–11. A germinal center within the secondary follicles of a lymph-node cortex. (original magnification ×240). (Specimen kindly provided by Dr. S. Yamashiro. From Tizard, I. Veterinary Immunology. 2nd ed. W. B. Saunders, Philadelphia, 1982. With permission.)

Spleen

The spleen has a number of important functions. Thus, just as lymph nodes serve to filter antigen from lymph, so the spleen filters blood. The filtering process removes both antigenic particles and aged blood cells. The spleen also stores erythrocytes and platelets and undertakes erythropoiesis in the fetus. This organ is also of major immunological significance since it is a major site for the production of antibodies and effector cells. It is, therefore, divided into two compartments: one compartment for storage of erythrocytes, for antigen trapping, and for erythropoiesis, called the red pulp, and one compartment in which the immune response occurs, known as the white pulp (Fig. 9–12).

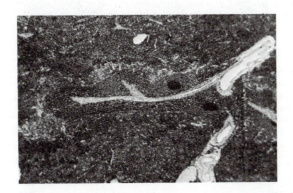

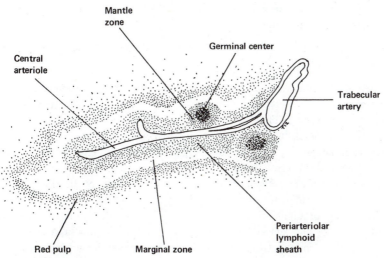

FIGURE 9–12. A histological section and diagram showing the structure of the spleen (original magnification ×50). (Specimen kindly provided by Dr. J. R. Duncan. From Tizard, I. Veterinary Immunology. 2nd ed. W. B. Saunders, Philadelphia, 1982. With permission.)

Structure of Splenic White Pulp

The white pulp of the spleen consists of lymphoid tissue intimately associated with its vasculature. Vessels that enter the spleen travel through muscular trabeculae before entering its functional areas. Immediately on leaving the trabeculae, each arteriole is surrounded by a lymphoid sheath. The arteriole eventually leaves this sheath and after branching opens, either directly or indirectly, into venous sinuses that drain into the splenic venules. The periarteriolar lymphoid sheath largely consists of T cells and is thus depleted following neonatal thymectomy. However, scattered through the sheath are round primary follicles containing B cells. On antigenic stimulation, these follicles may develop germinal centers and so become secondary follicles. Each follicle is surrounded by a layer of T cells in what is known as the mantle zone. The white pulp as a whole is separated from the red pulp by a marginal sinus, a reticulum sheath, and a marginal zone of cells, many of which are macrophages.

Response of the Spleen to Antigen

Intravenously administered antigen will be trapped, at least in part, in the spleen, where it is taken up by macrophages situated in the marginal zone and lining the sinusoids of the red pulp. These cells then carry antigen to the primary follicles of the white pulp from which, after a few days, antibody-producing cells migrate. These antibody-producing cells in turn colonize the marginal zone and the red pulp, and it is in these regions that antibody production is first detected. Germinal-center formation occurs within the primary follicles within a few days, although this formation is not directly associated with antibody production. In an animal already possessing circulating antibody, trapping by dendritic cells within the secondary follicles becomes significant. As in a primary immune response, the antibody-producing cells migrate from these follicles to the red pulp and to the marginal zone, where antibody production largely occurs. Some antibody may also be produced within the hyperplastic secondary follicles.

Lymphocyte Trapping

When antigen enters the spleen or lymph nodes, it initiates lymphocyte trapping. That is, lymphocytes that normally pass freely through these organs get trapped so that they cannot leave and the node begins to swell. The nature of the trapping process is not clear, but the process probably occurs as a result of the interaction between antigen and macrophages, leading to the release of biologically active factors (Chap. 12) that influence the movement of lymphocytes in some way. Presumably, trapping serves to concentrate antigen-sensitive cells in close proximity to sites of antigen accumulation and so increases the efficiency of the immune responses. Many adjuvants may also "spring" this trap, and it is possible that herein lies one explanation of adjuvanticity. After about 24 hours, the lymph node begins to release the trapped cells and shows increased cellular output for about seven days. Toward the end of this time, many of these released cells become antibody producers and memory cells.

The Bone Marrow as a Site of Antibody Production

Although its scattered nature makes it difficult to measure, the bone marrow constitutes the largest mass of secondary lymphoid tissue in the body. If antigen is given intra-

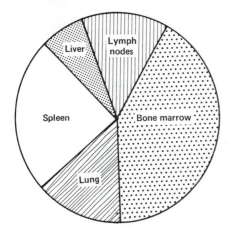

FIGURE 9-13. The relative contributions of the different lymphoid tissues to antibody production following a single intravenous dose of antigen. (From Tizard, I. Veterinary Immunology. 2nd ed. W. B. Saunders, Philadelphia, 1982. With permission.)

venously, much of it will be trapped not only in the liver and spleen but also in the bone marrow. During a primary immune response, however, the antibodies produced are derived only from the spleen and lymph nodes. Toward the end of that response, memory cells apparently leave the spleen and colonize the bone marrow. When a second dose of antigen is given, the bone marrow begins to produce very large quantities of antibody and is the major source of IgG antibodies in adult rodents. (Fig. 9–13) Up to 70 percent of the antibody produced to some antigens may be derived from the bone marrow.

Other Secondary Lymphoid Tissues and the Sites of Antibody Production

As the foregoing discussion indicates, antibodies are produced in the secondary lymphoid tissues. These tissues include not only the spleen, lymph nodes, and bone marrow, but also the lymphoid tissues scattered throughout the body, particularly in the digestive (Fig. 9–14), respiratory, and urogenital tracts.

Antigen administered orally, if it can penetrate the intestinal wall without being degraded, may stimulate the intestinal lymphoid tissues. As a result, sensitized lymphocytes

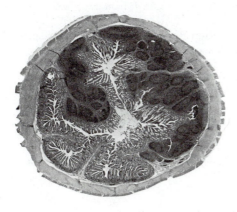

FIGURE 9-14. A section of a dog intestine showing a large Peyer's patch in the wall of the ilium (original magnification ×5). (Specimen kindly provided by Dr. S. Yamashiro. From Tizard, I. Veterinary Immunology, 2nd ed. W. B. Saunders, Philadelphia, 1982. With permission.)

leave the intestine, circulate in the bloodstream, and then colonize surfaces throughout the body. Antigenic stimulation of one part of the intestine may thus provoke antibody formation throughout the digestive tract as well as in the lung, the mammary glands, and the urogenital tract (Chap. 15). Antigen administered by inhalation stimulates local antibody production in the lymphoid tissues of the respiratory tract, and, if absorbed into the bloodstream, will provoke a systemic immune response.

Many adjuvants, such as those containing alum or water-in-oil emulsions, act by forming an insoluble antigen-containing depot. It is usual for this foreign material to stimulate chronic inflammation granulation-tissue formation. Antibody-forming cells may develop within this granulation tissue and may contribute a significant proportion of the antibody formed in these cases.

Sources of Additional Information

Anderson, N. D., et al. Specialized structure and metabolic activities of high endothelial venules in rat lymphatic tissues. Immunology, *31:* 455–473, 1976.

Butcher, E. C., Scollay, R. G., and Weissman, I. L. Organ specificity of lymphocyte migration: Mediation by highly selective lymphocyte interaction with organ-specific determinants on high endothelial venules. Eur. J. Immunol., *10:* 556–561, 1980.

Cahill, R. N. P., et al. Two distinct pools of recirculating T lymphocytes: Migratory characteristics of nodal and intestinal T lymphocytes. J. Exp. Med. *45:* 420–428, 1977.

Friedman, H., ed. Thymus factors in immunity. Ann. N.Y. Acad. Sci., *249:* 1–547, 1975.

Gowans, J. L., and Knight, E. J. The route of recirculation of lymphocytes in the rat. Proc. R. Soc. Lond (Biol.), *159:* 257–282, 1964.

Ham, A. W. Histology. J. B. Lippincott, Philadelphia, 1974.

Hay, J. B., and Hobb, B. B. The flow of blood to lymph nodes and its relation to lymphocyte traffic and the immune response. J. Exp. Med., *145:* 31–44, 1977.

Knowles, D. M., and Holck, S. Tissue localization of T-lymphocytes by the histochemical demonstration of acid α-naphthyl acetate esterase. Lab. Invest. *39:* 70–76, 1978.

Low, T. L. K., Mu, S-K, and Goldstein, A. L. Complete amino acid sequence of bovine thymosin B$_4$: A thymic hormone that induces terminal deoxynucleotidyl transferase activity in thymocyte populations. Proc. Natl. Acad. Sci., U.S.A., *78:* 1162–1166, 1981.

Owen, R. L., and Nemanic, P. Antigen processing structure of the mammalian intestinal tract: An SEM Study of lymphoepithelial organs. Scanning Electron Microscopy, *11:* 367–378, 1978.

Scollary, R. G., Butcher, E. C., and Weissman, I. L. Thymus cell migration. Quantitative aspects of cellular traffic from the thymus to the periphery in mice. Eur. J. Immunol., *10:* 210–218, 1980.

Weiss, L. Cells and tissues of the immune system: Structure, functions, interactions. Foundations of Immunology series. Prentice-Hall, Inc., Englewood Cliffs, NJ, 1972.

Weissman, I. L. Thymus cell migration. J. Exp. Med., *126:* 291–304, 1967.

Weissman, I. L., Gutman, G. A., and Fredberg, S. H. Tissue localization of lymphoid cells. Ser. Hematol., *8:* 482–504, 1974.

Wekerle, H., Ketelsen, V. P., and Ernst, M. Thymic nurse cells, lymphoepithelial cell complexes in murine thymuses. Morphological and serological characterization. J. Exp. Med., *151:* 925–944, 1980.

10
Lymphocytes

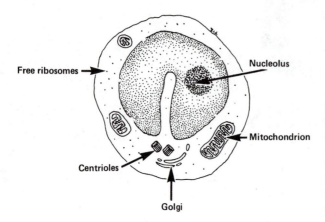

FIGURE 10–1. A diagram showing the basic structure of a lymphocyte. (From Tizard, I. Veterinary Immunology. 2nd ed. W. B. Saunders, Philadelphia, 1982. With permission.)

All lymphocytes are small, spherical cells, ranging from 7 to 15 μm in diameter. They possess a large, round nucleus that stains intensely and evenly with dyes such as hematoxylin. They possess a thin rim of cytoplasm containing some mitochondria, free ribosomes, and a small Golgi apparatus (Figs. 10–1 and 10–2). Their structure provides no clues as to their complex role within the body.

By scanning electron microscopy, the surface of some lymphocytes is observed to be smooth, while that of others is covered by a large number of villous processes (Fig. 10–3). These differences are, however, variable and probably reflect changes in the state of activity of each lymphocyte.

Since lymphocytes cannot be differentiated on the basis of morphology, it has proved necessary to attempt to define them in operational terms. Thus, lymphocytes are defined on the basis of their ontogeny, their surface receptors, their enzyme content, and their characteristic cell-surface antigens.

A subpopulation of large granular lymphocytes characterized by a rather more extensive cytoplasm and the presence of cytoplasmic granules has been identified with the natural killer cells (Fig. 10–9). The significance of these morphological differences is unclear.

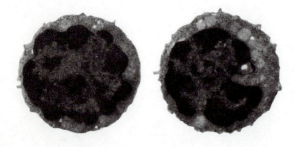

FIGURE 10–2. A transmission electron micrograph showing two lymphocytes obtained from the peritoneal cavity of a mouse (original magnification ×3000). (From Tizard, I. Veterinary Immunology. 2nd ed. W. B. Saunders, Philadelphia, 1982. With permission.)

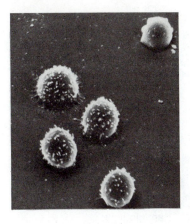

FIGURE 10-3. A scanning electron micrograph showing lymphocytes derived from a mouse mesenteric lymph node (original magnification ×1500). (From Tizard, I. Veterinary Immunology. 2nd ed. W. B. Saunders, Philadelphia, 1982. With permission.)

T and B Lymphocytes

As described in the previous chapter, those lymphocytes that undergo maturation within the thymus are known as T cells. The T cells that emigrate from the thymus accumulate within the paracortical zone of lymph nodes, in the periarteriolar lymphoid sheath of the spleen, and in the interfollicular areas of the gastrointestinal lymphoid tissues. All these areas are depleted of cells in neonatally thymectomized animals.

B lymphocytes are also of bone marrow origin but localize within the so-called thymus-independent regions; these include the lymph follicles and medulla of lymph nodes, follicles within the gastrointestinal lymphoid organs and spleen, as well as the marginal zone of the splenic white pulp. T cells are the predominant circulating lymphocytes, accounting for up to 80% of the lymphocytes seen in peripheral blood. These T cells, as discussed earlier (Chap. 9) recirculate through the high endothelial venules of the lymph-node paracortex and the lymphatic circulation.

T cells are relatively long-lived cells that probably survive for at least 6 months and possibly for as long as 10 years in man. B cells, in contrast, have a variable life span, some being long-lived and others short-lived. Their average life span in mice is 5 to 7 weeks.

A proportion of circulating blood lymphocytes are not readily classified as either T or B cells and are, therefore, generally referred to as **null cells.** Some investigators believe that these cells really belong to either the T- or B-cell pool (Table 10-1).

TABLE 10-1   Characteristics of Lymphocytes in Human Blood

Marker	Approximate % Positive	Probable Cell Type
Membrane Ig	21	B cells
Aggregated Ig (Fc receptor)		
E rosettes	70	T cells
Null cells	9	NK cells

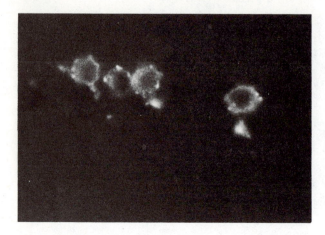

FIGURE 10–4.
Immunoglobulin on the surface of lymphocytes as revealed by the use of fluorescein-labelled antiglobulin.

Antigen Receptors

B-Cell Receptors

B cells have the ability to bind antigens because they possess antibody molecules on their surface that function as antigen receptors (Fig. 10–4). Each B-cell membrane is covered by about 20,000 to 200,000 immunoglobulin molecules that have identical antigen-binding sites. These B-cell surface immunoglobulins may belong to any class or subclass, although their distribution is by no means random.

Immature B cells usually carry only cell-membrane-bound IgM. This IgM is probably monomeric and the C_{H4} region of its heavy chains has a specific hydrophobic structure that enables it to bind to the cell membrane in such a way that the Fab regions are free to bind antigen. (See Chap. 8 for a discussion on the molecular basis of this phenomenon). As B cells mature, they synthesize cell-membrane IgD in addition to IgM as the cell translates its genes for μ and δ chains simultaneously. Thus mature B cells of this type possess both surface IgM and IgD.

When a mature B cell encounters antigen under appropriate conditions, it responds by division and differentiation. At this time, the responding cells lose their cell membrane IgD and produce and secrete IgM specific for the inducing antigen. As the immune response progresses, these B cells may switch their heavy-chain constant-region production from μ to γ, ϵ, or α, while retaining their original variable regions. As a result, they produce immunoglobulins of other classes without changing their antigen specificity.

Other B-Cell Receptors

Fc Receptors (FcR)   If sheep erythrocytes are treated with antisheep erythrocyte antibodies in low levels and, after washing, exposed to B cells, then the antibody coated erythrocytes will adhere to the lymphocytes (Fig. 10–6). The lymphocyte receptors that bind these erythrocytes attach to the Fc regions of the bound immunoglobulins and are, therefore, called Fc receptors (FcR). Fc receptors consist of a single polypeptide chain with a molecular weight of about 120,000, which bears no relationship to either the major histocompatibility antigens or the immunoglobulins. These receptors are specific for each immunoglobulin class or subclass. Fc receptors are closely bound to the cell-membrane lipids but may be released into the surrounding fluid and may bind to other cells, enabling them to fix immune complexes also. The number of Fc receptors appears to vary according to the degree of stimulation of a B cell and is probably related to the level of cyclic nucleotides within the cell. Free Fc fragments, presumably acting through these receptors, can serve as B-cell mitogens or as suppressor factors. (You can read more about Fc receptors and their activities at the end of Chap. 7).

Complement Receptors (CR)   Mouse B cells possess receptors for activated complement components (see Chap. 14). About 50 to 70% of mature B cells have a receptor called CR1, which binds C3b and C4b. CR1, a 205,000-dalton molecule, is found not only on lymphocytes but also on neutrophils, macrophages, and eosinophils. B cells from immature mice (less than 2–3 weeks old) lack CR1. A second complement receptor on B cells is CR2, a 75,000-dalton molecule that binds C3d and C3bi. B cells also possess receptors for factor H and for C1q. (You can read more about complement receptors on p. 251).

Insulin Receptors   The lymphocyte insulin receptor is a ubiquitous marker of cellular activation. It is found on both activated T and B cells.

T-Cell Receptors

The nature of the T-cell antigen receptor is by no means as well defined as that on B cells (Table 10–2). For example, it is clear that although T cells may passively adsorb some immunoglobulins, they do not possess intrinsic cell-membrane immunoglobulin of the type possessed by B cells. Nevertheless, T cells do possess antigen receptors, and it has been hypothesized that the specific molecule that binds antigen must have an "antibodylike" binding site. After all, it seems unlikely that two alternative and very complex sets of pro-

TABLE 10–2   Receptors on Human T and B Cells

Receptor for	B Cells	T Cells
Antigen	+ + + +	+ + +
Immunoglobulin Fc	+ + +	+
Complement		
CR1	+ +	+*
CR2	+	−
Insulin	+*	+*
Erythrocytes	−	+ + +
Histamine		
H-2	−	+ +
H-1	−	(+)
α-fetoprotein	−	+

*When activated

"−"—absent.

"+"—present in varying amounts from + (erratic) to + + + + (very large quantities).

teins would have evolved to recognize the same sets of antigenic determinants. There is now a considerable body of evidence to suggest that this is indeed the case. The T-cell antigen receptor probably possesses combining sites very similar, if not identical, to immunoglobulin heavy-chain variable regions, but the rest of the receptor structure appears to be rather different from immunoglobulin constant regions.

The evidence for the existence of heavy-chain variable regions on the T-cell receptor is generally based upon serologic cross-reactivity. For example, you may recollect that idiotypes are antigenic determinants located in the hypervariable regions of immunoglobulin variable regions (Chap. 6). When T cells are incubated in antisera made against specific V_H region idiotypes the response of the T cells to the corresponding antigen is blocked. In addition, antisera directed against F(ab')2 or against V_H-region framework determinants will bind to T-cell surfaces. Conversely, antisera made against isolated T-cell antigen receptors are able to react with determinants located within the Fab region of immunoglobulins.

By using antibodies directed against these combining-site determinants on T cells, it has proved possible to isolate the receptor molecules involved. They appear to have a molecular weight of 65,000 to 70,000 and to bear a superficial relationship to μ chains. Since they bind to some lectins, they probably contain carbohydrate. Some investigators have suggested that these molecules may consist of a unique immunoglobulin heavy chain named τ (tau) (Fig. 10–5).

Evidence also suggests that a second structure may be associated with the T-cell antigen receptor. Thus, antisera made against the products of the I region of the mouse MHC (Ia antigens) will also block the T-cell response to antigen. Although this activity may be interpreted to suggest that Ia antigens are an essential component of the T-cell antigen receptor, other evidence suggests that they probably are not. Thus, physical isolation of the V_H-bearing component does not isolate Ia and vice versa. Similarly, the two molecules appear to be unlinked on the cell surface, so that while one is "capped" (aggregated on the cell surface) by antisera, the other remains distributed over the cell surface. The V_H com-

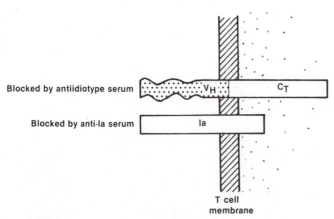

FIGURE 10–5. One possible structure of a T-cell antigen receptor. The precise degree of association between the Ia peptide and the V_H–C_T peptide is unclear. It may be that paired structures of this type can function as antigen-specific helper factors.

ponent and the Ia component may be noncovalently linked, such as occurs in the association between $\beta2$ microglobulin ($\beta2M$) and the heavy chains of Class I histocompatibility antigens (although these do co-cap).

> While there is probably a general consensus that a portion of the T-cell antigen receptor is associated with an immunoglobulinlike structure, it is only fair to point out that some investigators have voiced severe criticisms of this concept. Thus the immunoglobulins may be passively absorbed, the anti-idiotype serum may be cross-reacting with other determinants, and the lymphocyte surface is covered with many other structures that possess immunoglobulinlike structures, for example, the major histocompatibility antigens (see Fig. 6–10). It has also proved impossible to detect active V_H genes within T cells. Unfortunately, no one has yet been able to come up with a better hypothesis.

Owen and his colleagues have suggested that the mouse T-cell antigen receptor may be associated with three T-cell alloantigens called Tthy^d, Tsu^d and Tind^d coded for by genes located very close to the immunoglobulin heavy-chain allotype loci (Igh) on chromosome 12. The Tsu^d molecule is a peptide of 67,000 Mr, which may be the constant region of the T-cell antigen receptor.

Other T-Cell Receptors

Erythrocyte Receptors (E Receptors)   For unknown reasons, the T cells of man and all other animals tested possess the ability to bind directly to certain foreign erythrocytes and thus form rosettes similar to that seen in Figure 10–6. The erythrocyte receptor is a polypeptide of 40,000 to 50,000 Mr and specific antisera have been raised against this

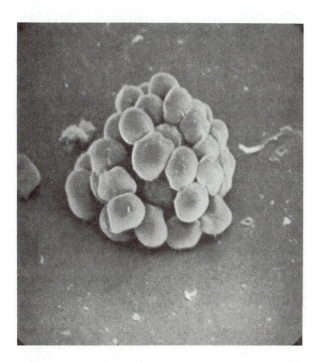

FIGURE 10–6.   A scanning electron micrograph of a "rosette" formed by allowing antibody-coated sheep erythrocytes to come into contact with a mouse lymphocyte. The lymphocyte is almost hidden by the erythrocytes (original magnification ×2250). (From Tizard, I. Veterinary Immunology. 2nd ed. W. B. Saunders, Philadelphia, 1982. With permission.)

structure, which is known as Leu-5 in mice and T 11 in man. These antisera can block T-cell division by preventing access of calcium ions to the cell. Their physiological role is probably that of a negative-signal receptor.

How to Make E Rosettes

Lymphocytes may be readily obtained from peripheral blood by careful centrifugation. The lymphocyte suspension is mixed with a suspension of washed sheep erythrocytes, centrifuged gently, and then held overnight at $+4°$. When gently resuspended, the E rosettes will remain intact and can be examined and counted under the microscope.

Fc Receptors   Some T cells possess Fc receptors but to a much lesser extent than B cells. About 60% of human peripheral-blood T cells have Fcμ receptors and may function as helper cells. Another 25 percent have Fcγ receptors and function as suppressor cells. Some T cells may have receptors for Fcα or Fc ϵ as well. The FcαT cells have helper activity specific for IgA.

Complement Receptors   T cells possess receptors for activated complement components, which probably only become expressed when the cells are activated by antigen.

Histamine Receptors   T cells possess H2 histamine receptors, while B cells do not. Stimulation of these receptors by exposure to histamine reduces T-cell activity through the elevation of cyclic AMP. T cells may also possess small numbers of H1 receptors, stimulation of which depresses intracellular cyclic AMP and thus promotes T-cell activity.

α-Fetoprotein Receptors   Some T cells have receptors for α-fetoprotein, a major fetal serum protein. Their function is unknown, but α-fetoprotein is a potent stimulator of suppressor T-cell activity.

Lymphocyte Enzymes

Hydrolytic Enzymes   T cells, when stained for hydrolytic enzymes such as neutral esterases or acid phosphatase, characteristically show a single enzyme-filled vesicle (lysosome) within the cytoplasm. B cells have no characteristic enzyme-staining patterns.

Terminal Deoxynucleotidyl Transferase   Terminal deoxynucleotidyl transferase (TdT) is a DNA polymerase that can add nucleotides to a DNA segment in the absence of a template. The enzyme TdT is found in some bone-marrow cells and in immature T cells, but not in mature T or B cells.

Purine-Salvage-Pathway Enzymes   Three enzymes, 5′-nucleotidase, adenosine deaminase, and purine nucleotide phosphorylase are all important in lymphocyte function, since a deficiency of any of them leads to an immunodeficiency (Chap. 18). 5′-nucleotidase is found in many cells, including T and B cells. Adenosine deaminase is present in higher concentrations in T cells than in B cells. Purine nucleotide phosphorylase can be found in the cytoplasm of T but not B cells.

Lymphocyte Mitogens

Certain natural compounds have the ability to provoke lymphocytes to divide. The most important group of molecules that do this are a family of proteins, usually isolated from plants, called **lectins.** Examples of such lectins include phyohemagglutinin (PHA) obtained from the red kidney bean *(Phaseolus vulgaris)*, concanavalin A (Con A) obtained from the jack bean *(Canavalis ensiformis)*, and pokeweed mitogen (PWM) obtained from the poke-weed plant *(Phytolacca americana)*.

These lectins have the ability to specifically bind sugars. For example, phytohem-agglutinin binds N-acetyl-D-galactosamine, while concanavalin A binds α-D-mannose and α-D-glucose (Table 10–3).

The binding of lectin to lymphocyte membranes stimulates nucleoside incorporation, phospholipid synthesis, DNA synthesis, and cell division. Not all lymphocytes, however, respond equally well to all lectins. Thus PHA primarily stimulates T-cell division, although it has a slight effect on B cells. Con A is also a T-cell mitogen, while PWM acts on both T and B cells and induces some B cells to synthesize immunoglobulin. One of the features of Con A that makes it very useful in immunological research is that it appears to exert a selective inducing effect on suppressor T cells (Chap. 13).

Mechanisms of Mitogenic Activity

Although lectins interact with carbohydrate residues on lymphocyte membranes, they are clearly insufficient by themselves to cause cell division, since Con A also binds to B cells, yet does not stimulate them to divide. In addition, some lectins, such as wheat germ agglutinin, can bind just as well as the mitogenic lectins but will not stimulate lymphocytes to divide, and nonmitogenic lectins can stimulate cell-membrane movement just as well as can the mitogenic lectins.

Although the mechanisms of mitogenicity involved are quite unclear, the plant lectins are known to open Ca^{++} channels in the cell membrane. They also enhance cell membrane phospholipid methylation as well as phosphatidylinositol turnover.

How to Measure Mitogenicity

In order to measure the effect of lymphocyte mitogens, it is first necessary to grow lymphocytes in tissue culture. These cells can be obtained either directly from the spleen in small rodents, or, more usually, from peripheral blood. The lymphocytes are usually incubated in tissue-culture fluid for at least 24 hours before the mitogen is

---

TABLE 10–3   Some Lymphocyte Mitogens

Lectin	Carbohydrate Specificity	Target
Phytohemagglutinin	D-N-acetylgalactosamine	T(B)
Wheat-germ agglutinin	N-acetylglucosamine, sialic acid	T
Concavalin A	D. mannose D. glucose	T
Lentil lectin	D. mannose, D. glucose	T
E. coli endotoxin	D. mannose	B
Helix pomata (garden snail)	N-acetylgalactosamine	T
Pokeweed mitogen	Not carbohydrate-specific	T,B
Lipopolysaccharide	Not carbohydrate-specific	B

added. Once this is done they begin to divide. In dividing, they are obliged to synthesize new DNA and will, therefore, take up any available nucleotides from the medium.
    It is usual to incorporate in the tissue-culture fluid a small quantity of the nucleo-
tide thymidine labelled with the radioactive isotope of hydrogen, tritium [^{3}H]. The tritiated thymidine is only incorporated in the DNA of cells that are dividing. About 24
hours after exposure to tritiated thymidine, the cultured cells are separated from the
tissue-culture fluid, either by centrifugation or filtration and their radioactivity counted
in a liquid scintillation counter. The amount of radioactivity in the lectin-treated cells
may be compared with that in an untreated lymphocyte culture. This difference may be
expressed as a ratio known as the stimulation index. As an alternative to the use of
tritiated thymidine, it is possible to use a radiolabelled amino acid such as ^{14}C-leucine.
Uptake of this substance is an indication of increased protein synthesis.

Other Lymphocyte Mitogens

Although the plant lectins are the most efficient lymphocyte mitogens, mitogenic
activity is also found in other unexpected sources. For example, an extract from the snail
Helix pomata stimulates T cells, while lipopolysaccharide from Gram-negative organisms
stimulates B cells to divide. Although this lipopolysaccharide can function as a very specific
B-cell mitogen, the presence of T cells is required for an optimal response. Other important
mitogens include neutral proteases, such as trypsin, that act as B-cell mitogens, Fc fragments of immunoglobulins that also stimulate B cells, and BCG vaccine (Bacille Calmette
Guérin—an avirulent strain of *Mycobacterium bovis* that is used as a vaccine against tuberculosis), which is a T-cell mitogen (although it may exert a slight effect on B cells).

These mitogens can be used to assist in the differentiation of T and B cells and, by
measurement of the response provoked, demonstrate the ability of the T- and B-cell systems
to respond to nonimmunologic stimuli.

Lymphocyte Motility

Lymphocytes are motile cells. T cells move relatively rapidly (about 7 to 12 μm per
minute), while B cells move more slowly (about 3 to 5 μm per minute). T cells are susceptible to chemotactic influences being attracted to B cells, activated macrophages, endotoxin-
treated serum, and plant lectins.

Lymphocyte Antigens

Since B and T cells are structurally indistinguishable, immunologists have sought to char-
acterize them by identifying characteristic antigens on their cell membranes.

Mouse-Lymphocyte Antigens

B-Cell Antigens   The major surface antigens of B cells are the immunoglobulins that
serve as antigen receptors. In addition, mouse B cells possess a variety of cell surface antigens. These include the Ia antigens and the lymphocyte antigens Lyb 1, 2, 3, 4, and 5, as
well as two plasma cell-specific antigens PC1 and PC2. Not all B cells are Lyb3$^+$ or
Lyb5$^+$. The Lyb3$^+$ cells appear to function as helper cells in some way. Lyb5$^-$ cells fail
to respond to a number of thymus independent antigens that Lyb5$^+$ cells can respond to.

T-Cell Antigens   In contrast to B cells, T cells have been shown to possess a great range of characteristic cell surface antigens, the most important of which is called Thy-1 or ⊖.

Thy-1   A 19,000-dalton glycoprotein, Thy-1 is found on the surface of brain cells (astrocytes), epidermal cells, fibroblasts, and T lymphocytes. Thy-1 is found in largest quantity on immature thymocytes, and the amount on cell surfaces declines rapidly once thymocytes leave the thymus (Fig. 10–7). It exists in two allelic forms, with genes Thy-1[a] and Thy-1[b] coding for alleles Thy-1,1 and Thy-1,2 respectively. Thy-1 is distributed evenly through the T-cell subsets.

TL   Thymocytes but not peripheral T cells or B cells possess TL antigens. These TL antigens are cell-surface proteins coded for by the Tla locus, a gene complex found on chromosome 17 of the mouse and associated with the MHC. There are five different TL specificities, TL-0, 1, 2, 3, and 5.TL-2 is present on all TL$^+$ cells. TL$^-$ mice can develop TL$^+$ leukemias, since the expression of TL is regulated, not only by regulatory genes, but probably also by the activities of the murine leukemia viruses. The structure of the TL antigens is almost identical to that of the Class I histocompatability antigens (See Chap. 3).

Qa   Qa-1 antigen is a glycoprotein with a molecular weight of 46,000. It is found on the surface of about 60% of T cells and is inherited through a genetic locus located close to H-2D. Qa-2 is found on T cells and on a proportion of IgM-positive B cells. Qa-3 is found on a subpopulation of peripheral T cells.

The TL, Qa-1, 2, and 3 antigens, as well as two minor histocompatability antigens

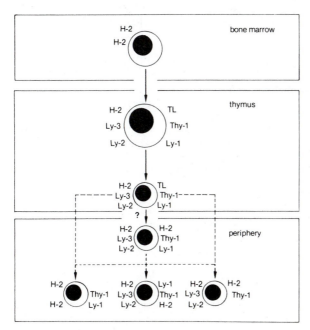

FIGURE 10–7.
Differentiation of mouse T cells with acquisition of differentiation antigens. Dotted lines indicate possible alternative routes of differentiation. TL, Ly-1, Ly-2,3, Ly-1,2,3, and Thy 1 are T-cell differentiation antigens found on the cell surface. H-2 antigens are found on cell surfaces in most tissues of the mouse. Boxes indicate distinct anatomical compartments. (Reprinted by permission from Hood, L. E., Weissman, I. L., and Wood, W. B. Immunology, Menlo Park, California, The Benjamin / Cummings Publishing Company, 1978, Fig. 1–11, p. 13.)

and an immune-response gene controlling the immune response to ferritin, together constitute the Tla gene complex (Fig. 3–5).

The Lyt Antigens While the antigens described previously either identify T cells as a whole or are associated with their degree of maturation, the Lyt antigens appear to be associated with certain functional characteristics of T cells (Table 10–4).

Lyt-1 antigen is a glycoprotein with a molecular weight of 67,000 coded for by a locus on chromosome 19. There are two alleles, Lyt-1^a and Lyt-1^b coding for antigens Lyt-1.1 and Lyt-1.2 respectively.

Lyt-2 and Lyt-3 are glycoproteins of 35,000 daltons coded for by loci on chromosome 6. They are found on two different polypeptide subunits linked by disulfide bonds and, consequently, are always paired. Each locus has two alleles, Lyt-2.1, -2.2, -3.1, and -3.2.

In the peripheral blood of mice, about 55% of the T cells are Lyt1$^+$23$^+$, about 10 percent are Lyt1$^-$23$^+$, and about 35% are Lyt1$^+$23$^-$. The Lyt1$^+$23$^-$ cells function as "helpers" in that they enhance the functional activities of other T cells, B cells, and macrophages. The Lyt1$^-$23$^+$ cells include supressor cells, which depress immune responses, and cytotoxic cells, which have the ability to lyse foreign (allogeneic) target cells. Lyt1$^+$23$^+$ are precursors of the other two subclasses and are thus relatively immature.

Ia Antigens As has been described in some detail in Chapter 3, genes located in the I region of the major histocompatibility complex (H-2) code for lymphocyte surface antigens. Genetically, these I-region genes fall into four subregions, I-A, I-C, I-E, and I-J.

Genes in the I-A subregion code for antigenic specificities Ia-1, 2, 7, 8, 9 and 15. These antigens are found on all B cells, where they are associated in some way with the Fc receptor, on macrophages, especially the dendritic and Langerhans cells, on sperm, and on certain T cells, most notably dividing T cells and those T cells that possess Fc receptors. The Ia specificities on T cells appear to be distinct from those on B cells. Less than 1% of normal T cells are Ia$^+$, but after exposure to a mitogen, such as PHA, up to 70% become Ia$^+$.

The genes of the I-J subregion code for an antigenic specificity Ia-4 found only on suppressor T cells, soluble suppressor factors, and on macrophages. I-J-positive T cells are the only T cells that can bind isolated free antigen.

The genes of the I-C subregion code for Ia-3 and Ia-6. They are found only on T cells and appear to be associated with helper activity.

TABLE 10–4 The Association of Lyt Antigens with T-Cell Function

Lyt Phenotype	Function
Lyt1	Helper cell production. Proliferation in response to antigens or mitogens. Production of helper factors.
Lyt23	Suppressor cell production. Production of suppressor factors. Cytotoxic effects.
Lyt123	Precursors of Lyt1 and Lyt23 cells. May also respond to allogeneic cells.

The I-E subregion genes code for Ia-5, 7, 22, and 23. Ia-7 is public, being found on all mice, 22 and 23 are private and are thus found only on some mice. Ia-5 is found on all B cells.

Other Lymphocyte Alloantigens in Mice   A very large number of other lymphocyte alloantigens have been identified in mice. These antigens include G1X, an antigen found on thymocytes and some mouse leukemia viruses, Leu-5, antibodies against which block E rosetting (p. 169) and Tsu and Tind, antigens on T suppressor cells, which may be associated with the T-cell antigen receptor.

Human Lymphocyte Antigens

The identification of human lymphocyte subsets has only recently been undertaken as a result of the availability of monoclonal antibodies derived from hybridomas. Their analysis does, however, remain somewhat confused as a result of conflicting terminology. One simple system uses hybridomas directed against antigens designated T-1, T-2, etc. Very early T cells have markers designated T9 and T10 (Fig. 10–8). As the cells mature, T9 is lost and the cells acquire T, 4, 6, and 8. T6 is probably the human homolog of murine TL antigens. Mature thymocytes then split into two subpopulations; one population is T $1^+3^+4^+$, which functions as a helper-cell population and accounts for 55 to 65% of peripheral blood lymphocyte. T4 is probably analogous to murine Ly1$^+$. The other population becomes T $1^+3^+8^+$. These cells are cytotoxic and immunosuppressive and account for 20 to 30% of peripheral blood cells. T8 is probably analogous to Ly23 in the mouse. The T4$^+$ cells are subdivided into Ia$^+$ cells, which seem to act as nonspecific helper cells, and the Ia$^-$ cells, which do not themselves appear to respond to antigen, yet are needed for optimal proliferation.

Human-T-Cell Antigen Receptor

The use of monoclonal antibodies has identified several surface structures on the surface of human T cells involved in antigen recognition. Like the mouse T-cell antigen receptors, they appear to consist of two units.

Antibodies to T3, T4, and T8 surface antigens block cytotoxic T-cell activities. How-

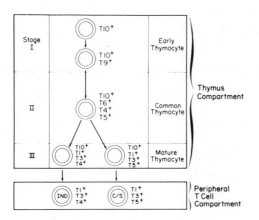

FIGURE 10–8. Stages of T-cell differentiation in human beings: Three discrete stages of thymic differentiation can be defined on the basis of reactivity with monoclonal antibodies. The most mature thymocyte population (Stage III) gives rise to the peripheral T-cell inducer (IND) and cytotoxic/suppressor (C/S) subsets. (T5 is identical to T8.) (From Reinherz, E. L., et al. Reprinted by permission of The New England Journal of Medicine, 303; 371, 1980.)

ever, anti-T3 blocks responses to all antigens, while anti-T4 blocks responses to Class II histocompatibility antigen, and anti T8 blocks responses to Class I histocompatibility antigen. Antisera to a fourth molecule, closely linked to T3 and specific for individual T-cell clones, only blocks the response of that clone.

On this basis, it is suggested that each receptor consists of two units. A complex of T3 with the clonally unique protein and either T4 or T8. The T3 complex recognizes specific antigen. The T4 or T8 component accounts for the MHC restriction of the cell (T4 recognizing Class II antigens, and T8 recognizing Class I antigens). Only when both antigens are recognized in association will a T cell respond by exercising its cytotoxic activity. $T4^+$ cells respond to soluble antigen; they respond to alloantigens, but not by producing cytotoxicity; they respond well to PHA; and they produce nonspecific helper factor (Interleukin-2, Chap. 11). $T8^+$ cells, in contrast, fail to respond to soluble antigen, produce cytotoxic cells in response to alloantigens, respond poorly to PHA, and function as suppressor cells.

In recent years, there has been a tendency to use the ratio of $T4^+$ to $T8^+$ cells as a measure of lymphocyte reactivity in clinical situations. An elevated T4 count implies increased lymphocyte reactivity while a high T8 level has an opposite effect and implies depressed lymphocyte reactivity. Although this is clearly an oversimplified analysis, it is a useful initial step in analyzing immune reactivity.

The Ontogeny of B Cells

B cells arise from pluripotent stem cells in the bone marrow, as may be shown by the fact that only bone-marrow cells can reconstitute a lethally irradiated animal. These pluripotent stem cells eventually develop to become specific B-lymphocyte precursors. These precursors can be identified, since they possess Fc receptors and contain μ heavy chains within their cytoplasm. As these cells further mature into immature B cells, they begin to synthesize light chains, and the complete molecules are transported to the cell surface. As the maturation process continues, these cells develop cell-surface IgD, and it is at this time that they develop complement receptors. It is only when they reach this stage of development that they are ready to encounter antigen and mediate an immune response.

The Ontogeny of T Cells

Mouse T cells also arise from precursors within the bone marrow, where they eventually develop into prothymocytes showing a trace of Thy-1 and TL. When these cells colonize the thymus, they immediately gain Lyt 1, 2, 3 and become sensitive to lysis by corticosteroids. The amount of Thy-1 on their surface increases greatly for a time. As maturation progresses, however, the amount of Thy-1 begins to drop, while the TL antigen disappears completely. These thymocytes, while maturing within the thymus, differentiate the same histocompatibiltiy antigens as those expressed on the thymic epithelium. Thus this differentiation does not depend upon the origin of the T cells but is entirely dependent on the nature of the epithelial cells.

When T cells leave the mouse thymus, they carry a persistent residue of Thy-1 but, as described earlier, differentiate into the major subpopulations on the basis of whether they possess Lyt 1, Lyt 2,3, or both.

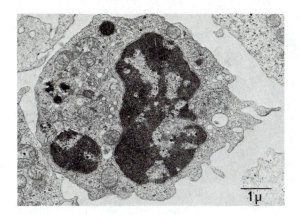

FIGURE 10–9. Morphology of the human NK cell: The nucleus is indented and rich in chromatin. Cytoplasm is abundant and characteristic osmiophilic granules, numerous mitochondria, centrioles, and Golgi apparatus are visible (original magnification ×17,000). (From Carpen O., Virtanen, I., and Saksela E. J. Immunol., *128:* 2691, 1982. With permission.)

Null Cells

When peripheral blood lymphocytes are examined for B- and T-cell markers, a small proportion fail to fall into these two categories. For example, some have T-cell surface antigens, but fail to make E rosettes. Others may be shown to possess very small quantities of cell-surface immunoglobulin if exquisitely senstive techniques are used. There are two possible reasons for this. They may either be atypical members of the two major subpopulations or they may represent a distinct third subpopulation. There is good evidence that a third population of non-T, non-B, "null" cells actually do exist. The presence of small quantities of immunoglobulin on their surface may reflect the fact that they possess Fc receptors that may bind free immunoglobulin.

The best-defined of the non T, non B (null) cells are known as **natural killer** or NK cells since they are found in unimmunized normal animals and have the ability to bind and destroy tumor cells, cells modified chemically or by viruses, and some bacteria and fungi.

NK cells are large, granular, nonadherent, nonphagocytic lymphocytes constituting about 5% of blood or splenic lymphocytes (Fig. 10–9). Because they have Fc receptors, they

TABLE 10–5   Properties of NK Cells

Surface Antigens	NK$_I$	NK$_T$	TK	NK$_M$	NC
Thy1	−	+	+	−	−
Lyt-2	−	−	+	−	−
Qa-5	+	+	−	−	−
Lyb-5	+	+	+	+	?
Regulated by interferon	+	?	−	−	?
Regulated by interleukins	−	+	+	−	?
Activity in beige mice	−	−	+	+	+
Activity in nude mice	+	+	−	−	?

Source: Minato N., et al. J. Exp Med, *154*:750–762, 1981. With permission.

NK$_I$ = classic NK cell; NK$_T$ = NK cells resembling classical cytotoxic T cells in expressing Thy-1; TK = Thy-1-positive cells resembling cytotoxic T cells; NK$_M$ = found only in bone marrow; NC = natural cytotoxic cells with specific activity against solid tumors

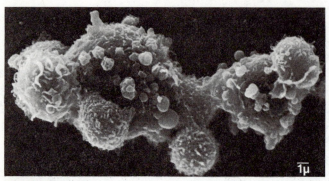

FIGURE 10-10. A cluster of NK effector cells and target cells after 4-hr incubation in the presence of IFN (1000 μ/ml). The effector cell in the middle is bound to two target cells. Bullous extrusions on the surface of the target cells indicate their impending demise. The cell on the extreme left is a monocyte. (From Carpen, O., Virtanen, I., and Saksela, E. J. Immunol., *128:* 2691, 1982. With permission.)

can bind IgG and thus function as the K cells that mediate ADCC. They show some relationship to T cells; for example, about half of the human NK cells form E rosettes, and most react with various monoclonal antibodies directed against T-cell-associated antigens. Nevertheless, NK cells also share markers with macrophages and neutrophils.

Because of this heterogeneity, it is generally believed that several distinct NK-cell populations exist (Table 10–5). These differ, not only in their serological phenotype, but also in their biological activities. Some, for example, act on lymphoma cell targets (NK cells), while others are more effective against solid-tumor targets (NC—natural cytotoxic cells) (Fig. 10–10).

The functions of NK cells are described in Chapter 19.

Sources of Additional Information

Ahmed, A., and Smith, A. H. Surface markers, antigens and receptors on murine T and B cells, parts 1 and 2. CRC Crit. Rev. Immunol. *3:* 331, 1982 and *4:* 19, 1983.

Cantor, H., and Boyse, E. A.: Functional subclasses of T lymphocytes bearing different Ly antigens. I. The generation of functionally distinct T cell subclasses in a differentiative process independent of antigen. J. Exp. Med., *141:* 1375–1399, 1975.

Cook, R. G., Rich, R. R., and Flaherty, L. The Qa-1 alloantigens. Identification and molecular weight characterization of glycoproteins controlled by the Qa-1[a] and Qa-1[b] alleles. J. Immunol., *127:* 1894–1898, 1981.

Greaves, M. F., Owen, J. J. T., and Raff, M. C. T and B lymphocytes. Origins, Properties, and Roles in Immune Response. Elsevier-North Holland, New York, 1975.

Howard, F. D., et al. A human T lymphocyte differentiation marker defined by monoclonal antibodies that block E-rosette formation. J. Immunol., *126:* 2117–2122, 1981.

Jannosy, G., and Greaves, M. F. Lymphocyte activation. I. Response of T and B lymphocytes to phytomitogens, Clin. Exp. Immunol., *9:* 483–498, 1972.

Klinman, N. R. The acquisition of B cell competence and diversity. Am. J. Pathol., *85:* 696–703, 1976.

Miller, R. G., and Phillips, R. A. Development of B lymphocytes. Fed. Proc., *34:* 145–150, 1975.

Minato, N., Reid, L., and Bloom, B. R. On the heterogeneity of natural killer cells. J. Exp. Med., *154:* 750–762, 1981.

Moller, G., ed. B cell differentiation antigens. Immunol. Rev., *69:* 5–159, 1983.

Moller, G., ed. Subpopulations of B lymphocytes. Transplant. Rev., *24:* 3–236, 1975.

Mosier, D. E., and Cohen, P. L. Ontogeny of mouse T lymphocyte function. Fed. Proc., *34:* 137–144, 1975.

Nadler, L. M., et al. Characterization of a human B cell-specific antigen (B2) distinct from B1. J. Immunol., *126:* 1941–1947, 1981.

O'Neill, G. J., anand Parrott, D. M. V. Locomotion of human lymphoid cells. I. Effect of culture and Con A and T and non-T lymphocytes. Cell. Immunol., *33:* 257–267, 1977.

Rowlands, D. T., and Daniele, R. P. Surface receptors in the immune responses. N. Engl. J. Med., *293:* 26–32, 1975.

Spurll, G. M., and Owen, F. L. A family of T-cell alloantigens linked to Igh-1. Nature, *293:* 742–745, 1981.

vanAgthoven, A., and Terhorst, C. Further biochemical characterization of the human differentiation antigen T6. J. Immunol. *128:* 426–432, 1982.

Wolters, E. A. J., and Benner, R. Different target antigens for T-cell subsets acting synergistically *in vivo*. Nature, *286:* 895–896, 1980.

11

The Response of
B Cells to Antigen

It is clear from our observations of immune responses that cells must exist that are able to recognize foreign antigenic determinants and then respond to them. It is also clear that the response of these antigen-sensitive cells must result either in the production of antibodies or in the production of cells that can participate in the cell-mediated immune responses (specific effector cells). In addition, cells must be generated that can respond even more effectively to a second exposure to the same antigen—in other words, memory cells.

The hypothesis that is generally held to account for the ability of animals to mount a specific immune response is known as the clonal selection theory. The basic postulates of the theory developed by F. M. Burnet in 1959 are as follows:

1. Lymphoid stem cells differentiate randomly to produce clones of lymphocytes, each of which is committed to respond to a single antigenic determinant.
2. Antigen binding to lymphocyte receptors triggers them to proliferate and differentiate into antibody-producing cells, effector cells, and memory cells.
3. The specificity of antibodies produced by a lymphocyte is identical to that of its antigen receptors.
4. Tolerance results when a clone of antigen-binding cells is destroyed or suppressed.

It is now recognized that antigen-sensitive cells do exist. There are two distinct populations: the B cells, which eventually give rise to antibody production; and the T cells, which give rise to cell-mediated immunity. Antigen binding to these cells induces them to proliferate and is the initiating event that triggers an immune response.

How to Demonstrate that the Binding of Antigen to Lymphocytes is Needed for an Antibody Response to Occur

This technique is based on negative selection because it relies on eliminating specific antigen-binding cells. A mouse is first primed with bovine serum albumin (BSA) and bovine gamma globulin (BGG). A lymphocyte suspension is then made from the spleen and divided in two. One half is passed through a column containing BSA chemically linked to dextran beads. The other half is passed through a column containing BGG linked to dextran beads. The two cell populations are then tested for their ability to make antibodies to bovine serum albumin or bovine gamma globulin by injecting the cell suspensions into X-irradiated mice and then testing these reconstituted mice for production of antibody after challenge with each antigen.

It is found that mice receiving cells passed through the BSA column will not make antibodies to BSA but will make them against BGG, while mice that received cells passed through the BGG column will make antibodies to BSA but not to BGG. Why? Because lymphocytes have receptors for antigen. The BSA column selectively binds and thus removes cells with receptors for BSA. The BGG column removes cells with receptors for BGG. In the absence of these cells with these receptors an immune response could not occur.

Cell Interactions

It has been pointed out previously that neonatal removal of the thymus or the bursa prevents the development of a normal immune response. Removal of the thymus prevents the development of both cell-mediated and antibody-mediated immunity, while removal of the bursa in birds blocks only the antibody-mediated responses.

Similarly, if animals, such as mice, are lethally irradiated, B (bone marrow) cells alone or T (thymus) cells alone will not reconstitute antibody formation. Cells from both populations are required and must, therefore, interact in order for an antibody response to occur (Table 11–1).

Cooperation between T and B Cells

By reconstituting lethally irradiated mice, as mentioned previously, it is possible to show that both T and B cells are needed for antibody formation to occur. It does not, however, show which cell makes the antibodies and which cell just "helps." By treating the cell suspensions with antibodies specific for histocompatibility antigens of each donor strain, it is possible to show that the helper cell possesses the histocompatibility antigens of the T-cell donor. By using specific antisera, the helper T cell in a primary immune response can be shown to be Thy-1^+, Lyt 1^+23^-.

If chromosome markers are used, it is possible to demonstrate that the bone-marrow-derived cells produce antibody.

In order for cooperation to occur, T and B cells must also have certain histocompatibility antigens in common. When this requirement is investigated, it is found that compatibility between T and B cells at the Class II loci is considerably more significant than compatibility at the Class I loci. The Class II locus is, of course, the location of the genes that control immune responsiveness—the Ir genes.

Because of this requirement for histocompatibility between cooperating T and B cells, it has been suggested that some form of like–like interaction occurs and that the role of the Class II antigens is to identify and cooperate with other identical histocompatibility antigens. Unfortunately, things are probably not quite this simple.

For example, it is possible to make chimeric mice (**chimeras** are animals possessing a mixture of cells from different individuals) by mixing together the cells of eight-cell

TABLE 11–1   Demonstration that B and T Cells Collaborate in Antibody Formation

Reconstituted with	Anti-Sheep-Cell Plaque-Forming Cells
10^7 Bone Marrow (B cells) + 10^8 sheep erythrocytes	310 ± 45
10^9 Thoracic duct (T cells) + 10^8 sheep erythrocytes	No significant response
10^7 Marrow + 10^9 Thoracic duct + 10^8 sheep erythrocytes	2103 ± 261

Source: Mitchell, G. F., and Miller, J. F. A. P., 1968. Immunological significance of the thymus and thoracic duct lymphocytes. Proc. Nat. Acad. Sci. USA, *59:* 296–303, 1968. With permission.

Mice were lethally irradiated in order to remove all their lymphocytes. They were then reconstituted by syngenic bone-marrow cells (B cells) or thoracic-duct lymphocytes (T cells) or both. The mice were then challenged with sheep erythrocytes and the response monitored using the Jerne plaque assay (see p. 194) with the following results.

It was possible to selectively kill the antibody-producing cells by anti-sera directed against the bone-marrow donor. Thus, the B cells make antibody. The T cells "help."

embryos from allogeneic mouse strains and permitting the resulting allophenic chimeras to grow in surrogate mothers. These mice actually consist of a mixture of allogeneic cells of different haplotypes. When the T and B cells of these animals were tested for cooperation they were found to interact normally in spite of their obvious histoincompatibility.

Another way of making chimeras is to reconstitute irradiated F1 (first-generation cross between inbred strains) mice with a mixture of parental B cells and F1 T cells. In these mice, antibody production is normal and cooperation can be shown to take place between T and B cells of different haplotypes. Some ideas on how this cooperation might occur are discussed in the next chapter.

Antigens and T-Cell–B-Cell Cooperation

It was pointed out in Chapter 2 that for a hapten to provoke an antibody response, it must be bound to an immunogenic carrier molecule. It was also pointed out that this carrier does not function just as a transport mechanism for the hapten, since a secondary immune response to the hapten will only occur if it is attached to the same carrier as was used for priming. The same hapten on a different carrier will only provoke another primary response. (This experiment is described in Chapter 2). If two groups of mice are primed, one with the hapten bound to a carrier (H-A) and the other with an unrelated carrier, B, then transfer of cells from both donors to a single recipient will enable the recipient to mount a secondary response to the hapten linked to carrier B (H-B). If the cells responding to this unrelated B carrier are treated with anti-Thy-1 and complement, then the secondary response to H-B is blocked. Similar treatment of cells obtained from the donor mouse responding to H-A will not block the response to H-B. Thus, the response to the carrier is mediated through the T cells. Since the antibodies are directed against the hapten, presumably they are derived from B cells.

Cooperation between Macrophages, B Cells, and T Cells

If absolutely pure suspensions of T cells and B cells are mixed together with antigen and cultured, antibodies are not produced. If, however, a crude mixed-cell suspension, such as can be derived from the spleen, is mixed with antigen and cultured, then antibody production will readily occur. The difference between these two experiments lies in the fact that the crude spleen-cell population contains macrophages, and these macrophages are needed for optimal T-cell–B-cell interaction. Macrophages can be selectively removed from a spleen-cell suspension by allowing them to bind to a glass or plastic surface. (Lymphocytes are nonadherent cells and will not be removed in this way.) When this is done, the nonadherent cells are no longer able to mediate an in vitro immune response. (Another experiment that also demonstrates the necessity of macrophages for an immune response is described on p. 206.)

When the requirement for macrophages is studied further, it can be shown that these macrophages must also be compatible with the helper T cells at the Class II locus of the major histocompatibility complex. It has been pointed out earlier that macrophages are required to process antigen in order that it may provoke an immune response. This macrophage-processed antigen is present on the macrophage surface. We may, therefore, consider that, in order for an antigen-sensitive cell to cooperate with a macrophage, it probably recognizes antigen or its fragments associated with a Class II antigen.

The continuous presence of these macrophages is required for an ongoing B-cell response.

The Mechanisms of T-Cell–B-Cell–Macrophage Cooperation

Two general theories have been developed in an attempt to account for T-cell–B-cell–macrophage cooperation. One suggests that soluble helper substances are produced by the interacting cells, the other suggests that direct cell-to-cell contact is required. It is probable that both mechanisms are involved. Clearly, the recognition of cell-membrane-bound antigens by lymphocytes will involve direct cell-to-cell contact (Fig. 11–1). On the other hand, helper effects have been observed to occur when T and B cells are separated across a cell-impermeable membrane, thus implying the existence of soluble helper substances. Several different helper substances have been identified. Some are antigen-specific and will promote only the response of B cells responding to the same antigen as the T cells. Others are non-antigen-specific and promote the responses of any B cell encountering antigen (Table 11–2).

Non-Antigen-Specific Helper Factors

Allogeneic Effect Factor

It has already been explained how compatibility at the Class II region of the MHC is needed for T-cell–B-cell cooperation to occur. However, if allogeneic T cells are given to mice while they are in the process of responding to an antigen, they will mount a much greater immune response than normal. This occurs irrespective of the antigen to which the B cells are responding and seems to be related to the occurrence of a transient graft-versus-host reaction (see Chap. 19.) This so-called allogeneic effect is very dependent upon the dose of foreign cells administered, and excess allogeneic T cells may overcome it.

It has proved possible to induce the allogeneic effect in vitro by using supernatant

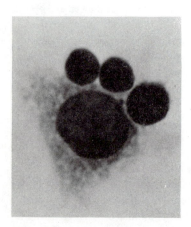

FIGURE 11–1. Lymphocytes bound to an antigen-bearing macrophage: The initial stage of the B-cell response. (From Tizard, I. Veterinary Immunology, 2nd ed. W. B. Saunders, Philadelphia, 1982. With permission.)

TABLE 11–2 Immunoregulatory Lymphokines

Non-Antigen-Specific Factors	Antigen-Specific Factors
Suppressor factors	Suppressor factors
IgE specific suppressor factors	$V_H^+Ia^+$ two-chain factors
Haplotype-specific suppressor factors	$V_H^+Ia^+$ one-chain factors
Immunoglobulin binding factors	$V_H^+Ia^-$ one-chain factors have also been reported
Others	
Helper factors	Helper factors
Interleukin 2	$V_H^+Ia^+$ two-chain factors
T-cell replacing factor	
Allogeneic effect factor	
Interleukin 1	
Immune interferon	
Factors acting on hematopoetic cells	

fluids from suspensions of allogeneic T cells. These supernatants can substitute for T cells in generating helper activity. The active factors in this supernatant fluid are called allogeneic effect factors and are not antigen-specific. They have molecular weights ranging from 30,000 to 45,000 and, while they do not contain any immunoglobulin antigenic determinants, they may contain H-2, Ia, and β-2 microglobulin determinants. They are produced by Lyt 1^+23^- T cells.

How to Show the Allogeneic Effect

In this experiment, a group of strain-13 inbred guinea pigs were primed with dinitrophenol conjugated to ovalbumin (DNP-OA). Three weeks later, when the level of anti-DNP antibodies in these guinea pigs had fallen to low levels, the guinea pigs were given an intravenous dose of strain-2 guinea-pig lymphocytes. (Guinea-pig strains 2 and 13 differ primarily at the Class II region of the guinea-pig MHC.) By six days after lymphocyte transfer (Fig. 11–2), there was a sharp rise in the level of serum anti-DNP antibodies, anti-OVA antibodies, and total gammaglobulins. This stimulation is a result of the allogeneic effect.

Katz, D. H., et al. J. Exp. Med., 133: *169–186, 1971.*

Interleukins and T-Cell-Replacing Factor

The supernatant fluid obtained when lymphocytes are cultured in the presence of antigen or mitogens, such as phytohemagglutinin and concanavalin A, contains a number of non-specific promoters of T- and B-cell activities. The factor that stimulates T cells is called interleukin 2. The factors that stimulate B cells are collectively called T cell replacing factor (TRF or B-cell growth factor.) (Table 11–3).

Interleukin 2 (IL-2) is a glycoprotein with a molecular weight of 15,000 (rat and human) or 30,000 (mouse) derived from Thy 1^+, Lyt 123^+ cells. It has the ability to bind to a receptor on T cells and enhance their response to mitogen, to enhance the generation of cytotoxic T cells, and to promote interferon production; it promotes B-cell functions by

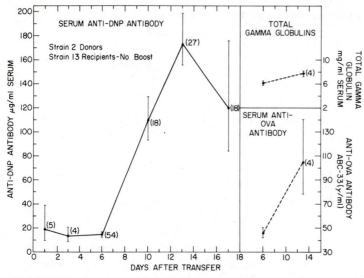

FIGURE 11-2. 2×10^8 lymphocytes from strain-2 guinea pigs were administered intravenously to strain-13 recipients three weeks after the strain-13 animals had been primed by DNP-ovalbumin (DNP-OVA). The allogeneic effect results in a sharp jump in levels of anti-DNP and anti-OVA antibodies in the serum of these animals. (From Katz, D. H., et al. J. Exp. Med., *133:* 169–186, 1971. With permission.)

enhancing helper-cell activities. TRF is a mixture of glycoproteins with molecular weights of 17,000 and 50,000. They act synergistically on B cells to promote division and immunoglobulin synthesis.

Normal serum contains an IL-2 inhibitor, a 50-Kdal protein derived from Lyt 1^-23^+ cells. This inhibitor has relatively high activity and, as a result, IL-2 will only act in close physical proximity to a T_H cell.

Interleukin 1 (IL-1) is a peptide with a molecular weight of 12,000 to 16,000 Mr derived from Ia^+ macrophages. It acts on immature T_H cells to promote their differentiation and the release of IL-2. IL-1 can replace macrophages in the in vitro immune response,

TABLE 11-3   The Properties of the Non-Antigen-Specific Helper Factors*

	Allogeneic Effect Factor (AEF)	T Cell Replacing Factor (TRF)	Interleukin 1 (IL-1)	Interleukin 2 (IL-2)
Size (daltons)	45,000	30–50,000	15,000	30,000
Source	T cells	T cells	Macrophages	T cells
Target	Resting T cells	Resting and Activated T cells	T cells	Activated T cells
Ia content	Ia^+	Ia^-	Ia^-	Ia^-

*In mice.

and it will enhance E-rosette formation by T cells. IL-1 may also modulate their expression of the IL-2 receptor. Interleukin-1 acts on the liver to stimulate the synthesis of acute-phase proteins.

It is suggested that the release of IL-1 from macrophages accounts for some of the macrophage-mediated promotion of the immune response, while the release of IL-2 by T_H cells accounts at least in part for T-helper-cell activity.

The name interleukin 3 has been given to a lymphokine produced by antigen activated Lyt 1^+23^- T_H cells, which also promotes T-cell maturation and proliferation.

Antigen-Specific Helper Factors

The factors that enhance the response of B cells to a specific antigen (the same antigen to which the T_H cell is responding) are much less well defined than the nonspecific factors. Some antigen-specific factors, but not all, have been claimed to possess both idiotypic determinants and V_H determinants. Other antigen-specific factors appear to lack any immunoglobulin determinants. Many of those described contain antigenic determinants coded for by the genes of the major histocompatibility complex. Thus, in mice, they may contain $\beta2$ microglobulin, I-J gene products, or I-A gene products. Other antigen-specific factors appear to lack MHC-coded determinants. If, however, antigen-specific helper factors do contain MHC-coded determinants, it could explain how histocompatibility-restricted cooperation could occur in the absence of direct cell–cell contact.

Thymus-Independent Antigens

Certain antigens appear to be able to provoke antibody formation in the absence of T cells. These so-called T-independent antigens are usually relatively simple repeating polymers, such as, for example, *E. coli* lipopolysaccharide, polymerized salmonella flagellin, pneumococcal capsular polysaccharide, dextrans, levans and polyglutamic acid (Table 11–4).

Characteristically, T-independent antigens only trigger IgM responses in B cells and fail to generate memory cells. It is probable that they cannot trigger the B-cell subpopulation that initiates memory-cell formation. The identification of some characteristic morphological features in the B cells that respond to these antigens tend to support this suggestion. In addition, if T-dependent and T-independent forms of the same antigen are given simultaneously, the response tends to be additive, again implying that different B-cell subpopulations are being triggered.

TABLE 11–4 Some Thymus-Independent Antigens

Polymerized flagellin
Bacterial lipopolysaccharide
Pneumococcal polysaccharide
Polyvinyl pyrollidone
Dextrans
Polyglutamic acid
Hyaluronic acid

Recent evidence has indicated that the T independence of many of these antigens is not absolute. In addition, T-independent antigens can be subdivided according to their ability to induce responses in CBA/N mice. CBA/N mice are deficient in some B cell subsets especially Lyb 5^+ cells. TI-1 antigens, such as TNP linked to lipopolysaccharide, can induce an immune response in these mice. TI-2 antigens, such as pneumococcal polysaccharide, will not. The biological significance of this phenomemon is unclear.

What Does it Take to Trigger a B Cell?

For the foregoing discussion, it appears that B cells can be triggered into responding to antigen in two distinct ways (Fig. 11–3). In the case of the T-independent antigens, it may well be that these act by cross-linking a relatively large number of B-cell surface immunoglobulin receptors. Since these antigens are repeating polymers, they possess an array of identical antigenic determinants, and the effective dose of these determinants is thus relatively large. Supporting evidence comes from the observation that haptens arranged in repeating arrays become less T-dependent. It may well be that the matrix of antigenic determinants in these molecules provides a sufficient stimulus for the proliferation of at least some B cells.

Most antigens, however, do not possess repeating arrays of antigenic determinants. As a result, B cells are presented with a much lower "dose" of any specific determinant. It is the function of the helper T cell to provide on additional stimulus in order to provoke the B cell to respond. This second stimulus probably comes from helper T cells in form of TRF.

In order to release TRF, helper T cells need to receive a stimulus from macrophages. This stimulus probably involves IL-1 since IL-1 can replace macrophages in some in vitro immune systems. From studies on the carrier effect, it is also clear that helper T cells must also recognize carrier determinants in a hapten-carrier complex.

Finally, all the interactions require that these cell populations must be compatible with respect to antigens coded by the Class II gene loci. There are a number of alternative

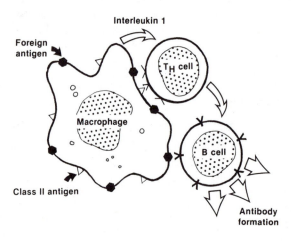

FIGURE 11–3. One possible way in which B cells respond to antigen: The antigen must be presented to a T helper cell in association with a Class II histocompatibility antigen. Under the influence of interleukin 1 from macrophages, the helper cell releases lymphokines that act on the B cells to trigger their response to antigen.

models of the interactive process that may account for all these processes. However, bearing in mind the growing number of soluble helper factors that may be either antigen-specific or non-specific, it may well be that a number of simultaneous alternative interacting networks are possible.

The Response of B Cells to Antigen

The clonal selection theory, as outlined at the beginning of this chapter, suggests that cells specific for a single antigenic determinant are generated at random. When antigen enters the body, it must be processed by macrophages and then presented to a B cell capable of responding to it specifically. It is important to get an idea of just how many B cells are available to react with a given antigenic determinant. The term clonotype is used to describe a clone of B cells capable of responding to a single antigenic determinant.

In a normal mouse, there exist at any one time about 3×10^8 B cells. In the newborn mice, there are about 10^4 different clonotypes, but their numbers increase as the mouse matures and may reach 10^8. Presumably this increase reflects increased use of alternative sets of V genes and somatic mutation. In an adult mouse, the numbers of cells within a given clonotype varies as a result of exposure to different antigens over the animal's lifetime. For some antigens, there may be as few as 10 responsive cells in the spleen or bone marrow, while, for others, there may be as many as 10^4 cells.

T and B cells must interact very closely to ensure that an antibody response occurs. Since each clonotype is present at a very low average frequency, there is clearly a very low probablility for effective contact. Indeed, as discussed in Chapter 9, T and B cells have different migration patterns and tend to segregate in different locations. It is unclear, therefore, just how these cells encounter each other. It is assumed that activated T cells circulate until they encounter the "correct" B cell. This seems to be a very inefficient process, especially in young animals in which clonotype frequency is low. As an individual ages, however, the most "used" clonotypes will expand and the process will increase in efficiency.

Each B cell carries 20,000 to 200,000 identical IgM and IgD receptor immunoglobulin molecules on its surface, whose half-life is about 24 hours. These unstimulated B cells may secrete a small quantity of 7S IgM into the medium spontaneously. When antigen binds to the immunoglobulin receptors of a B cell, the molecules, which are normally free to diffuse across the plane of the lipid membrane, aggregate in one area on the cell surface. This phenomenon is called **capping** (Fig. 11–4). Capping is not energy-dependent, but is associated with the contractile elements of the cell such as myosin. Microvilli also form on the cell surface at the site of cap formation. After capping, the B cell exhibits transient "restlessness" before the capped immune complexes are taken into the B cell through endocytosis and destroyed (although in some cases, they may be shed into the medium). After a further period, the cell receptors regenerate.

Provided a B cell, at the time it encounters antigen, receives other appropriate stimuli from helper T cells and macrophages it will commence to divide repeatedly (Fig. 11–5). Some of these progeny cells begin to develop a rough, endoplasmic reticulum (Fig. 11–6) increase their synthesis of immunoglobulin and start to secrete it. The half-life of immunoglobulins in or on the cells eventually drops from 20 to 30 hours to 2 to 4 hours.

In the unstimulated, mature B cell, the surface immunoglobulins consist of both IgM and IgD. When a B cell responds to antigen, the IgD disappears and IgM synthesis is

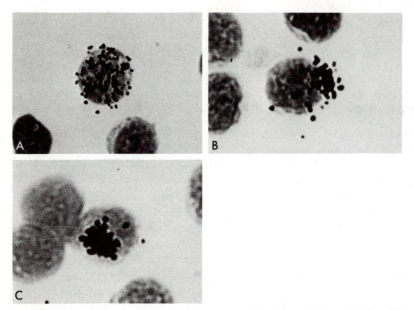

FIGURE 11–4. The capping phenomenon: Autoradiographs of lymph-node cells from an immunized mouse incubated with bound, tritiated, polymerized flagellin. **A)** Uniform distribution of antigen after incubation at 0°C for 30 minutes. **B** and **C)** Aggregation of antigen at a polar region after incubation at 37°C for 15 minutes. (A, B and C, original magnification x2400.) (From Diener, E., and Paetkau, W. H. Proc. Nat. Acad. Sci., 69: 2364, 1972. With permission. Courtesy of Dr. Diener.)

enhanced. Within a few days, however, the cell switches to synthesizing another immunoglobulin class. This switch can occur at any time during a B cell's lifespan and results in a change from IgM to IgG, IgA, or IgE production. As discussed in Chapter 8, this switch occurs as a result of deletion of unwanted heavy-chain gene segments and the joining of variable-region genes to the next available constant-region genes. The specificity of the antibody produced remains unchanged. The presence of T_H cells is probably not necessary for this switch to occur.

Plasma Cells

Plasma cells arise by differentiation from B cells responding to antigen. As a result, it is possible to identify a series of cells, intermediate in morphology between lymphocytes and plasma cells (Fig. 11–5). These so-called plasmablasts develop in secondary lymphoid tissues in the areas where T- and B-cell cooperation can occur. They are found, therefore, at the margin between the lymph-node cortex and paracortex and in the mantle zone in the spleen. Once developed, the fully mature plasma cells usually migrate away from these areas and may eventually be found distributed throughout the body. They are found in greatest numbers in the spleen, the medulla of lymph nodes, and in the bone marrow (Chap. 9).

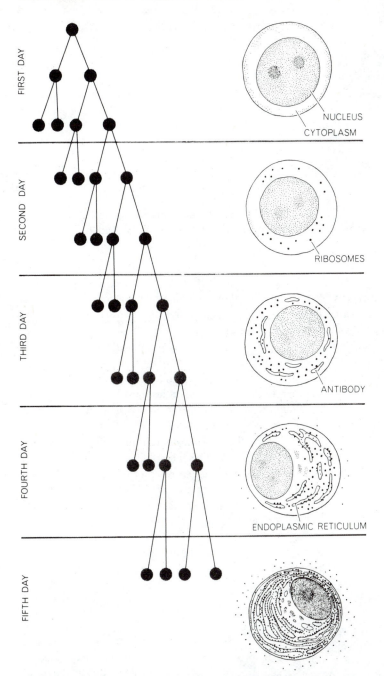

FIGURE 11–5. The progressive development of mature plasma cells after lymphocyte triggering by antigen: This process takes about five days and eight cell generations. The mature plasma cell has a small nucleus and extensive rough endoplasmic reticulum. It is almost totally devoted to immunoglobulin production. (From the complement system by G. J. V. Nossal. Copyright © 1964 by Scientific American, Inc. All rights reserved.)

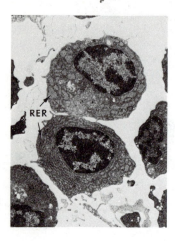

FIGURE 11–6. An electron micrograph of two plasma cells. (Courtesy of Dr. A. O. Anderson.)

Plasma cells are ovoid, 8 to 9 μm in diameter (Fig. 11–7). They possess a round, eccentrically placed nucleus with unevenly distributed chromatin. As a result, the nucleus may resemble a clockface or cartwheel (Fig. 11–8). They have an extensive cytoplasm that is very rich in rough endoplasmic reticulum. It stains strongly with basic dyes and pyronin. Plasma cells are capable of synthesizing up to 300 molecules of immunoglobulin per second. The heavy and light chains are synthesized on the polyribosomes and secreted into the intracellular pool where they combine to form complete immunoglobulins. Normally, a slight excess of light chains is produced. Because these molecules must be secreted, plasma cells possess a large, pale-staining Golgi apparatus. However on occasion, the production of immunoglobulins may be so rapid that they accumulate within cells to form vesicles known as Russell bodies. Normally, however, the immunoglobulin molecules are secreted by reversed pinocytosis soon after they are formed. The immunoglobulin produced by a plasma cell is of identical specificity to the original antigen receptor on the parent B cell. Once fully differentiated, plasma cells die in three to six days. This loss of plasma cells does not immediately result in decreased serum antibody levels since the immunoglobulins once formed decline slowly through catabolism (Fig. 11–9).

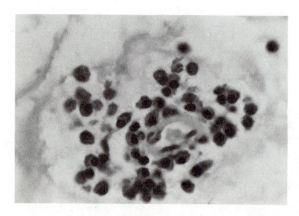

FIGURE 11–7. Plasma cells in the medulla of a lymph node. (Hematoxylin and eosin stain; original magnification x450.) (Specimen kindly provided by Dr. S. Yamashiro. Tizard, I. Veterinary Immunology, 2nd ed. W. B. Saunders, Philadelphia, 1982. With permission.)

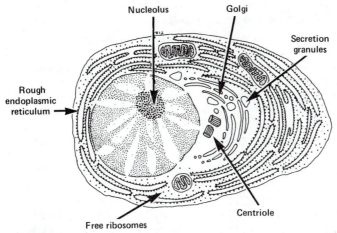

FIGURE 11-8. The major structural features of a plasma cell. (From Tizard, I. Veterinary Immunology, 2nd ed. W. B. Saunders, Philadelphia, 1982. With permission.)

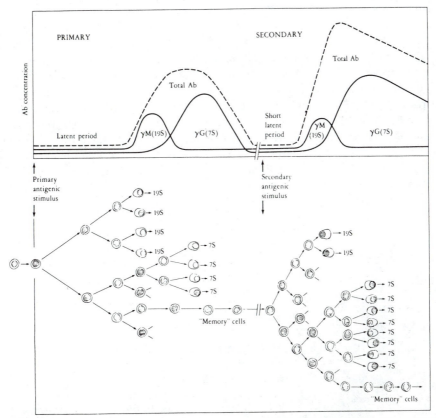

FIGURE 11-9. The response of antigen-sensitive B cells to antigen. (From Bellanti, J. A., Immunology II. W. B. Saunders, Philadelphia, 1979. With permission.)

How to Detect Individual Antibody-Forming Cells

It is now a relatively simple matter to identify individual cells producing antibody against sheep erythrocytes. The test (known as a Jerne plaque assay, after its originator) can be performed by mixing a suspension of antibody-producing cells (usually spleen cells from an inoculated animal) with sheep erythrocytes and stabilizing the mixture in an agarose gel (agarose is a purified form of agar). When the mixture is incubated at 37°C, antibodies released from the producing cells diffuse into the agarose and combine with nearby red blood cells. If hemolytic complement is incorporated in the agarose, and if the antibody being produced is IgM, then antibody-coated red blood cells will by lysed. As a result, there appears a clear zone or plaque owing to the local lysis of red blood cells around each antibody-producing cell (Fig. 11–10). These are known as plaque-forming cells (PFC). The test may be modified to detect cells producing antibodies of other immunoglobulin classes by incorporating specific antiglobulins in the agarose. Thus anti-IgA will reveal IgA-producing cells, and so on. It may also be employed to detect antibodies to soluble antigens, if these antigens are first chemically linked to the erythrocytes.

Memory Cells

Two populations of cells develop from B cells responding to antigen. The first is the plasma cell population described above. The second population consists of memory B cells. These form a reserve of antigen-sensitive cells to be called upon on subsequent exposure to an antigen. These memory cells may develop from the same B cells that give rise to plasma cells or alternatively they may develop from a special subclass of B cells. Their precise origin is unclear. Memory cells, unlike plasma cells, do not have a characteristic morphology, but resemble other small lymphocytes. Memory B cells accumulate within germinal centers. Their development requires the presence of C3, and their persistence probably requires the presence of antigen in the form of immune complexes on the surface of dendritic cells. The specificity of the memory B cells remains unchanged from that of their parent cells. Many of these memory cells or their precursors migrate from the spleen and lymph nodes to colonize the bone marrow.

If a second dose of antigen is given to a primed animal, it will be met by a large

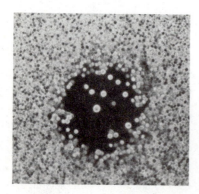

FIGURE 11–10. A zone of hemolysis surrounding a mouse spleen cell secreting antibodies against sheep erythrocytes—the Jerne plaque technique. (From Tizard, I. Veterinary Immunology, 2nd ed. W. B. Saunders, Philadelphia, 1982.)

number of memory B cells, which respond in the manner described previously for antigen-sensitive B cells. As a result, a secondary immune response is much greater than a primary immune response. The lag period is shorter since more antibody is produced and it is detected earlier. There is also a tendency for IgG to be produced in preference to the IgM so characteristic of the primary response.

Changes in Antibody Affinity

As was described in Chapter 7, as an IgG immune response progresses, there is a gradual increase in antibody affinity. This increase is probably not due to changes in individual B cells but reflects progressive somatic mutation and selection occurring within the responding B-cell population (Chap. 8).

When Things Go Wrong—Myelomas

Malignant transformation of a single B cell may give rise to the development of a clone of immunoglobulin-producing tumor cells. The morphological features of these cells may vary, but they are usually recognizable as plasma cells (Fig. 11–11). Plasma-cell tumors are known as myelomas or plasmacytomas. Because myelomas apparently arise from a single precursor cell, they produce a homogeneous immunoglobulin product known as a myeloma protein or M protein.

Terminology

Myeloma proteins are also known as *paraproteins* and their presence in serum is termed *paraproteinemia*. The term *gammopathy* or *hypergammaglobulinemia* is used to denote any condition in which a pathological increase in immunoglobulin levels occur. In general, the gammopathies are of two types. *Monoclonal gammopathies,* as are found in myelomas, are characterized by a great rise in a single molecular type of immunoglobulin (Fig. 11–12). This is readily seen as a very narrow, sharp peak on an electrophoretic scan. *Polyclonal gammopathies* are characterized by an overall rise in gamma globulin levels, which may be readily identified on electrophoresis, since there is a rise in all the proteins in the globulin region, thus producing a broad peak on the electrophoretic scan.

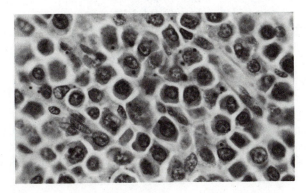

FIGURE 11–11. A photomicrograph of a section of a myeloma (original magnification x900). (From a Specimen kindly provided by Dr. R. G. Thomson. From Tizard, I. Veterinary Immunology, 2nd ed. W. B. Saunders, Philadelphia, 1982. With permission.)

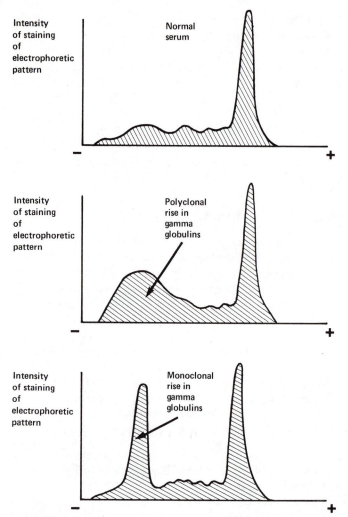

FIGURE 11–12. Serum electrophoretic patterns showing the normal pattern and the differences observed in monoclonal and polyclonal gammopathies. A monoclonal gammopathy is characteristic of serum from patients with myeloma since the tumor-derived immunoglobulin is perfectly homogeneous. (From Tizard, I. Veterinary Immunology, 2nd ed. W. B. Saunders, Philadelphia, 1982. With permission.)

Myeloma proteins may belong to any immunoglobulin class. In general, the prevalence of the various immunoglobulin classes in myeloma proteins correlates well with their relative quantities in normal serum, suggesting that the condition arises as a consequence of a random mutation of a single plasma-cell clone. Light-chain disease is a condition in which light chains alone are produced or the production of light chains is greatly in excess of the production of heavy chains. Similarly, there is a very rare variant of this condition in which fragments of heavy chains are produced. This condition is termed heavy-chain disease.

Myelomas have been reported to occur in humans, mice, dogs, cats, horses, cows, pigs, and rabbits. Because myeloma cells also break down bone, the presence of tumor masses in bone may lead to the development of multiple bone lesions that may result in pathological fractures. Light chains, being relatively small (22,000 daltons), pass through the glomerulus and are excreted in the urine. Unfortunately, these molecules appear to be toxic for renal tubular cells, and, as a result, myelomas may be associated with renal failure. These light chains may also be detected in urine by electrophoresis of concentrated urine or, in some cases, by heating the urine. Light chains may precipitate when heated to 60°C but redissolve as the temperature is raised to 80°C. Proteins possessing this curious property are known as Bence-Jones proteins (Dr. Bence-Jones first described them), and their presence in urine is suggestive of a myeloma.

Because of the overwhelming commitments of the body's immune resources to the production of neoplastic plasma cells as well as to the replacement of normal marrow tissue by tumor cells and the negative feedback induced by elevated serum immunoglobulin, individuals with myelomas are profoundly immunosuppressed. As a consequence, they commonly suffer from pyogenic bacterial infections. In humans, renal failure and overwhelming infection are the commonest causes of death in this disease.

Hybridomas

Although myeloma cells secrete vast quantities of homogenous immunoglobulin, this material is usually of unknown antigen specificity and has only been found useful by biochemists seeking to analyze the fine structure of immunoglobulin molecules. Clearly, it would be extremely useful to have available myeloma cells that would secrete an immunoglobulin product directed against a known antigenic determinant.

In 1975, George Kohler, a postdoctoral student at Cambridge University in Dr. Cesar Milstein's laboratory, was examining cell hybrids made between different lines of cultured myeloma strains by using Sendai virus to induce the cells to fuse together. (Sendai is an influenza virus that characteristically causes cell fusion). He also attempted to make the myeloma cells fuse with normal lymphocytes. However, in order to provide a "marker" for the normal cells, he first immunized the donors with sheep erythrocytes. After making the hybrids, he tested them to see if they still made antibodies to the sheep erythrocytes. To his surprise (and delight) he found that some of his hybrids were indeed making large quantities of specific antisheep erythrocyte antibodies. These hybrid cells are called **hybridomas.** Hybridoma cells can be cloned—that is, single cells can be selected and grown up. As a result, their products are derived from a single clone of cells and are thus called **monoclonal antibodies.**

The method for producing these monoclonal antibodies developed by Kohler and Milstein has since been refined and currently may be summarized thus (Fig 11-13).

Mice are first immunized with the antigen of interest and then boosted several times to ensure that they mount a good immune response. Two to four days later, the spleens of these animals are removed and broken up to form a spleen-cell suspension. These spleen cells are then mixed with cultured mouse myeloma cells that have been adapted to grow in culture. It is usual to use myeloma cell lines that do not secrete immunoglobulins, since this simplifies purification later on.

Polyethylene glycol is added to the cell mixture where it promotes cell-membrane fusion. (Polyethylene glycol is much more reliable than Sendai virus.) Only one in every

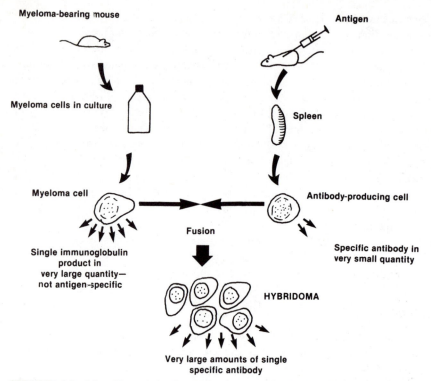

FIGURE 11–13. The production of monoclonal antibodies from hybridoma cells: Hybridomas are generated by the fusion of specific antibody-producing cells, with neoplastic myeloma cells.

200,000 spleen cells actually forms a viable hybrid with a myeloma cell. Because of this it is important to get rid of unfused normal spleen cells and unfused myeloma cells. The normal spleen cells do not survive in culture and soon dissappear. The unfused myeloma cells have to be selectively destroyed by a biochemical trick. Myeloma parent cells are selected so that they lack the enzyme hypoxanthine phosphoribosyl transferase. These cells cannot utilize hypoxanthine derived from the culture medium to manufacture purines and pyrimidines. The fused-cell mixture is, therefore, placed in a medium containing Hypoxanthine, Aminopterin, and Thymidine (HAT medium). Aminopterin is a drug that prevents myeloma cells from making their own purines and pyrimidines and, since they cannot use hypoxanthine from the culture medium either, they soon die. Hybrids between spleen cells and myeloma cells, however, contain the transferase since it is provided by the normal spleen cells. As a result, the hybridoma cells are able to use the hypoxanthine and thymidine in the culture medium and thus survive.

The hybridomas divide rapidly in the HAT medium doubling their numbers every 24 to 48 hours. On average, about 300 to 500 different hybrids can be generated from the cells of a single mouse spleen, although, of course, not all will be making antibodies of interest.

If a mixture of spleen and myeloma cells is plated on a 96-well plate with about 5

$\times~10^4$ myeloma cells per well, it is usual to obtain about one hybrid in every three wells. After growing them for two to four weeks, the growing cells can be seen on gross examination, and the supernatant fluid can be screened for specific antibody. It is important to use a good, sensitive, and specific assay at this time. Radioimmunoassays are favored, but ELISAs may also be employed.

Clones that produce the desired antibody are grown to mass culture and recloned to eliminate non-antibody-producing cells.

Unfortunately, antibody-producing clones tend to loose this ability after being cultured for several months. Thus, it is usual to make large stocks of hybridoma cells and store them frozen in small aliquots. These can be thawed as required. They may then be grown up in mass culture. Alternatively, they can be injected intraperitoneally into mice. Being tumor cells, hybridomas grow rapidly and induce the effusion of large quantities of fluid into the peritoneal cavity. This ascites fluid is rich in monoclonal antibody and can be readily harvested.

Monoclonal antibodies have been raised against a wide variety of antigens. Their greatest impact has been on the analysis of cell-membrane antigens. Mammalian cells possess hundreds of different cell-membrane antigens. By the use of conventional immunization procedures, a few of the most immunogenic cell membrane antigens have been characterized. However, the hybridoma technique enables investigators to inoculate crude antigen mixtures into mice and then select clones producing exquisitely specific antibodies, each directed against a single cell-surface antigen.

Similar techniques have enabled investigators to identify specific subcomponents in complex mixtures of lymphokines. Monoclonal antibodies to antigens on bacteria and viruses have enabled investigators not only to identify specific antigenic components, but also to subclassify groups of organisms that had hitherto been thought to be homogeneous.

Within the past few years, monoclonal antibodies have become the preferred source of antibodies for immunological research. They are very pure, absolutely specific for individual antigenic determinants and are available in unlimited amounts. Because of their uniformity, they function as standard chemical reagents. As a result, they are rapidly being incorporated in clinical diagnostic technics where large amounts of antibody of consistent quality are required. The widespread availability of monoclonal antibodies has transformed many areas of immunology and has the potential to significantly influence other related disciplines, including biochemistry, genetics, bacteriology, virology, endocrinology, and parasitology. Monoclonal antibodies provide a method for identifying characteristic tumor-cell antigens and, coupled to cytotoxic drugs, may well transform tumor therapeutic technics.

Rarely has such a "simple" and elegant technique had such a profound influence over so many areas of scientific investigation.

Sources of Additional Information

Burnet, F. M., and Fenner, F. The Production of Antibodies. MacMillan, Melbourne, London, and New York, 1949.

Chestnut, R. W., and Grey, M. M. Studies on the capacity of B cells to serve as antigen-presenting cells. J. Immunol., *126:* 1075–1079, 1981.

Feldman, M., and Basten, A. Cell interactions in the immune response: specific collaboration across a cell impermeable membrane. J. Exp. Med., *136:* 49–67, 1972.

Katz, D. M., et al. Carrier function in anti-hapten antibody responses. III Stimulation of antibody synthesis and facilitation of hapten-specific secondary antibody responses by graft-versus-host reactions. J. Exp. Med., *133:* 169–186, 1971.

Kohler, G., and Milstein, C. Continuous cultures of fused cells secreting antibody of predefined specificity. Nature, *256:* 495–497, 1975.

Mitchell, G. F., and Miller, J. F. A. P. Cell-to-cell interaction in the immune response II. The source of hemolysin-forming cells in irradiated mice given bone marrow and thymus or thoracic duct lymphocytes. J. Exp. Med., *128:* 821–837, 1968.

Mitchell, G. F., and Miller, J. F. A. P. Immunological significance of the thymus and thoracic duct lymphocytes. Proc. Natl. Acad. Sci. USA, *59:* 296–303, 1968.

Mosier, D. E. A requirement for two cell types for antibody formation *in vitro*. Science, *158:* 1573–1575, 1967.

Potash, M. J. B lymphocyte stimulation. Cell, *23:* 7–8, 1981.

Potter, M. Immunoglobulin-producing tumor and myeloma proteins of mice. Physiol. Rev., *52:* 631–719, 1972.

Robertson, M. The life of a B lymphocyte. Nature, *283:* 332–333, 1980.

Schreiner, G. F., and Unanue, E. R. Membrane and cytoplasmic changes in B lymphocytes induced by ligands—surface immunoglobulin interactions. Adv. Immunol., *24:* 38–165, 1976.

Unanue, E. R. Cooperation between mononuclear phagocytes and lymphocytes in immunity. N. Engl. J. Med., *303:* 977–985, 1980.

Waldman, T. A., and Broder, S. Polyclonal B-cell activators in the study of the regulation of immunoglobulin synthesis in the human system. Adv. Immunol., *32:* 1–63, 1982.

12

The Response of
T Cells to Antigen

In contrast to the B-cell response, T cells serve a large number of different functions that collectively result in **cell-mediated immunity** (Table 12–1). Thus, T cells are essential for protection against intracellular bacteria, against viruses and virus-infected cells, against foreign-tissue grafts and against some tumor cells. They also mediate the characteristic inflammatory response known as **delayed hypersensitivity.** In addition to these effector functions, T cells also function as regulators of the immune system. We have already discussed the requirement for T helper cells in the B-cell response. These responses are also regulated by cells known as **suppressor T cells.** Clearly, we have to establish therefore, not only how T cells respond to antigen, but also the factors that determine the specific type of T-cell response.

TABLE 12–1   The Activities of T Cells

Effector cells	Lymphokine secretors
	Cytotoxic T cells
	Delayed-hypersensitivity T cells
Regulatory cells	Helper T cells
	Suppressor T cells
Memory cells	Memory T cells

Antigens that Provoke T-Cell Responses

MHC Antigens

Since cell-mediated immune mechanisms predominate in graft rejection, in destruction of virus-infected or chemically modified cells, and in the destruction of some tumor cells, it is clear that T cells can respond well to foreign or altered tissue cells. These T-cell responses are directed against the major histocompatibility antigens expressed on the target cells (Table 12–2). Indeed, as discussed earlier, these antigens not only stimulate T-cell responses but also regulate them.

For example, if lymphocytes from two genetically dissimilar (allogeneic) individuals are mixed together in culture, the cells from each individual will respond to the presence of the foreign cells. This response is reflected by cell proliferation, and the amount of proliferation reflects the intensity of the response. By selecting cells from individuals of different haplotypes it can be readily shown that the best proliferative response is obtained when

TABLE 12–2   The MHC Determinants Recognized by T Cells

T-cell function	Syngeneic reactions	Allogeneic reactions
Help	Class II	Class II
Proliferation	Class II > Class I	Class II > Class I
Cytotoxicity	Class I	Class I > Class II
Suppression	Class I + I-J	Class I > Class II

the two cell populations differ at the Class II locus (that is the I region in mice and the DR region in man).

If the cell mixture is cultured for several days, the lymphocytes from each individual will begin to attack and destroy each other. When the amount of cytotoxicity is measured, it is found that the best results are obtained if the cell population differs, not at the Class II locus but at the Class I locus (K and D in mice, A, B, and C in man). Clearly, therefore the response of the proliferating cells is provoked by a different group of histocompatibility antigens than is the response of the cytotoxic cells.

We can go even further in defining the specificity of cytotoxic cells. Cytotoxic T cells have the ability to destroy virus-infected tissue cells. The production of these cells is clearly provoked by the exposure of T cells to virus antigen. However, most T cells, unlike B cells, are unable to bind virus antigen when it is in free solution or even when insolubilized. T cells only recognize virus antigen when it is associated with a nucleated cell membrane.

Recognition of virus antigen and the subsequent killing of virus-infected cells is regulated by the interacting cell surfaces. Thus cytotoxic T cells generated against cell-bound virus will only kill virus-infected cells if both the T cells, and their targets, are of an identical haplotype. When this restriction is analyzed, it can be shown that the cells must, in fact, be identical at the Class I locus.

The reader who has managed to follow this so far will immediately be aware of an inconsistency here. The destruction of allogeneic cells is due to a response directed against *foreign* Class I antigens. The destruction of virus-infected cells (and also, incidentally, chemically modified cells) only occurs if the Class I antigens are *not* foreign. How can these facts be reconciled? The most probable explanation is that these techniques measure the activities of two distinct cytotoxic T-cell subpopulations. Thus, in mice, those cytotoxic T cells that are restricted to attacking histocompatible targets possess a surface antigen called Qa4, while those T cells that attack allogeneic targets do not.

The importance of histocompatibility antigens in provoking a T-cell response is emphasized by the observation that up to 10 percent of the T cells in a mouse spleen will divide in response to an allogeneic cell population, but that only one in 10^4 to 10^5 cells will respond to a more conventional antigen. This responsiveness to histocompatibility antigens is determined during the maturation of T cells within the thymus. For example, if a lethally irradiated mouse is reconstituted using allogeneic fetal bone-marrow cells, the transplanted cells will mature in a foreign environment. Lethal irradiation does not kill thymic epithelial cells. As a result, some of the transplanted bone-marrow cells will mature within the thymus of the recipient animal. The T cells that eventually develop in these animals recognize the histocompatibility antigens of the recipient as self. It can be shown that the haplotype of the thymus in which T-cell maturation occurs determines which histocompatibility antigens are recognized as "self" by the maturing T cell. This is independent of the origin of the maturing T cell.

Non-MHC Antigens

By the use of appropriate adjuvants, for example Freund's complete adjuvant, it is possible to provoke a T-cell response to conventional antigens. In general, T cells appear to respond to a narrower range of these antigens than do B cells.

The experiments that demonstrated the carrier effect (see p. 18) showed that T helper cells clearly responded to a different set of antigenic determinants than those that provoked a B-cell response. When the properties of carrier determinants are studied, it is possible to show that the T cells are able to respond to denatured antigen, and it is probable that this denaturation is brought about by macrophage processing. Additional evidence for the importance of this macrophage processing comes from studies on protein antigens. Antibodies formed against protein molecules can be shown to be directed against conformational determinants (i.e., the intact molecule). On the other hand, the delayed-hypersensitivity skin response, a T-cell-mediated reaction, is directed against sequential determinants (i.e., chains of amino acids in specific order rather than of specific shape). These sequential determinants are usually generated after partial denaturation.

While T cells therefore recognize a different repertoire of antigenic determinants than B cells, they are additionally required to recognize these antigens in close association with Class II histocompatibility antigens on macrophage membranes. This association acts to regulate T-cell responsiveness.

Genetic Regulation of the T-Cell Response

In Chapter 3, guinea pigs and mice were shown to possess immune response (Ir) genes. Experiments with inbred animals showed that some strains were specifically unresponsive to certain defined antigens. This unresponsiveness was shown to be inherited and specifically associated with genes at the Class II locus within the MHC. It was also described in Chapter 3 how these Ir genes coded for Ia protein molecules expressed on the surface of some macrophages and lymphocytes.

The phenomenon of **MHC restriction** suggested that part of the explanation for the action of Ir genes could be that T cells only recognize antigen in close association with specific MHC products. For example, since only Ia$^+$ macrophages can present antigen in order to provoke a T-cell response, it is believed that T helper cells are only activated by foreign antigenic determinants associated with Ia molecules on the surface of macrophages (Table 12–3).

TABLE 12–3   Effects of Spleen Cells on C3H Strain Targets

Mouse Strain Donating Cytotoxic Cells	Haplotype	%^{51}Cr Release from C3H Targets (H-2^k)
CBA	k	65.1
Balb/c	d	17.9
C57Bl	b	22.7
CBAXC57Bl	k/b	56.1
C57BlXBalb/c	b/d	24.8

The Phenomenon of MHC Restriction

In 1974, Rolf Zinkernagel and Peter Doherty were studying the cytotoxicity of mouse spleen cells for macrophages infected with lymphocytic choriomeningitis virus. They first tested the cytotoxic effect of spleen cells from several mouse strains on C3H strain targets. C3H mice are of the H-2^k haplotype (see p. 36). Their results are summarized in Table 12–3.

From these results it was clear that maximum cytotoxicity only occurred when the cytotoxic cells and the target cells had identical haplotypes. Subsequently, the researchers confirmed that the cytotoxicity was also specific for virus-infected cells, that is, Balb/c spleen cells attacking virus-infected Balb/c targets gave 61.8 percent ^{51}Cr release while on normal Balb/c targets chromium release was only 27.6 percent.

Thus, these cytotoxic cells identify two features of their target: virus-derived antigenic determinants *and* its haplotype.

Zinkernagel, R. M. and Doherty, P. C. Restriction of in vitro *T cell-mediated cytotoxicity in lymphocytic choriomeningitis within a syngeneic or semiallogeneic system. Nature, 248: 701–702, 1974.*

Two theories have been put forward to account for the action of Ir genes. One theory suggests that the foreign antigen must bind to a specific Ia molecule. In nonresponder animals, this binding may not occur. Alternatively, it might be that T cells capable of responding to a specific antigen-Ia complex are absent from nonresponder animals. This absence of responding T cells might be due to the absence of a gene coding for the required T-cell receptor. Alternatively, it may be due to selection against responding T cells of a certain phenotype. For example, if self-reactive T cells are deleted in order to generate tolerance, then nonresponsiveness to a foreign antigen might be due to the fact that a certain antigen-Ia complex mimicked a self determinant. On the other hand, if T cells are selected for the ability to identify self-MHC, then nonresponder animals may not develop the clones of T cells capable of recognizing the antigen-Ia complex. Recent experiments have tended to favor the last possibility.

Autoreactivity in the T-Cell Response

It has been implicit in the discussions on immune responses to this point that the body does not normally mount immune responses to self. It has been pointed out many times, however, that the cell interaction involved in the immune responses usually involves the recognition of self-histocompatibility antigens. Because identity at the Class I or II loci of both responding cell populations was required for cell cooperation, it was generally assumed that some form of "like–like" interaction was required. However, several experiments suggested that this was not an absolute requirement and that, in some situations, cooperation took place between cells of different MHC haplotypes. (These are described in the previous chapter.)

An alternative explanation for the requirement for histocompatibility is that the T cell may have receptors with anti-self MHC reactivity that interacts with the MHC products on macrophages (and also, in the case of an antibody response, with MHC products on B cells). Thus, the cell interactions in the immune response may be "self–antiself" rather than "like–like." This hypothesis implies that T cells possess two sets of antigen receptors, one for conventional antigen and one for self-MHC. A T cell will be triggered to respond only if both receptors receive signals at the same time. This is probably the most favored explanation for the phenomenon of MHC restriction at the present time.

The Relationship between Ly Phenotype and MHC Restrictions

It has long been realized (see Chap. 10) that Lyt 1^+23^- cells are T_H cells, while Lyt 1^-23^+ cells are cytotoxic T cells. As pointed out earlier in this chapter, T_H cells are restricted in their activities by Class II MHC antigens, while cytotoxic T cells are restricted by Class I MHC antigens. Recently, however, this differentiation has been questioned. T_H activity has been found in some Lyt 1^-23^+ cell populations, and this is restricted by Class I antigens, while cytotoxic activity restricted by Class II antigens has been demonstrated in some Lyt 1^-23^- cell populations.

Thus, there is a clear association between MHC restriction and the Ly phenotype, but the function of the T cell probably depends on some other factor associated with antigen stimulation.

Cell Interactions in the T-Cell Response

The T-cell system, like the B-cell system is primarily regulated through cell interactions. Thus, in order for a T cell to respond optimally to antigen, it requires the assistance of helper T cells and Ia$^+$ antigen-processing cells. The level of the T-cell response is moderated by the activities of suppressor T cells.

There are several methods of demonstrating T helper-cell activity in the cell-mediated responses. For example, one type of response is known as the graft-versus-host reaction since it involves an attack on host cells by transplanted lymphocytes. If, instead of using a cell suspension from a single organ or tissue to inject into a recipient animal, cells from two sources, such as a mixture of thymus cells and peripheral blood cells are used, it can be shown that the GVH reaction is up to ten times greater than the response would be if the effect of mixing the cells were merely additive.

Another simple method of demonstrating helper-cell interactions in the T-cell system is to use cell mixtures in cytotoxic assays. Thus, if pure Lyt 1^+23^- T cells are exposed to allogeneic targets, they are not cytotoxic. If pure Lyt 1^-23^+ cells are used, they are only weakly cytotoxic. However, if a mixture of both cell types is employed, it can be shown to be potently cytotoxic. In this system, the Lyt 23^+ cells are the cytotoxic cells, while the Lyt 1^+ cells appear to act as helpers. It is probable that the helper cells release non-antigen-specific helper factors such as interleukin 2 which stimulates the cytotoxic cell population.

Although, as discussed earlier, T cells preferentially respond to foreign histocompatibility antigens, they are also well capable of responding to more conventional foreign antigens, if presented in association with Class II MHC antigens. The most effective way of accomplishing this is through the use of Ia^+ macrophages or dendritic cells (Table 12–4).

It is likely that these cells are required, not only to process and present antigen to the responding T cells, but also to serve as a source of interleukin 1 (Fig. 12–1). Unlike the B-cell response, however, in which the continuous presence of presenting cells is required, the T-cell response appears to become independent of these cells once it is initiated.

The Response of T Cells to Antigen

T cells probably only respond to antigen in association with MHC antigens. These antigens, together with the additional stimulus provided by the interleukins and other soluble

TABLE 12–4 Evidence that T-Lymphocyte Activation Requires Macrophage Presentation of Antigen

Addition to Culture	Column Purified Lymph-Node Lymphocytes*	
	Control	Antigen-pulsed
None	0.6 ± 0.1	0.8 ± 1.0
Macrophages	1.4 ± 0.3	2.4 ± 0.2
Macrophages pulsed with antigen	10.1 ± 0.1	10.8 ± 0.9

Source: Rosenthal, A. S., et al. Function of macrophages in genetic control of immune responsiveness. Fedn. Proc., *37:* 79–85, 1978. With permission of the publisher and courtesy of Dr. A. S. Rosenthal.

*Lymphocytes depleted of endogenous macrophages were pulsed with media (control) alone or with 10 µg/ml PPD for 60 min. at 37C in a humidified 95% air, 5% CO_2 incubator, washed four times and cultured with or without further addition to culture. After 4 hr, 3 µCl of [^{3}H]TdR (6.7 Ci/mMO were added for an additional 1 hr. [^{3}H] TdR incorporation, indicated as cpm $\times 10^3$, was assessed and the data of four experiments expressed as the mean cpm $\pm$ SE.

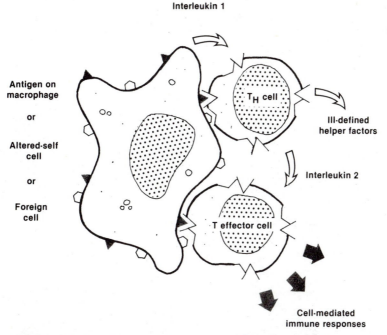

FIGURE 12–1. One possible way in which T cells respond to antigen: The antigenic stimulus is provided by cell-associated antigen from a number of alternative sources. This is recognized by T helper cells in association with either Class I or Class II histocompatibility antigens. The stimulated helper cell acts on the T effector cell population through the activities of interleukin 2 to induce the effector cell to mediate an immune response.

helper factors, stimulate the antigen-sensitive T cell to divide and differentiate (Fig. 12–2). The responding T cells eventually generate both memory-cell and effector-cell populations. The effector cells are larger than unstimulated lymphocytes, and their cytoplasm may become pyroninophilic, suggesting the ability to synthesize proteins (Fig. 12–3). It is these "lymphoblasts" that synthesize and secrete various non-antigen-specific regulatory glyco-proteins known as **lymphokines,** and generate antigen-specific, biologically active proteins called **transfer factors.** Additionally they can participate in direct cytotoxic reactions in contact with either allogeneic target cells or with virally or chemically modified syngeneic cells.

Lymphokines

Lymphokines are lymphocyte-derived, regulatory glycoproteins with molecular weights between 10,000 and 200,000. They are released mainly from activated T cells in the pres-ence of macrophages and helper cells, but B cells may produce them in response to poly-clonal stimulants, such as bacterial lipopolysaccharides or PPD tuberculin. Lymphokines possess a wide range of biological activities (Table 12–5) and at least 90 different lympho-kine-mediated activities have been recognized. Unfortunately, it is not yet clear whether

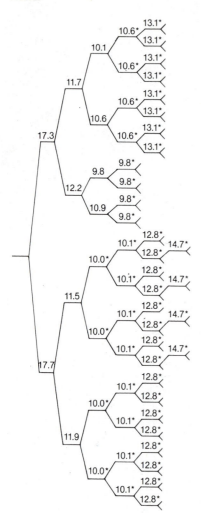

FIGURE 12-2. Reconstruction of the fate of a single lymphoblast through the 64-cell stage after exposure of tuberculin-sensitive human lymphocytes to tuberculin: Generation times shown in hours over appropriate lines; those marked with an asterisk are average times for a group of cells where it was impossible to follow the fate of a single cell but where the mitoses within the group were clearly seen. (From Marshall, W. H., Valentine, F. T., and Lawrence, H. S. J. Exp. Med., *130:* 327, 1969. With permission.)

these activities are a true reflection of their heterogeneity or, as may be more likely, of the many different methods used to assay them. In general, lymphokines are neither antigen-binding nor antigen-specific.

Lymphokines and Macrophages   The lymphokine that was discovered first and that has been most thoroughly studied acts in vitro to prevent macrophages from migrating out of capillary tubes. It is, therefore, known as macrophage migration inhibition factor (MIF). The activity of MIF can be demonstrated by packing a glass capillary tube with a suspension of macrophages and lymphocytes. (This suspension is easily obtained by washing out the peritoneal cavity of a laboratory animal with tissue-culture fluid). If the capillary tube is then placed horizontally on a flat surface immersed in tissue-culture fluid and incubated, the macrophages will migrate out to form a fan of cells on the surface (Fig. 12-4). This migration will occur if cells from an unsensitized donor are allowed to migrate in the presence of antigen. Similarly, cells from a sensitized donor migrate normally in the absence of

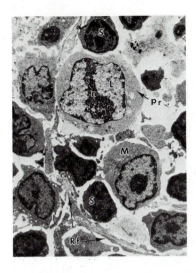

FIGURE 12-3. This electron micrograph of lymph-node paracortex includes an "immunoreactive" lymphoblast (L) containing a giant nucleolus (n) and numerous polyribosomes (Pr); abundant cytoplasm and a prominent nucleolus distinguish intermediate-sized lymphocytes (M) from small lymphocytes (S), which have little cytoplasm and a dense heterochromatic nucleus. Reticular fibrils (Rf) can also be seen. (Reprinted by permission of the publisher from Cellular Functions in Immunity and Inflammation, by J. J. Oppenheim, D. L. Rosenstreich, and M. Potter, eds. Copyright 1981 by Elsevier Science Publishing Co., Inc. Courtesy of Dr. A. O. Anderson.)

TABLE 12-5 Some of the Non-Antigen-Specific Lymphokines Produced by T Cells Following In Vitro Antigenic Stimulation

Type of Factor	Factor	Characteristic
Factors affecting macrophages	Migration inhibition factor (MIF)	Prevents migration of macrophages
	Macrophage aggregating factor (MAF)	Causes macrophages to aggregate
	Macrophage disappearing factor (MDF)	Makes peritoneal macrophages adhere to serosa
	Macrophage chemotactic factor (MCF)	Attracts macrophages
	Specific macrophage-arming factor (SMAF)	Stimulates macrophage cytotoxic activity
	Macrophage stimulating factor (MSF)	Stimulates macrophage migration
Chemotactic factors for:	Neutrophils	
	Eosinophils	
	Basophils	
Cytotoxic and growth inhibitory factors:	Lymphotoxins (LT)	Kill target cells
	Inhibitor of DNA synthesis (IDS)	Inhibits target-cell division
	Proliferation inhibiting factor (PIF)	Inhibits target-cell proliferation
	Suppressor factors	Suppress immune reactivity
Growth stimulating factors:	Mitogenic factor (MF)	Stimulates the lymphocyte division
	Lymphocyte activating factor (LAF)	Stimulates the lymphocyte response to antigen
	Interleukin 2 (IL2)	Required for T helper activity
	Helper factors	Mediate T helper activity
	Interferon (IFN)	Promotes immune reactivity

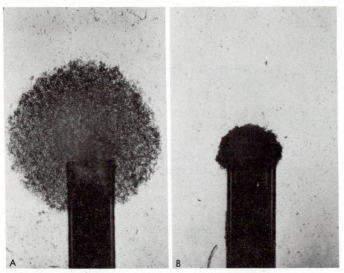

FIGURE 12-4. The macrophage migration inhibition test using bovine MIF: **A)** Normally, guinea-pig peritoneal macrophages are free to migrate from a glass capillary tube. MIF was produced by exposing peripheral blood lymphocytes from a sensitized calf to appropriate antigen. **B)** In the presence of this factor, macrophage migration is inhibited. (Courtesy of Dr. B. N. Wilkie. From Tizard, I. Veterinary Immunology, 2nd ed. W. B. Saunders, Philadelphia, 1982. With permission.)

antigen. Cells from a sensitized animal, however, do not migrate when incubated in the presence of antigen. The inhibition of macrophage migration is due to the release of MIF from Lyt 1$^+$ T cells exposed to antigen. The MIF acts by increasing the level of intracellular cyclic AMP, which in turn causes microtubule polymerization. As a result, the macrophages are prevented from migrating. In humans, mice, and guinea pigs, MIF is a mixture of glycoproteins that range in size from 35,000 to 65,000 daltons. They can be isolated and the purified material used to prevent the migration of normal macrophages in the absence of antigen. MIF may be detected in vivo in the lymph draining the sites of delayed-hypersensitivity skin reactions (a form of localized cell-mediated immune response occurring when antigen is injected intradermally into a sensitized animal). MIF is also secreted by B cells in response to antigens or to mitogens. A related but distinct lymphokine that has been described is leukocyte inhibitory factor, so-called because it prevents neutrophil migration in a manner similar to MIF.

When T cells are exposed to allogeneic cells or certain bacteria such as *Listeria monocytogenes* or *Mycobacterium tuberculosis*, they may release lymphokines that can enhance macrophage activities. The lymphokines that do this are called macrophage-activating factors and are a mixture of glycoproteins with molecular weights in the region of 30,000 Mr. Interferons are also capable of inducing macrophage activation (Chap. 13).

These macrophage-activating factors exercise many important functions. First, they enhance the cytotoxic properties of macrophages by promoting their binding to target cells and by enhancing their release of proteolytic enzymes. There is some evidence to suggest that in the initial stage of activation, the enhanced macrophage cytotoxicity is immunologically specific. As the activation proceeds, however, the enhancement becomes nonspecific.

Second, macrophages activated by lymphokines in this way show enhanced bactericidal activity. Normally, organisms such as *Listeria monocytogenes, Mycobacterium tuberculosis, Legionella pneumophilia,* and *Toxoplasma gondii* are facultative intracellular parasites (Table 12–6) and thus are able to survive and multiply within macrophages (Fig. 12–5). The reasons for this are unclear, but it appears that these organisms prevent the fusion of lysosomes with the phagosome by releasing cyclic AMP into the macrophage cytoplasm. They are thus not exposed to macrophage hydrolytic enzymes.

Activated macrophages can destroy ingested organisms by overcoming this block in phagosome–lysosome fusion (Figs. 12–6 and 12–7). These cells also show increased spreading, enhanced random locomotion, and chemotactic responsiveness. They contain elevated levels of hydrolytic enzymes and respiratory-burst metabolites and they are more avidly phagocytic than normal cells.

Activated macrophages also show enhanced secretory activity. They release large quantities of proteinases, which can act locally to activate the complement components also secreted by the macrophages. They release **monokines.** Monokines are regulatory glycoproteins derived from macrophages. They include molecules such as interferon and interleukin 1 as well as thromboplastin, prostaglandins, fibronectins, and plasminogen activator. It is also of interest to note that activated mouse macrophages generate increased quantities of Ia antigen on their surface and thus show an enhanced ability to process antigen for the immune response. This Ia antigen may be released into the surrounding fluid and be taken up by nearby T cells. Because activated macrophages show a nonspecific enhancement of their microbicidal activities, they confer enhanced resistance to bacteria in general.

Other lymphokines that modify macrophage behavior include macrophage chemotactic factors, which attract these cells to sites of antigen–T-cell interaction, macrophage stimulating factor, which promotes the random motility of macrophages, macrophage com-

TABLE 12–6   Some Facultative Intracellular Pathogens

Protozoa	*Toxoplasma gondii*
	Leishmania donovani
	Trypanosoma cruzi
Bacteria	*Mycobacterium tuberculosis*
	Legionella pneumophilia
	Brucella abortus
	Salmonella typhimurium
	Listeria monocytogenes
	Corynebacterium ovis
	Francisella tularensis
	Nocardia asteroides
Fungi	*Candida albicans*
	Histoplasma capsulatum
	Cryptococcus neoformans

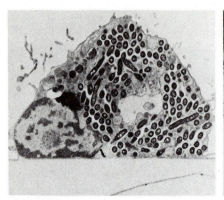
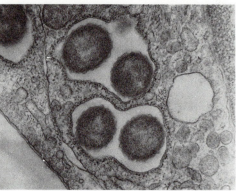

FIGURE 12–5. *Left:* An electron micrograph of a cultured monocyte heavily infected with *Legionella pneumophila* (original magnification x5,400). *Right: L. pneumophilia* in vacuoles (phagosomes?) within monocyte cytoplasm. The walls of these vacuoles are studded with ribosomelike structures whose significance is unknown. (Original magnification x32,400.) (Reproduced from *The Journal of Clinical Investigation,* 1980, Vol. *66,* p. 441, by copyright permission of The American Society for Clinical Investigations. Courtesy of Dr. M. A. Hurwitz.)

plement activator, which enhances macrophage synthesis of C2, and macrophage mitogenic factors and macrophage fusion factors. (These molecules promote giant-cell formation.)

The precise relationships between these factors is unclear and, many of these biological activities may well reside in the same molecule.

Immunoregulatory Lymphokines   Many of the proteins released by activated T cells have the ability to influence immune responses. Some, such as the allogeneic-effect factor and interleukins 2 and 3 act as antigen-non-specific helper factors; we have noted the prob-

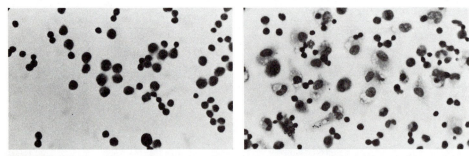

FIGURE 12–6. Giemsa-stained monolayers of mouse peritoneal macrophages grown under identical conditions: *Left:* from a normal mouse; *Right:* from a mouse infected 10 days previously with a sublethal dose of *Listeria monocytogenes.* These macrophages have been "activated" in a form of cell-mediated immune response (original magnification x450). (From Tizard, I. Veterinary Immunology, 2nd ed. W. B. Saunders, Philadelphia, 1982. With permission.)

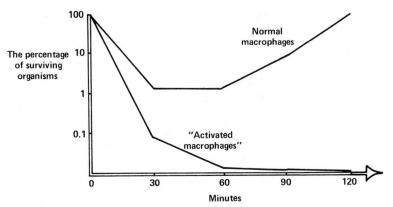

FIGURE 12-7. The destruction of *Listeria monocytogenes* when mixed with cultures of normal macrophages and "activated" macrophages from *Listeria*-infected mice. (From Tizard, I. Veterinary Immunology, 2nd ed. W. B. Saunders, Philadelphia, 1982. With permission.)

able existance of other, antigen-specific helper factors. Among the most important of the immunoregulatory lymphokines are the interferons.

Interferons

Many cells, when invaded by viruses release glycoproteins known as **interferons.** These interferons (IFN) have potent anti-viral and immunoregulatory activity (Table 12-7).

Interferons may be classified according to their origin although they all appear to have very similar biological activities. Virus-infected leukocytes produce a family of proteins, known as the α interferons, of which there are at least ten different members. These interferons are acid-stable and are only weakly species-specific. Fibroblasts, when infected

TABLE 12-7 The Effects of Interferons

Target	Effect
Virus-infected cells	Blockage of viral replication
Cytotoxic T cells	Enhancement of cytotoxicity
NK cells	Enhancement of cytotoxicity and recruitment
K cells	Enhancement of ADCC
Macrophages	Activation and promotion of phagocytosis
	Enhancement of expression of Fc receptors
Suppressor T cells	Enhancement of suppressive activity
Tumor cells	Enhancement of expression of histocompatibility antigens
	Possible protection against NK cells
T cells	Modulation of expression of Fc receptors and histocompatibility antigens. Blockage of capping
B cells	Modulation of responses to antigen and immunoglobulin production
Lymphocytes	Induction of release of ACTH and endorphins

by viruses, release up to five proteins known as the β interferons. These are also acid-stable, but are relatively species-specific. T cells, on the other hand, release a characteristic interferon called γ interferon on exposure to mitogens or to antigen in the presence of macrophages and interleukin 2. Otherwise known as immune-interferon, γ interferon is acid-labile and has a somewhat wider antiviral spectrum than either α or β interferon. It can also act on the cells of the immune system to either enhance or depress their reactivity to antigen.

If given late in the immune response, γ interferon enhances the antibody response; but, if given before antigen, it can act as an effective immunosuppressant. It acts on macrophages, K cells, and neutrophils to enhance the expression of FcγR and thus promotes ADCC. It also enhances the expression of both Class I and Class II histocompatibility antigens, β2 microglobulin, and the T-cell-differentiation antigens Lyt 1 and Lyt 23. It acts on T cells to enhance their cytotoxicity and promotes the release of interleukin 2, ACTH, and α endorphin. (Both ACTH and α endorphin are potently immunosuppressive.) It can activate macrophages and thus enhance their phagocytic activities, anti-tumor activity, and the destruction of intracellular parasites such as *Toxoplasma gondii*. γ interferon acts on NK cells, enhancing their activity by promoting the production of new NK cells. However, it also acts to block the activation of B cells and inhibits antibody synthesis and release. It also enhances the resistance of target cells to cell-mediated lysis, depresses the mixed lymphocyte reaction, graft-versus-host disease and allograft rejection (Chap. 19), and inhibits delayed hypersensitivity reactions.

Given all these alternative effects of the interferons on the immune system, it may well be that they represent the net effect of a mixture of different molecules. Interferon γ is produced largely by T cells (Lyt 23$^+$ in mice, Fcγ^+ in man), but it may also be produced by B cells. Macrophages may produce either IFN α or IFN γ, while NK cells produce IFN γ. The production of interferon by T cells also requires the presence of macrophages. It is probable, therefore, that, in the interferon system, we have an interacting network of reactions, a pattern observed in several other areas of immune regulation.

Lymphokines that Act on Other Cells   A form of inflammatory reaction induced by the inoculation of certain antigens into the skin of sensitized animals is known as **cutaneous-basophil hypersensitivity,** since the inflammatory lesion is extensively infiltrated with basophils. This reaction is caused, in some cases, by the release of a basophil-chemotactic lymphokine from sensitized T cells.

In certain systemic helminth infestations, such as trichinosis, it is probable that the massive eosinophilia so characteristic of these conditions may be mediated, at least in part, by eosinophil-mobilizing lymphokines.

T-Cell-Mediated Cytotoxicity

Some activated T cells develop the ability to bind and destroy allogeneic or altered cells. The mechanisms of this cytotoxic process are unclear, but antibodies and complement are not involved. The cytotoxic process is very rapid. Less than a minute after the T cell touches its target, the organelles and the nucleus of the target cell disrupt. The T cell may then disengage itself and move on to find another target.

This process of T-cell-mediated cytotoxicity may be divided into a number of stages.

The first stage involves direct and intimate contact between a T cell and its target. This interaction requires Mg^{2+} and can be inhibited by drugs such as colchicine implying that cellular microfilaments and microtubules are involved in the interaction. Cytotoxic T cells must recognize antigens on the target cell, although they do so fairly nonspecifically. Thus, T cells directed against one type of influenza-A virus will destroy T cells infected by any of the influenza-A viruses, even though antibodies easily discriminate between these. When two cytotoxic cells meet each other, only one is triggered. Perhaps the one with highest affinity for antigen.

The second stage in the cytotoxic process is the programming of the T cell to lyse the target. We know only that it is influenced by the level of cyclic AMP within the T cell. Thus, drugs that stimulate cAMP levels to rise tend to inhibit cytolysis.

The "lethal hit"—the name given to the mechanism whereby the T cell kills the target—may, in some cases, be due to the release of soluble cytotoxic lymphokines. Lymphotoxins, however, cannot account entirely for the cytotoxic process, since drugs, such as colchicine, which block the cytotoxic process, have no effect on lymphotoxin production. An alternative theory suggests that the cytotoxic T cells set up intracytoplasmic connections between themselves and their targets. Since the lytic event commonly takes less than a minute to occur, however, there is probably insufficient time for the connections to be established. The third hypothesis suggests that the cytotoxic T cells may possess membrane-associated lytic enzymes, such as phospholipases or proteases. Determination of which of these hypotheses is correct must await further experimentation. The process is clearly fundamentally different from lysis due to osmotic shock, such as that mediated by complement.

How to Measure Cell-Mediated Cytotoxicity

Viable cells of any sort have the ability to take up sodium chromate. If the cell dies or is disrupted in any way, however, the chromium is released into the extracellular fluid. Radioactive ^{51}Cr may be used in this way to measure cell death (Table 12–8).

　　　Thus lymphocytes from an immune animal are mixed in an appropriate ratio with ^{51}Cr-labelled target cells. The mixture is centrifuged gently to ensure that all the cells are in contact and incubated for between 4 and 24 hours. At the end of this time, the cell suspension is centrifuged and the presence of ^{51}Cr in the supernatant measured.

TABLE 12–8　Comparison of Methods of Measuring Cell-Mediated Cytotoxicity

Cytotoxic Cells	Target Cells	Test Read At	Mechanism
Normal lymphocytes	^{51}Cr-labelled allogeneic cells	24 hr	NK activity
Normal lymphocytes + specific antibody	^{51}Cr-labelled allogeneic cells	6 hr	ADCC activity
Cells from animals immunized against target cells	^{51}Cr-labelled allogeneic cells	1 hr	T-cell–mediated cytotoxicity

> The amount of chromium released is related directly to the amount of cytotoxicity occurring. However, some of the chromium taken up by cells is released spontaneously. Therefore, the chromium release in the absence of cytotoxic cells must also be measured and subtracted from that released in the presence of cytotoxic cells in order to get a true reading.

Lymphotoxins

Lymphokines with cytoxic activity have been isolated from supernatant fluids of mouse, human, and guinea-pig T-cell cultures.

In the mouse, the lymphotoxins have been shown to be a complex family of proteins (Table 12–9). Thus, there are seven different α lymphotoxins, two different β lymphotoxins, and a γ lymphotoxin. These molecules aggregate around a nontoxic core to produce a complex lymphotoxin with a molecular weight of more than 200,000 Mr. Another lymphotoxin is termed αH (alpha heavy) with a molecular weight of 140,000 to 160,000 Mr. Both complex lymphotoxin and αH bind to lymphocyte membranes in association with $F(ab')_2$-like receptors, and they are capable of activating lymphocyte phospholipases. As discussed earlier, their relationship to classic T-cell-mediated cytotoxicity is unclear.

Macrophage-Mediated Cytotoxicity

Macrophages may be spontaneously cytotoxic although this is enhanced in the presence of lectins or antibodies. Cytotoxic macrophages may be either antigen-specific or nonspecific. Macrophages activated by *Listeria* or *Toxoplasma* infections, by BCG vaccination, or by exposure to muramyl dipeptide tend to be non-antigen-specific, although they selectively lyse some tumor cells as opposed to normal cells. Similarly, normal macrophages can be rendered nonspecifically cytotoxic by exposure to supernatants from antigen-stimulated T cells. Macrophages that develop after allogeneic stimulation exert an antigen-specific cytotoxic effect. However, it is very likely that this phenomenon, when carefully analyzed, will be found to be antibody-mediated. Some of the non-specific macrophage cytotoxicity may be attributable to the release of C3b, cytotoxic peroxides, or proteases.

Transfer Factor

The classic method of demonstrating that an immune reaction is cell-mediated is to show that it can be passively transferred to nonsensitized syngeneic animals by means of a washed

TABLE 12–9 The Lymphotoxins of Mice

Name	Molecular Weight	
α–LT	70–90,000	} may be divided further
β–LT	35–50,000	} into subclasses
γ–LT	12–15,000	
$LT_{\alpha H}$	140–160,000	} blocked by specific
LT_{Cx}	> 200,000	} antiserum
	possibly a complex of α, β, & γ–LTs	

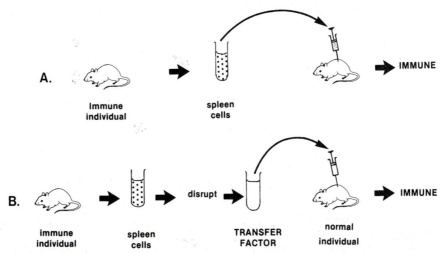

FIGURE 12–8. Cell-mediated immune responses may be transferred between normal animals by means of a suspension of spleen cells (Remember the animals must be histocompatible!). However, an extract of spleen cells may also be able to confer cell-mediated immune reactivity under some circumstances. The active factor in this cell extract is known as transfer factor or dialyzable leukocyte extract.

suspension of lymphocytes (Fig. 12–8). Although, normally, these transferred cells must be viable, it is possible under some circumstances, to transfer the response to a normal recipient using an extract of lymphocytes. The active material in the cell extract is dialyzable and is known as **transfer factor** (**dialyzable leukocyte extract** is a term preferred by many investigators). This transfer factor contains some of the biological properties of the cells from which it is derived. As a result it is capable of transferring some cell-mediated responses to normal recipients.

Some studies have shown that the transfer of cell-mediated responses by transfer factor is antigen-specific, while others have shown it to be nonspecific. These results may reflect two different components. The specific activity has generally been associated with the transfer of delayed skin hypersensitivity reactions. The nonspecific activities have included augmentation of the activities of macrophages and neutrophils, and effects on the responses of lymphocytes to antigens and mitogens.

It has been suggested that transfer factor activity may result from the transfer, in the leukocyte extract, of very small quantities of antigen together with a nonspecific stimulant. However, since the biological activity is dialyzable, it probably has a molecular weight of less than 10,000 daltons. In such a case, only a fragment of antigen could be present in the factor.

Many investigators have studied the chemical composition of transfer factor. It appears, at least in some cases, to consist of a peptide linked to a nucleotide (Fig. 12–9). It may be that the peptide contains information concerning antigen specificity. Recently, it has been shown that the antigen specificity of some transfer factor preparations may be absorbed out, using antigen bound to polystyrene, suggesting that it possesses antigen-binding specificity. Since it has also been claimed that transfer factor contains Ia antigenic deter-

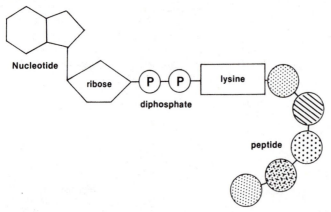

FIGURE 12-9. One of the possible structures of transfer factor: Any specific information transferred must be contained within the peptide portion of the molecule.

minants, it may be that antigen-specific transfer factor may be related to the T-cell antigen receptor or to some of the antigen-specific helper factors.

In view of the great disparity of activities ascribed to dialyzable leukocyte extracts, it is most probable that a great range of active factors are found in these extracts, some antigen-non-specific and some specific.

How to Make Transfer Factor

Before harvesting transfer factor, it is necessary to ensure that the donor exhibits delayed hypersensitivity to a specific antigen. The original experiments were conducted using tuberculin-positive individuals (Chap. 23), but volunteers specifically sensitized to other antigens have also been used.

Leukocytes (as many as possible) are obtained from the blood of the donor usually by leukapheresis (i.e., the red blood cells and plasma are returned to the donor after the leukocytes are removed). After extensive washing, the cells are frozen and thawed several times and then dialyzed. The dialyzate contains the transfer-factor activity and can be freeze-dried. One transfer-factor unit is the material obtained from 5×10^8 lymphocytes.

In order to test for activity, the transfer factor is injected into unsensitized volunteer recipients. Four to seven days later, they are skin-tested, using both the specific and unrelated antigens given by intradermal injection. A positive reaction to the specific antigen implies that cell-mediated immune activity has been transferred.

Burger, D. R. et al. Human transfer factor: structural properties suggested by HPRP chromatography and enzymic snesitivities. J. Immunol, 122: 1091–1098, 1979.

Tumors of T Cells

When lymphocytes become cancerous they can give rise to thymomas, lymphomas, or leukemias. Most lymphomas and leukemias are of B-cell origin but up to 20% of acute lymphoblastic leukemias may be due to malignant proliferation of T cells. The majority of these T-cell tumors do not secrete soluble mediators. Sometimes, however, they secrete immunosuppressive factors; these tumors, therefore, are probably composed of suppressor cells. Severe immunosuppression is a common feature of many T-cell leukemias. Infection with human T-cell leukemia virus (HTLV) may give rise to T-cell leukemia in some individuals. However, HTLV has been found in AIDS patients (Chap. 18) and may, therefore, be immunosuppressive in its own right.

T-Cell Hybridomas

By fusing specifically immune T lymphocytes with cultured thymoma cells, it has proved possible to generate T-cell hybridomas. Some of these hybridoma cell lines secrete large quantities of non-antigen specific lymphokines including interleuken 2, T-cell replacing factor, allogeneic effect factor, and macrophage activating factors. Hybridomas have also been produced that secrete antigen-specific helper or suppressor factors. These factors generally express both idiotypic and Ia-coded determinants (Table 11-2) and provide a very convenient source of material for structural and biological analysis.

Sources of Additional Information

Altman, L. C. Chemotactic Lymphokines: *In* Gallin J. I. and Quie, P. G., Eds. Leukocyte Chemotaxis—Methods, Physiology and Clinical Implications. Raven Press, New York, 1978, pp. 267–287.

Altman, A., and Katz, D. H. The biology of monoclonal lymphokines secreted by T cell lines and hybridomas. Adv. Immunol., *33:* 73–166, 1982.

Binz, H., and Wigzell, M. Shared idiotypic determinants on T and B lymphocytes reactive against the same antigenic determinants. J. Exp. Med., *142:* 197–211, 1975.

Bloom, B. R. Interferons and the immune system. Nature, *284:* 593–595, 1980.

Bloom, B. R. *In vitro* approaches to the mechanism of cell-mediated immune reactions. Adv. Immunol., *13:* 101–208, 1971.

Burger, D. R. et al. Human transfer factor: structural properties suggested by HPRP chromatography and enzymatic sensitivities. J. Immunol., *122:* 1091–1098, 1979.

Cantor, H., and Asofsky, R. Synergy among lymphoid cells mediating the graft-versus-host response III. Evidence for interaction between two types of thymus derived cells. J. Exp. Med., *135:* 764–779, 1972.

Clark, W. R., and Golstein, P., eds. Mechanisms of cell-mediated cytotoxicity. *In* Advances in Experimental Medicine and Biology, vol. 146. Plenum Press, New York, 1982.

Doherty, P. C., Blanden, R. B., and Zinkernagel, R. M. Specifity of virus-immune effector T cells for H-2K or H-2D compatible interactions; implications for H-antigen diversity. Transplant. Rev., *29:* 89–124, 1976.

Huber, B., et al. Cell-mediated immunity: delayed type hypersensitivity and cytotoxic responses are mediated by different T-cell subclasses. J. Exp. Med., *143:* 1534–1539, 1976.

Katz, D. H., and Benacerraf, B. The function and interrelationships of T-cell receptors, Ir genes, and other histocompatibility gene products. Transplant. Rev. *22:* 175–195, 1974.

Klesius, P. H., Fudenberg, H. H., and Smith, C. Comparative studies on dialyzable lymphocyte extracts containing transfer factor: a review. Comp. Immun. Microbiol. Infect. Dis., *3:* 247–260, 1980.

MacKaness, G. B. The immunological basis of acquired cellular resistance. J. Exp. Med., *120:* 105–120, 1964.

Matter, A. Microcinematographic and electron microscopic analysis of target cell lysis induced by cytotoxic T lymphocytes. Immunology, *36:* 179–180, 1979.

Matzinger, P. A one receptor view of T cell behavior. Nature, *292:* 497–501, 1981.

McCluskey, R. T., and Cohen, S. Mechanisms of Cell-Mediated Immunity (Basic and Clinical Immunology series). John Wiley and Sons, New York, 1974.

Paetkau, V. Lymphokines on the move. Nature, *294:* 689–690, 1981.

Rosenthal, A. S., and Shevach, E. M. Function of macrophages in antigen recognition by guinea pig T lymphocytes. 1. Requirement for histocompatible macrophages and lymphocytes. J. Exp. Med., *138:* 1194–1212, 1974.

Zinkernagel, R. M., and Doherty, P. C. Restriction of in vitro T cell-mediated cytotoxicity in lymphocytic choromeningitis within a syngeneic or semiallogeneic system. Nature, *248:* 701–702, 1974.

13

Regulation of the Immune Responses

The interaction between T cells, B cells, and macrophages is a complex network of cellular interactions. Students studying this area for the first time may find its complexity discouraging. It should, however, be borne in mind that all physiological processes are the subject of careful and rigorous control mechanisms. The immune system is by no means unique in its complexity, and the patterns of interaction which we are now uncovering are only a reflection of the superb sophistication of biological systems in general.

Physiological Control of Cellular Activity

The activities of all cells in the body, including those of the immune system, are regulated through a number of common mechanisms. The most important of these mechanisms modulate the intracellular ratio of two cyclic nucleotides, adenine 3'5'–cyclic monophosphate (cyclic AMP or cAMP) and guanosine 3'5'–cyclic monophosphate (cyclic GMP or cGMP) (Fig. 13–1). If the relative levels of intracellular cAMP and GMP are changed, then cellular activities are modified. As a general rule, elevated cAMP tends to depress cellular activities, while elevated cGMP enhances them. Most, if not all, of the mechanisms that regulate immune responses described later in this chapter, do so by directly or indirectly modulating the cAMP/cGMP ratio within cells.

A second physiological regulator of cellular function is the hormone insulin. Insulin has a general effect on metabolic processes, generally promoting anabolic pathways. It enhances cell-mediated cytotoxicity and concanavalin-A-induced mitogenicity. The presence of an insulin receptor on cell membranes is associated with a state of cell activation. It can thus be found on activated T and B cells.

A third group of regulators of cellular function are the prostaglandins. These are a group of related hydroxyaliphatic fatty acids with many different biological activities. Prostaglandins of the E series, for example, appear to be particularly effective in modulating T-cell-mediated immune reactivity. Thus PGE_1 inhibits the production of lymphokines, it induces nonspecific suppressor-T-cell activity, and it inhibits the response of T cells to

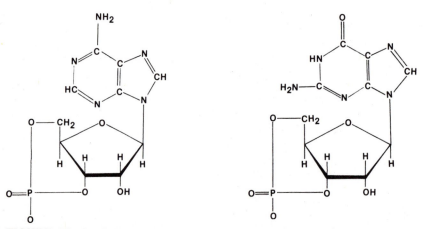

FIGURE 13–1.   The structure of the regulatory cyclic nucleotides: *Left,* cyclic adenosine monophosphate (cyclic AMP); *Right,* cyclic guanosine monophosphate (cyclic GMP).

mitogens. It may well be that the immunosuppression observed in graft-versus-host disease and in tumor-bearing animals (Chap. 19) is mediated by prostaglandins. Certainly, it is well recognized that macrophages may function as suppressor cells by releasing prostaglandins.

Significance of Regulation

The immune responses, both cell- and antibody-mediated, while essential for the protection of the body, have the potential to cause severe damage if permitted to act in an uncontrolled fashion. Thus, failure to control the specificity of immune responses may result in the production of autoantibodies and autoimmune disease. Failure to mount an adequate immune response may lead to immunodeficiency and increased susceptibility to infection. On the other hand, an excessive immune response may cause a disease such as amyloidosis (Chap. 18). Failure to control the burst of lymphocyte proliferation that occurs during immune responses may lead to the development of lymphoid neoplasia. Failure to control the immune response to the fetus may lead to abortion (Chap. 19).

It is obvious, therefore, that the immune responses must be very carefully regulated to ensure that they are appropriate with respect to both quality and quantity. As might be anticipated, a number of different control mechanisms exist in order to accomplish this regulation (Fig. 13–2).

Antigen Regulates Immune Responses

Immune responses are antigen-driven. They will commence only on exposure to antigen, and once antigen is eliminated, the responses terminate. If antigen persists, then the stimulus persists and, as a consequence, the immune response is prolonged. This type of prolonged response is observed after immunization with poorly metabolized antigens, such as the bacterial polysaccharides, or with antigen incorporated in oil or insoluble adjuvants so that it cannot be rapidly eliminated.

The quantity of antigen also influences the nature of the immune response. We have already discussed in Chapter 7 the phenomenon of affinity maturation in which high doses of antigen tend to provoke low-affinity antibody, while low doses selectively induce the formation of high-affinity antibody. Antigen-sensitive lymphocytes will only respond to an antigenic determinant if the antigen is presented to them at an appropriate time, dose and manner. If the antigen is encountered at the wrong period in a cell's development, or if the dose of antigen is either excessive or inadequate, or if the antigen is presented to the cells in an inappropriate fashion, then, instead of responding to antigen by division and differentiation, cells may become unreactive or even be eliminated, and a state of tolerance will therefore result.

Tolerance is a state in which an animal becomes specifically unresponsive to a particular antigen (Table 13–1).

Tolerance Due to Presentation of Antigen at an Inappropriate Time

The ability of the immune system to recognize foreign antigen automatically implies that it has the ability to recognize and avoid responding to self-antigens. This inability to respond to self-antigens is, of course, essential, if damage to normal tissues is to be avoided.

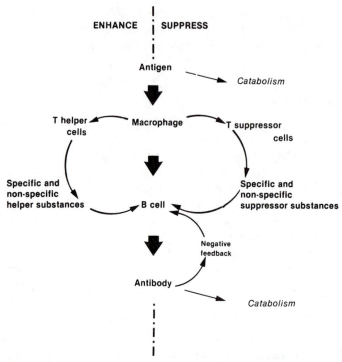

FIGURE 13-2. A schematic diagram depicting the major control mechanisms for the immune responses. (From Tizard, I. Veterinary Immunology, 2nd ed. W. B. Saunders, Philadelphia, 1982. With permission.)

Burnet and Fenner suggested in 1948 that this self-tolerance could be associated with the stage of development of antigen-sensitive cells at the time when they first encounter antigen. They proposed that antigen-sensitive cells became specifically unresponsive if exposed to antigen during fetal life, but that they eventually mature to a stage where they can respond to newly encountered antigens by mounting conventional immune responses. As evidence for this suggestion, they pointed to the existence of chimeric calves. When cattle

TABLE 13-1   A Classification of Tolerance

Induced by	Mechanism	Target
Macrophage avoidance Neonatal immunization High or low doses of antigen Soluble immune complexes	Suppressor T cells	Helper cells or B cells
High doses of antigen	Exhaustive differentiation	B cells
Passive antibody	Antibody feedback	B cells
Polymeric antigen	Receptor blockage	B cells
Neonatal immunization	Clonal abortion or deletion	T or B cells

have dizygotic (nonidentical) twin calves, the blood vessels in the two placentas commonly fuse. As a result, the blood of these calves is free to intermingle, and hematopoietic stem cells from one animal can colonize the other. When these calves are born, each is found to possess a mixture of red blood cells—some originating from the other calf. In spite of being genetically and thus antigenetically dissimilar, the foreign cells persist indefinitely. Thus, each calf may be considered to be a chimera, fully tolerant to the presence of foreign red blood cells. Burnet and Fenner suggested that this could only happen because each calf was exposed to the foreign cells early in fetal life at a time when antigen-sensitive cells become tolerant on exposure to foreign antigens. Cells from an unrelated calf would be rejected normally if administered after birth.

Medawar conducted a variation of this "natural" experiment by inoculating the cells from mice of one inbred strain (A) into the embryos of a second inbred strain (CBA). When the CBA mice grew to maturity, they were found to accept skin grafts from strain-A mice, but not from unrelated strains. This experiment also helped to support Burnet and Fenner's hypothesis.

Further evidence that prenatal exposure causes tolerance is seen in guinea pigs with a congenital deficiency of the fourth component of complement (C4). If injected with guinea pig C4, these animals make excellent anti-C4 antibodies. Thus, guinea pigs have the "ability" to make antibodies to their own C4—not, however, in the presence of natural C4.

The timing of this switch from tolerance induction to normal immune responsiveness varies between species. In laboratory rodents, it occurs soon after birth. In the other domestic mammals and man, it occurs during the first third of gestation.

The precise mechanisms involved in inducing this neonatal tolerance are unclear. On a cellular basis, it can be shown that immature B cells are rendered tolerant more easily than mature cells. Thus, a B-cell population that is at the transitional stage between pre-B and B cells can be rendered tolerant by one-millionth of the dose of antigen required to render a mature B-cell population tolerant.

The "tolerizability" of B cells appears to be inversely related to their possession of IgD. The cells of very young animals are low in IgD, and removal of IgD from a lymphocyte surface renders it readily tolerized. In addition, immature B cells may be unable to regenerate cell-surface immunoglobulins after capping, and macrophages of newborn animals present antigen very poorly to lymphocytes.

Tolerance Due to Specific Suppressor Determinants

The existence of suppressor determinants has been demonstrated on several different antigenic proteins. For example, myelin-basic protein, when injected into guinea pigs normally provokes an autoimmune disease called experimental allergic encephalomyelitis (EAE) by stimulating the production of cytotoxic T cells against myelin. This basic protein, however, can be cleaved into two distinct fragments. One fragment retains the ability to induce the encephalitis. Presumably, it is this fragment that stimulates the production of cytotoxic T cells. On the other hand, the other fragment of the molecule containing about 45 amino acids will, if given before inoculation of the basic protein, render guinea pigs insusceptible to EAE. This suppressive peptide appears to carry a determinant that provokes the development of suppressor T cells (T_S cells), which then act to block the immune response to myelin-basic protein.

Another example of a "suppressor" determinant is seen when β-galactosidase is used as an antigen. Normally, the immune response to this protein is regulated by a wave of helper-cell activity, which is then terminated by a wave of suppressor-cell activity. A peptide consisting of approximately 10 percent of the molecule has the ability to selectively promote suppressor-cell activity to such an extent that the response to β-galactosidase, or indeed to haptens conjugated to β-galactosidase, is completely abrogated.

An antigenic molecule may, therefore, carry up to three different classes of antigenic determinant: determinants that stimulate B cells and thus antibody formation (for example, most haptens), determinants that stimulate helper cells (for example, most carrier molecules), and determinants that stimulate suppressor cells. The net response to any antigen will depend upon the balance between these three groups of determinants.

Tolerance Due to Presentation of Antigen in an Inappropriate Fashion

Normally, any protein solution will contain a quantity of spontaneously aggregated molecules. These aggregated molecules are readily taken up by macrophages and are thus highly immunogenic. If a solution of an antigen, for example, bovine gamma globulin, is ultracentrifuged so that the aggregates are removed, then the aggregate-free solution will induce tolerance when injected into adult rabbits. This tolerance is specific, since it is directed only against the bovine gamma globulin. It is believed that it occurs as a result of the antigen-sensitive cells being exposed to free (nonmacrophage-bound) antigen.

Another method of inducing tolerance by inappropriate-antigen presentation is through the use of a nonimmunogenic carrier. Thus, if a normally effective hapten, such as DNP, is linked to a nonimmunogenic carrier such as a co-polymer of D-glutamic acid and D-lysine, then it will provoke tolerance. In this case, the tolerized animal will specifically fail to respond to the same hapten bound to an immunogenic carrier. Thus, the B cells must be specifically tolerant.

Tolerance Due to Inappropriate Antigen Dose

If a range of different doses of antigen ranging from very low to very high, are given to mice, it is found that very high doses of antigen induce a form of tolerance known as **immune paralysis,** and very low doses induce what is known as **low-zone tolerance** (Fig. 13–3).

Some Other Ways to Induce Tolerance

Experimentally, several other techniques have been used to induce tolerance. While they may have little physiological significance, they do point to ways in which the immune response may be effectively manipulated. One method involves giving immunosuppressive drugs simultaneously with antigen. If, for example, cyclophosphamide (a drug that destroys dividing lymphocytes) is given at the same time as sheep erythrocytes, then specific tolerance, rather than a normal immune response, will result. This is probably due to the presence of the drug at a time when the cells are dividing in response to the antigen and thus very vulnerable to destruction.

Another type of tolerance can be provoked by high doses of certain polysaccharide antigens, such as pneumococcal polysaccharides. These antigens can bind tightly to B-cell-antigen receptors and thus effectively freeze the cell membranes and block any further responses by these cells.

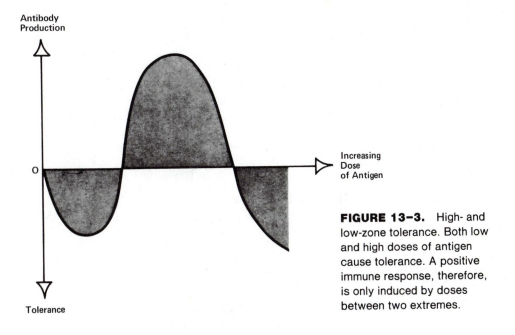

FIGURE 13–3. High- and low-zone tolerance. Both low and high doses of antigen cause tolerance. A positive immune response, therefore, is only induced by doses between two extremes.

The Mechanisms of Tolerance

Since tolerance can be induced by such a wide variety of stimuli, it is not at all surprising that several different mechanisms have been identified as causing it. There are, however, certain basic features of tolerance.

Tolerance can be shown to occur in both T- and B-cell populations by reconstituting lethally irradiated mice with T and B cells from normal and tolerant syngeneic donors. The susceptibility of these two populations to tolerance induction differs considerably. Thus, T cells are rapidly and easily tolerized by both low and high doses of antigen, and they remain in that state for a relatively long period of time (more than 100 days). In contrast, B cells develop tolerance much more slowly (about 10 days as compared with 24 hours for T cells) and return to normal within 50 days. Of course, since T cells acting as helpers are required for both cell- and antibody-mediated immune responses, an animal may remain functionally tolerant even though its B cells may have long returned to normal.

Three major groups of mechanisms have been associated with the development of tolerance. Probably of most importance are those due to suppressor cells. In low-zone tolerance, in immunological paralysis, and in tolerance induced by deaggregated antigen, suppressor cells appear to be involved, since the tolerance may be transmitted to syngeneic recipients by lymphocytes from tolerant donors. It is also highly probable that suppressor cells play a critical role in the induction and maintenance of self-tolerance. Thus, normal individuals possess cells with the ability to respond to self-antigens, but these are normally maintained in a quiescent state by suppressor cells (Chap. 21). If suppressor-cell function is depressed, as occurs in diseases such as systemic lupus erythematosus (Chap. 24), and in certain strains of mice, especially the New Zealand Black × New Zealand White hybrid, then autoimmune diseases tend to develop.

The second major mechanism of tolerance probably involves physical blockage of antigen receptors. It has already been noted, for example, how certain polysaccharide antigens can induce tolerance by irreversibly blocking B-cell-antigen receptors. High doses of antigen may also interfere with B-cell surface functions in immune paralysis.

The third major mechanism involves some form of functional elimination of B cells. The simplest hypothesis involving tolerance was put forward by Burnet when he proposed his clonal selection theory. He simply suggested that B cells were physically eliminated as a result of interaction with antigen during embryonic life. While this elimination may occur, it is almost impossible to differentiate this process from one in which the B cells are produced but are nonfunctional and thus undetectable, or from a process in which B-cell clones simply fail to develop.

Tolerance May Not Last Forever

When an animal is rendered tolerant, the duration of tolerance will depend upon the persistence of antigen and upon the ability of the bone marrow to generate fresh antigen-sensitive cells.

If the antigen is persistent (such as occurs in calf chimeras or with an animal's own tissue antigens) then tolerance will also persist. When the antigen is metabolized, the tolerance will fade. This is because, in the presence of antigen, newly formed antigen-sensitive cells will be tolerized immediately as they are produced. Treatment that promotes bone-marrow activity, such as low doses of radiation, will hasten the fading of tolerance, while immunosuppressive treatment will have the opposite effect.

In situations in which T cells but not B cells are tolerized, it is possible to stimulate antibody production by using either cross-reacting antigenic determinants or a new carrier molecule to stimulate nontolerant helper T cells. Thus, tolerance to a hapten can be broken by administering it on a carrier that is unrelated to the carrier originally used to provoke tolerance—the new carrier molecule stimulates a new and unsuppressed population of helper T cells. Similarly, one can break tolerance to an antigen by administering a cross-reactive antigen, since the determinants on the molecule will act as new carrier determinants and recruit new helper cells. Finally, it is possible to break tolerance to some self-antigens, such as thyroglobulin or myelin basic protein (Chap. 24) by administering the antigen with a potent adjuvant (such as Freund's complete adjuvant).

Regulation of Immune Responses by Antigenic Determinants

Determinants that Stimulate B Cells

The antigenic determinants that serve to trigger antibody formation are, as described earlier, located on the surface of antigenic molecules. For example, if the case of sperm-whale myoglobin, B cells recognize five prominent structures on the surface of the molecule (Fig. 2–1). We know quite a lot about the basic features of these determinants through Landsteiner's extensive studies with haptens, and Sela's with synthetic antigens (Chap. 2). Thus, the determinants must be exposed and the antibodies directed against them must conform topographically to their structure. As a result, the ability of a determinant to bind to specific B cells is critically dependent on its conformation. If a determinant is treated so that its shape is altered (even although its amino-acid sequence is unchanged), then it loses its ability to bind to specific antibody. This loss implies that B cells must recognize these determinants before the antigen is significantly modified by the activities of macrophages.

Determinants that Stimulate Helper Cells (T_H Determinants)

One simple method of characterizing T_H determinants is to attempt to make antibodies against them (i.e., determine whether they can also function as B cell-stimulating determinants), and then attempt to block the T-cell response with these antibodies.

This technique has been used to study the immune response to tetanus toxoid. Antibodies made against the pure toxoid cannot block T-cell proliferation induced by the toxoid bound to macrophages. In addition, when tetanus toxoid was denatured using urea, the denatured toxoid stimulated T-cell proliferation in the absence of macrophages. The responding T cells belonged to the same population that responded to the macrophage-processed toxoid. These results suggest that T cells respond to determinants on denatured antigen. In vivo, this denaturation probably occurs as a result of antigen processing by macrophages.

Additional evidence for the importance of macrophage processing in inducing a T-cell response comes from studies using ribonuclease as an antigen. Antibodies formed against ribonuclease are, as might be expected, directed against conformational determinants on the surface of the molecule, while the delayed-hypersensitivity skin response, a T-cell-mediated reaction (Chap. 23), is directed against sequential determinants (i.e., chains of amino acids in specific order rather than of specific shape). These sequential determinants are usually generated after partial denaturation within macrophages.

Determinants that Stimulate Suppressor Cells (T_S Determinants)

The characterization of T_S determinants is much less advanced than that of B and T_H determinants. It is clear, however, that these T_S determinants vary in their suppressive potency. For example, mice of the $H-2^b$ haplotype are unresponsive to chicken lysozyme but will respond to quail lysozyme. The difference appears to lie in a peptide on the chicken lysozyme consisting of about six amino acids. Thus lysozymes with a tyrosine at position 3 in the peptide are immunogenic for $H-2^b$ mice, while those with a phenylalanine at this position are suppressive. If this peptide is cleaved off using cyanogen bromide, then underlying T_H determinants are revealed. In the case of β-galactosidase, described earlier, there is also a single T_S determinant readily cleaved off by cyanogen bromide.

The T_S determinant on myelin basic protein described earlier does not function to suppress the response to this molecule when the complete molecule is administered. The T_S activity is only revealed if the suppressive peptide is administered before the encephalitogenic peptide and is not seen, if both are given simultaneously. In contrast, the T_S determinant on β-galactosidase does function when attached to the intact molecule, but only in the later stages of the immune response.

Since T_S cells, like B cells, have the ability to bind free antigen, it is possible that T_S determinants are conformational in nature.

Mechanisms of Action of Determinants

Several hypotheses may be put forward to account for the different properties of B, T_H, and T_S determinants. At one level, it is obvious that they must differ in some basic chemical feature. As a result, they are recognized in very different ways. In the case of B determinants, the recognition process involves direct linkage of the determinant to a B-cell immunoglobulin receptor. This does not involve histocompatibility antigens and occurs even if the stimulating determinant is attached to a suppressive carrier. As noted earlier, however, the recognition of T_H determinants is not determined by their configuration and involves the actions of Class II histocompatibility antigens.

The differences observed between T_H and T_S determinants may relate to the way in which antigen is processed. In a normal antibody response it is necessary for antigen to be processed by macrophages. These macrophages not only denature the antigen, so generating T_H determinants, but present it to the T_H cells in conjunction with the appropriate Class II histocompatibility antigens. Thus, as a result of macrophage processing, the T cells will receive a "helper" signal. On the other hand, if the antigen succeeds in reaching the T cells without having been processed by macrophages, it appears to cause the T cells to generate suppressor activity. This probably accounts for the tolerogenic effect of deaggregated gamma globulin in rabbits, and may also be demonstrated using myelin-basic protein. Myelin-basic protein produces a good immune response if presented to T cells by way of syngeneic macrophages (they must be syngeneic in order to deliver the signal from the histocompatibility antigen). However, this response can be effectively prevented if the antigen is present in soluble form at the time when the T cells meet the macrophages. What we have here, therefore, is an in vitro model of macrophage avoidance. It is probable that tolerance to many self-antigens is maintained in a similar manner.

Antibody Regulates Immune Responses

Antibodies or immune complexes generally exert a negative influence on immune responses. This influence can be shown by removing the antibody from an animal by plasmapheresis while it is mounting an immune response (plasmapheresis is a technique by which blood is removed from an animal, the cells and plasma are separated, and the cells returned to the donor). As a result, the immune response proceeds indefinitely, and the total quantity of antibody produced during the immune response is very many times greater than normal.

In general, IgG antibodies depress the production of IgM and IgG antibodies while IgM antibodies tend to depress the further synthesis of IgM. Specific antibody tends to suppress a specific immune response better than nonspecific immunoglobulin. This suppression can be very clearly seen in the method used in women to prevent hemolytic disease of the newborn. The administration of a very small quantity of anti-Rh blood-group antibody to a woman at the time of exposure to this antigen (Chap. 21) can completely prevent anti-Rh antibody formation.

Although the negative feedback exerted by specific antibody may be due to masking and destruction of antigen, this is likely to be only a minor mechanism since the inhibitory immunoglobulin molecules must have intact Fc regions. Both B cells and suppressor T cells possess Fc receptors, and it is probable that the binding of immune complexes to these receptors inhibits the antibody response. Immune complexes block B-cell differentiation into plasma cells but do not affect cell proliferation. (On the other hand, free Fc fragments can act as B-cell mitogens and promote polyclonal antibody formation. In addition, they bind to Lyt 1^+23^- cells to promote the release of a nonspecific helper factor. A tetrapeptide derived from the immunoglobulin in Fc region [tuftsin] also promotes the macrophage-mediated presentation of antigen to T cells.)

In conditions in which serum immunoglobulin levels are abnormally elevated, as in patients with myelomas (plasma cell tumors—Chap. 11), these feedback mechanisms depress normal immunoglobulin in synthesis. As a result, patients with myelomas are very susceptible to secondary infections. A similar phenomenon occurs in newborn animals that have acquired immunoglobulins passively from their mother. The presence of this maternal antibody, while conferring protection, also prevents the successful vaccination of newborn animals, since it effectively inhibits their own immunoglobulin synthesis (Fig. 13–4).

It is also of interest to note that once generated, antibody-producing cells promptly migrate from the lymph-node cortex and the lymphoid follicles of the spleen sites, where antigen-sensitive cells normally react with antigen (Chap. 9). Presumably, if this emigration did not take place, then the production of high levels of immunoglobulin in close proximity to cells responding to antigen might turn them off and thus make an immune response terminate prematurely.

The class, as well as the quantity, of immunoglobulin produced during an immune response is also effectively regulated. Most unstimulated B cells have both IgM and IgD surface immunoglobulin receptors. During the course of an immune response, these cells switch to the production of IgM, IgG, IgA, or IgE, and this switch is controlled by the activities of T cells. In animals, given T-independent antigens, there is no switch from IgM to IgG production, and a persistent low level IgM response ensues. Neonatal bursectomy may also result in a failure of the IgM-to-IgG switch, suggesting that the bursa of Fabricius is responsible for this process in birds.

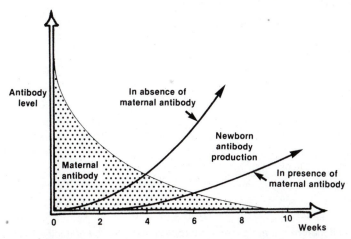

FIGURE 13–4. In the absence of maternally derived antibody, newborn animals produce their own antibody earlier than they would if the maternal antibody were present, reflecting the inhibitory effect of immunoglobulins on the antibody response.

How Antibody Controls the Immune Response

Henry and Jerne demonstrated the negative-feedback effect of antibody by giving mouse antisheep erythrocyte IgG at various times before and after an injection of sheep erythrocytes, and then measuring the antisheep erythrocyte response. It was clear from their results (Fig. 13–5) that IgG antibody given one hour before or up to four hours after injection of antigen effectively reduced the immune response. The simplest explanation for this is that the passively administered antibody prevents recognition of antigen by B cells. Gordon and Murgita conducted a similar experiment, however, in which they used not only purified immunoglobulin subclasses but also F(ab')$_2$ fragments. They found that while some subclasses, especially IgG1 were inhibitory, IgG2 in fact enhanced the antisheep cell response, while the F(ab')$_2$ fragments had no effect at all.

This finding implies that simple blocking of antigen cannot be the mechanism involved, not only because F(ab')$_2$ was without effect, but because IgG1 and 1gG2 differ only in their heavy-chain Fc region. It is this part of the immunoglobulin molecule that must exert the controlling influence.

Henry, C., and Jerne, N. K. Competition of 19S and 7S antigen receptors in the regulation of the primary immune response. J. Exp. Med., 128: 133–152, 1968.

Gordon, J., and Murgita, R. A. Suppression and augmentation of the primary in vitro immune response by different classes of antibodies. Cell. Immunol., 15: 392–402, 1975.

A Complex Interacting Network

It was originally suggested by Dr. Nils Jerne, and there is a growing body of evidence to show that the immunoglobulins generated during the course of an antibody response may themselves carry new antigenic determinants (idiotypes). Prior to immune stimulation,

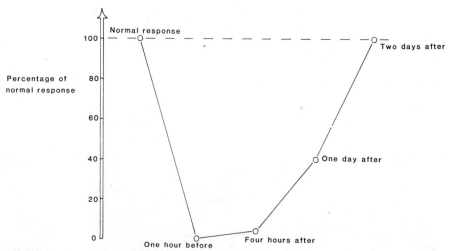

FIGURE 13–5. The inhibition of the antisheep erythrocyte response by administration of antisheep erythrocyte antibody. Each point represents the percentage of the maximum number of plaque-forming cells in the spleens from ten mice relative to the number in untreated mice (From Henry, C., and Jerne, N. K. J. Exp. Med., *128:* 133–152, 1968. With permission.)

any specific idiotype will be found only on a very small number of B cells and will probably be present in insufficient quantity to generate tolerance. During an immune response, large quantities of immunoglobulin molecules each carrying idiotypic determinants will be produced. These idiotypes, not having been recognized previously, will be perceived by antigen-sensitive cells as foreign antigenic determinants and will stimulate the production of anti-idiotype antibodies. The idiotypes on these new anti-idiotype antibodies will also be recognized as foreign and so provoke anti-anti-idiotypes! As this process continues, a complete network of interacting idiotype–anti-idiotype reactions may develop (Fig. 13–6). The significance of this lies in the fact that these reactions may modify the course of an immune response by enhancing or suppressing antibody responses. For example, anti-idiotypes may enhance lymphocyte responses by acting somewhat like antigens. That is, they bind and so trigger the antigen receptor of B cells. Anti-idiotypes can also inhibit an immune response by triggering the production of specific suppressor cells. The suppressive effect of anti-idiotype antibodies probably predominates under normal conditions and thus effectively terminates an immune response.

The reader will also recollect that the T-cell antigen receptor probably contains an idiotypic determinant on its V_H region. This suggests that T cells may also be subject to regulation by anti-idiotype antibodies and cells.

Complement Regulates the Immune System

In recent years, it has become difficult to escape the conclusion that the complement system plays a significant role in regulating the immune system. As might be expected, C3 plays a dominant role. Thus C3 appears to be necessary, at least in part, for some T-cell–B-cell cooperation, since deprivation of C3 will prevent the IgM-to-IgG switch. On the other hand, the C3a fragment is immunosuppressive, blocking T-helper-cell activity and inhibiting NK-cell activity. In contrast, C5a stimulates the immune response by enhancing interleukin 1 production by macrophages.

Immune Response Genes

The genes inherited at the Class II loci of the major histocompatibility complex regulate immune responsiveness (see Chap. 3 and Chap. 11).

Regulatory-Cell Networks

The regulatory cells of the body include populations of helper and suppressor T cells and macrophages. (Helper cells are discussed in Chapter 11.)

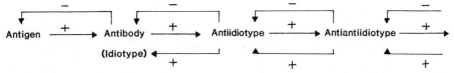

FIGURE 13–6. A schematic diagram showing an interacting idiotype–anti-idiotype network.

TABLE 13–2   Properties of Suppressor Cells

Cell Type	Antigen Specificity	Suppressor Factors	Target
Macrophages	nonspecific	prostaglandins monokines	B cells, T_H cells
T cells	nonspecific	lymphokine 40–70,000 Mr	macrophages
	specific	V_H–Ia complex 200,000 Mr	B cell, T_H cells
B cells	nonspecific	Fc γ receptors	B cells

Suppressor cells fall into three major groups: non-antigen-specific suppressor T (T_S) cells; antigen-specific T_S cells; and suppressor macrophages (Table 13-2). These cells may inhibit T-helper-cell activity, T-effector-cell activity, or even antigen-presenting-cell activity.

Non-Antigen-Specific Suppressor T Cells

There are two types of non-antigen-specific T_S cells. Following severe trauma or burns, a population of Lyt 1^-23^- suppressor cells are generated. In contrast, suppressor cells induced in mice by concavalin A are normally Lyt 1^-23^+. A simple way of generating non-specific suppressor-cell activity is to treat a mouse T-cell culture with the mitogen concanavalin A. As a result, nonspecific suppressor activity is released into the supernatant fluid. The activity is due to glycoproteins with a molecular weight range of 48,000 to 67,000. It has been argued that the nonspecificity of these supernatants is artifactual and may be the result of polyclonal production of a mixture of antigen-specific factors. However, at least some nonspecific suppressor factors act by blocking the production of interleukin 2 from helper T cells. The cell population that generates this activity is relatively radioresistant as compared with the cells that participate in antigen-specific suppression.

How to Demonstrate Non-Specific Suppressor-Cell Activity

Concanavalin A, the lectin obtained from the jackbean, can, in low doses, promote mouse helper-cell activity, but in slightly higher doses promotes suppressor-cell activity. If Con A is given intravenously to mice, these suppressor cells can be generated.

Thus, Con A was given to mice, and after 24 hours, their spleens were removed and added to in vitro antisheep erythrocyte systems. Five days later, the primary PFC was assayed. The results are seen in Figure 13-7. High doses of cells from the Con-A-treated mice were potently suppressive. It should be noted, however, that low doses of cells or cells from mice that had received a low dose of Con A were somewhat immunoenhancing.

Rich, R. R., and Pierce, C. W., Biological expressions of lymphocyte activation I. Effects of phytomitogens on antibody synthesis in vitro. J. Exp. Med. 137: 205–223, 1973.

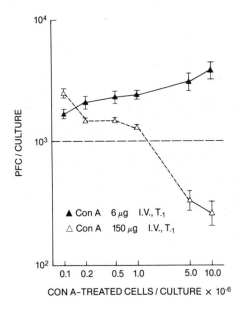

FIGURE 13–7. The suppression or enhancement of the five-day primary IgM plaque-forming-cell (PFC) response to sheep erythrocytes by addition of graded numbers of spleen cells from normal or concanavalin-A-treated mice. The Con A in high doses promotes nonspecific suppressor-cell activity. (From Rich, R. R., and Pierce, C. W. J. Exp. Med., *137*:205, 1973. With permission.)

In the figure: PFC / CULTURE (y-axis), CON A-TREATED CELLS / CULTURE × 10^{-6} (x-axis), ▲ Con A 6 μg I.V., T_{-1}; △ Con A 150 μg I.V., T_{-1}

Antigen-Specific T_S Cells

Antigen-specific T_S cells are radiosensitive cells with the phenotype Lyt 1^-23^+, I-J$^+$ FcγR$^+$. They are unique among the T cells in that they can recognize antigen unassociated with major histocompatibility antigens. Nevertheless, their production is enhanced by Lyt 1^+ helper cells and inhibited by other T_S cells.

Antigen-Specific Suppressor Factors

It is generally agreed that any antigen-specific suppressor molecule must have two distinct regions: one portion that is capable of binding and thus recognizing antigen, and one portion that exerts the suppressive activity.

Most studies have, indeed, shown that lymphocyte-derived suppressive molecules consist of two polypeptide chains. One chain binds antigen but is not suppressive, while the other chain is potently immunosuppressive but is not antigen-specific. Both chains may be synthesized by a single cell type but secreted in an associated form. Alternatively, they may be synthesized and secreted by distinct cell populations and subsequently associate to form antigen-specific suppressor factors.

The antigen-specific portion of the molecule has a molecular weight of 24,000, its activity is blocked by anti-idiotype serum, and it is coded for by a gene located close to the Igh allotype gene cluster on chromosome 12 of mice. It may, therefore, be an isolated V_H region, although most investigators have been unable to show that it possesses other immunoglobulin antigenic determinants.

The suppressor portion of the molecule has a molecular weight of about 45,000, binds antibodies to I-J-coded determinants, and is coded for by a gene located within the H-2 complex on chromosome 17. It is probably an isolated I-J-coded molecule. Its activity is genetically restricted, since it will only suppress I-J-compatible T_H target cells.

It is of interest to note the similarities in apparent structure between the T-cell antigen receptor (V_H associated with Ia), the antigen-specific helper factor (V_H attached to Ia) (Chap. 12), and the antigen-specific suppressor factor (V_H attached to I-J).

Macrophage-Mediated Suppression

The glycoproteins released by concanavalin-A treatment of thymic cell cultures also act on macrophages. They appear to act in two ways. First, they provoke the macrophages to release prostaglandins, which, as has been discussed earlier, cause a rise in lymphocyte cAMP and hence inhibition of blastogenesis.

The second suppressive mechanism involves the release of peroxides by the macrophages. These peroxides then act on a lymphocyte-derived nonspecific suppressive factor to enhance its activity.

Immunological Agnosis

Under some circumstances, T_S cells may act on antigen-presenting macrophages to prevent actual recognition of antigen. In these cases, the T_S cells and their targets must also be syngeneic at the Class I region. The mechanism of action of these is unclear, but it is postulated that these suppressor cells block a metabolic pathway within the antigen-presenting cells.

When Do Suppressor Cells Work?

Suppressor-cell activities have been described as involving almost all aspects of immune reactivity. Non-antigen-specific T_S cells are responsible for antigenic competition, lack of immune responses in the newborn, immunosuppression following trauma, burns, or surgery, prevention of autoimmunity, some cases of hypogammaglobulinemia, and blocking of responses to mitogens. Antigen-specific suppressor cells are responsible for tolerance provoked by low doses of antigen and by nonaggregated antigen. They have been found to be responsible for immunological unresponsiveness mediated by some Ir genes. These specific cells are found in some tumor-bearing animals where they block tumor rejection, and in pregnant animals where they block rejection of the fetus. They also occur in individuals unresponsive (anergic) to tuberculosis infection.

Since T_S cells are themselves regulated by the interactions of other T_H and T_S cells, and since T cells bear idiotypes as part of their antigen receptors, a regulatory T-cell idiotype–anti-idiotype network exists as a functional counterpart to the antibody network. For example, there appears to be a suppressor-cell cascade, in which one suppressor cell releases suppressor factors that act on other cell populations, that in turn suppress a third suppressor-cell population. Each of the suppressor factors released by these subpopulations has either idiotype or antiidiotypic specificity, and different suppressor-cell stimuli can stimulate the chain at different levels. Each suppressor-cell population can act at different points in the immune response. The complexity of the system is further compounded by an interlocking series of positive and negative feedback loops that ensure that the system functions only at its appropriate level.

Some Other Immunoregulatory Factors

In recent years, it has been shown that many normal body components may have the ability to regulate immune reactivity. In some cases, subsequent investigation has shown that this regulation is due to an ability to influence suppressor-cell populations. For example, α-fetoprotein, a protein that is synthesized in large amounts by the fetal liver, is potently immunosuppressive for T cells and probably contributes to the immunological acceptance of the fetus by the mother. α-Fetoprotein is a stimulator of suppressor-cell activity and preferentially inhibits responses to Class II MHC antigens.

Another immunoregulatory factor is C-reactive protein. C-reactive protein is an acute-phase protein of 135,000–140,000 daltons that is found at very low levels in normal serum. Its level increases rapidly within hours after infection, inflammation, or tissue damage. In addition to being immunosuppressive, CRP can promote phagocytosis, inhibit platelet aggregation, and activate complement. Its function is unknown, but it has been suggested that CRP may prevent the development of autoimmunity to intracellular antigens released from damaged tissue. C-reactive protein is closely related to the immunoglobulin molecules (Chap. 6).

Histamine, the vasoactive amine released from mast cells and basophils, has the ability to bind to T cells through specific receptors. There are two types of histamine receptor: H2 receptors, which predominate on T cells, and H1 receptors, found in blood vessels and on smooth muscle. Binding of histamine to the H2 receptors on T cells raises intracellular cyclic AMP levels. As a result, it blocks T-cell-mediated cytotoxicity, E-rosetting (Chap. 10), and lymphocyte blastogenesis and stimulates the T cells to release suppressor factors (Table 13–3). Histamine binding to H1 receptors stimulates contrasuppressor cell function (i.e., suppressors of suppressors)! Histamine also influences a number of other immunological activities. Thus, it inhibits the production of complement components from macrophages; it reduces eosinophil mobility but it enhances neutrophil mobility. Soluble Fcγ receptors released from lymphocytes may act as non-antigen-specific suppressor factors by adsorbing to FcR$^-$cells and binding IgG.

It should be clear to the reader who has managed to survive this far that many interacting control systems act to regulate immune reactivity. Consideration of this suggests that

TABLE 13–3   The Role of Histamine Receptors on Lymphocytes in Influencing Immune Reactivity

	H-1 Receptors	H-2 Receptors
Location	Unclear	On T_S cells
Effect of stimulation	Probably depresses cyclic AMP	Elevate cyclic AMP levels
Result	Enhance lymphocyte mitogenicity	Suppress lymphocyte mitogenicity
		Inhibit E rosette formation
		Promote release of a suppressor factor that suppresses MIF production
		Block T-cell-mediated cytotoxicity

this is an inevitable feature, not only of the immune system, but probably of all body systems. The immune system is almost certainly not unique in this respect. It happens to be the first of the body systems to be analyzed in detail. It may safely be predicted that other body systems that involve cell interaction will be found to be equally complex.

Sources of Additional Information

Auerbach, R., and Clark, S. Immunological tolerance: Transmission from mother to offspring. Science, *189:* 811–812, 1975.

Calderon, J., et al. The modulation of lymphocyte function by molecules secreted by macrophages. J. Exp. Med., *142:* 151–164, 1975.

Cantor, H., et al. Immunoregulatory circuits among T-cell sets: identification of a subpopulation of T-helper cells inducing feedback inhibition. J. Exp. Med., *148:* 871–877, 1978.

David, C. S. Role of Ia antigens in the immune response. Transplant. Proc., *11:* 677–682, 1979.

Dresser, D. W., and Mitchison, N. A. The mechanisms of immunological paralysis. Adv. Immunol., *8:* 129–181, 1968.

Geha, R. S. Regulation of the immune response by idiotypic-antiidiotypic interactions. N. Engl. J. Med., *305:* 25–28, 1981.

Gershon, R. K. A disquisition on suppressor T cells. Transplant. Rev. *26:*170–185, 1975.

Gordon, J., and Murgita, R.A. Supression and augmentation of the primary *in vitro* immune response by different classses of antibodies. Cell. Immunol., *15:*392–402, 1975.

Henry, C., and Jerne, N. K. Competition of 19S and 7S antigen receptors in the regulation of the primary immune response. J. Exp. Med., *128:* 133–152, 1968.

Jerne, N. K. Towards a network theory of the immune system. Ann. Immunol. (Paris), *125C:* 373–389, 1974.

Miller, J. F. A. P. T-cell regulation of immune responsiveness. Ann. NY Acad. Sci., *249:* 9–26, 1975.

Raff, M. Immunological networks. Nature, *265:* 205–207, 1977.

Rich, R. R., and Pierce, C. W. Biological expressions of lymphocyte activation. I Effects of phytomitogens on antibody synthesis *in vitro.* J. Exp. Med., *137:* 205–223, 1973.

Rosenthal, A. S. Determinant selection and macrophage function in genetic control of the immune response. Immunol. Rev., *40:* 126–152, 1978.

Rosenthal, A. S. Regulation of the immune response—role of the macrophage. N. Engl. J. Med., *303:* 1153–1156, 1980.

Taniguchi, M., Takai, I., and Tada, T. Functional and molecular organization of an antigen specific suppressor factor from a T-cell hybridoma. Nature, *283:* 227–228, 1980.

Unanue, E. R., et al. Regulation of immunity and inflammation by mediation from macrophages. Am. J. Pathol. *85:* 465–478, 1976.

Weigle, W. A. Immunological unresponsiveness. Adv. Immunol., *16:* 61–122, 1973.

14

The Complement System

Antigen–Antibody Interaction as an Initiating Event in Physiological Processes

The properties of antibody molecules complexed with antigen are very different from those of free antibody (Fig. 14–1). For example, antigen-bound antibody acquires the ability to bind to phagocytic cells and thus functions as an opsonin. Similarly, new antigenic determinants appear on antigen-bound antibody. These determinants are regarded by the immune system as foreign and therefore provoke the formation of autoantibodies known as rheumatoid factors (Chap. 24). The development of these new antigenic determinants and biological activities are a function of the immunoglobulin Fc region. Normally, the Fc region is masked by the Fab regions. When the antibody binds antigen through the Fab regions, the shape of the molecule changes and the Fc region is exposed. The active sites on the Fc region thus become available and free to exert their biological functions (Fig. 7–21).

A second mechanism involved in the development of the biological activity of immunoglobulins probably relates to the number of available active sites. A single immunoglobulin-active site may be unable to initiate reactions by itself. Only when several antibody molecules bind closely together on an antigen and multiple active sites exposed is the combined stimulus sufficient to initiate subsequent reactions.

Complement

There are a number of biochemical reactions that, if activated in the absence of effective controls, could lead to disastrous consequences. The clotting system, the fibrinolytic system,

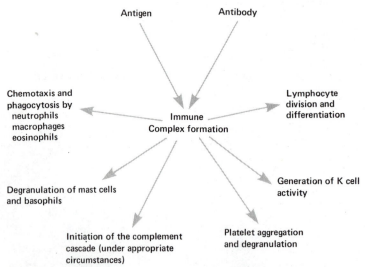

FIGURE 14–1. Some of the biological consequences of immune complex formulation. (From Tizard I. Veterinary Immunology, 2nd ed. W. B. Saunders, Philadelphia, 1982. With permission.)

and the kinin system all consist of a series of such reactions. Uncontrolled activation of these systems has the potential to cause uncontrollable hemorrhage, extensive intravascular thrombosis, or severe disturbance in vascular permeability, respectively. In order to ensure that uncontrolled activation does not occur, these systems are regulated by mechanisms that involve a series of linked enzyme reactions. The general principle of these reactions is that the products of one reaction catalyze a second reaction, whose products then catalyze a third reaction and so on (Fig. 14–2). Since many of the intermediate products either are present in limiting quantities, have a very short half-life, or are easily inhibited, it is possible to ensure that the system does not proceed to completion in an uncontrolled fashion.

How to Detect and Measure Complement

Complement components are normal serum proteins. They are therefore present in all normal sera. If antibody-coated erythrocytes (sheep erythrocytes are commonly used) are added to normal serum, the complement cascade is activated by the classical pathway. This eventually results in lysis of the erythrocytes. The hemolytic activity of serum varies between species. Thus, guinea pig complement is highly hemolytic. As a result guinea pig serum is commonly used as a source of complement. On the other hand, horse serum is nonhemolytic.

The level of "complement" in a serum may be quantitated by using CH_{50} units. One CH_{50} is the amount of complement required to lyse 50% of a standard preparation of sheep erythrocytes.

Hemolysis of antibody-coated sheep erythrocytes detects the activity of the classical complement pathway. In the presence of calcium-chelating agents such as EDTA, C1 is inactivated, and the classical pathway is blocked. The alternate pathway may then be measured by measuring hemolysis of xenogeneic erythrocytes or after activating the cascade with endotoxin or aggregated immunoglobulins.

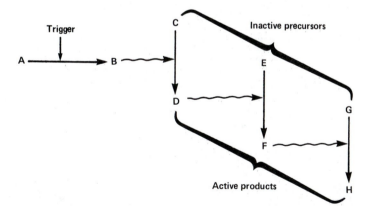

FIGURE 14–2. The principle of cascade reactions. The process is started by a trigger that initiates the conversion of an inactive proenzyme A to an active enzyme B. This enzyme B acts to convert proenzyme C to an active enzyme D. Enzyme D in turn converts proenzyme E to enzyme F, and so forth. (From Tizard, I. Veterinary Immunology, 2nd ed. W. B. Saunders, Philadelphia, 1982. With permission.)

Chain reactions of this type are known as "cascade" reactions and usually require some form of "trigger" to initiate the reaction chain. For example, in the case of the blood-clotting system, activation of Hageman factor by altered surfaces serves as the initiating event that sets the system in motion.

There also exists a system whose activation can result in the disruption of cell membranes and, therefore, may destroy cells or invading organisms. The system, termed **complement,** must be carefully regulated, since uncontrolled generation of the products of the system may lead to massive cell destruction. Complement was discovered in 1893 when the German scientist Buchner showed that serum that was heated at 56° lost its ability to kill certain bacteria. He called the heat-labile component alexine. Nationalist sentiments at the end of the 19th century, however, were such that the French introduced the rival term "complement" for this activity.

Complement is now known to be a system of interlinked enzyme-mediated reactions consisting of three distinct pathways. Two of these pathways represent alternative procedures for the activation of the third component of the cascade. The third, or terminal, pathway is not a true cascade reaction but a series of molecular aggregations by which a membrane-damaging complex is generated from the activated third component.

Components

Complement components are either labelled numerically with the prefix C—for example, C1, C2, C3—or designated by letters of the alphabet—B, D, P, and so forth. There are at least 17 of these components; they are all serum proteins and together they make up about 10% of the globulin fraction of serum. The molecular weights of the complement components vary between 80,000 daltons for C9 to 400,000 daltons for C1q. Their serum concentrations in humans vary between 3 mg/100 ml of C2 to 130 mg/100 ml of C3 (Table

TABLE 14–1   The Components of the Complement Cascade

Component	MW $\times 10^3$	Main Sources	Concentration in Serum μg/ml
C1q	390	G. I. epithelial cells, fibroblasts, macrophages	190
C1r	83	G. I. epithelial cells, macrophages	
C1s	83	G. I. epithelial cells, macrophages	110
C4	209	Macrophages, liver	430
C2	117	Macrophages	30
D	23.5	Macrophages, platelets	2
B	100	Macrophages, liver	240
P	186	Macrophages	23
C3	190	Macrophages, liver	1300
C5	206	Macrophages	75
C6	95	Liver	60
C7	120		55
C8	163	Liver	80
C9	71	Liver	58
I	88	Macrophages	34
H	160	Macrophages, platelets	500

14–1). Complement components are synthesized at various sites through the body. Thus most C3, C6, C8, and B are made in the liver, and C1 is synthesized in intestinal epithelium, while C2, C3, C4, C5, B, D, P, and I are synthesized by macrophages. As a result, these components are readily available at sites of inflammation where macrophages accumulate.

The levels of B, C1, C4, and C2 are regulated by genes found within the Class III locus of the major histocompatibility complex (Chap. 3).

The Classical Pathway for the Activation of C3 Convertase

C1 The first component of complement consists of three subcomponents C1q, C1r, and C1s bound together by calcium.

C1q is a molecule, which, on electron microscopy looks like a six-stranded whip (Fig. 14–3). The strands have a typical collagen structure with a glycine molecule at every third position and are rich in hydroxyproline and hydroxylysine. The tips of each strand have the ability to bind to antibody bound to antigen but not to free antibody. The site on an immunoglobulin that binds C1q is found in the Fc region probably associated with positively charged residues 316 to 340 on the surface of the C_{H2} region. This complement-activating site is present on unbound immunoglobulin molecules but is probably masked by the Fab regions. Only when the antibody binds to the antigen is the site exposed to the C1q molecule (Fig. 14-4).

The binding of C1q to an immunoglobulin results in a conformational change that is transmitted to C1r. As a result, the C1r undergoes a change to reveal an active proteolytic site, which cleaves a peptide bond in C1s to convert that molecule to an enzymically active form.

The stimuli that provoke activation of C1 include single, antigen-bound molecules of IgM or paired, antigen-bound molecules of IgG. (Since the two IgG molecules must be located very close together, IgG is very much less active than IgM in activating complement). C1 may also be activated directly by certain virus surface proteins, by some bacteria such as *E. coli* and *Klebsiella pneumoniae,* by C-reactive protein, or by myelin.

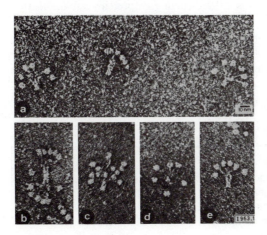

FIGURE 14–3. Different aspects of the C1q molecule shown by electron microscopy (final magnification x500,000). (From Knobel, H. R., Villiger, W., and Isliker, H. Eur. J. Immunol., *5*:78–82, 1975. With permission.)

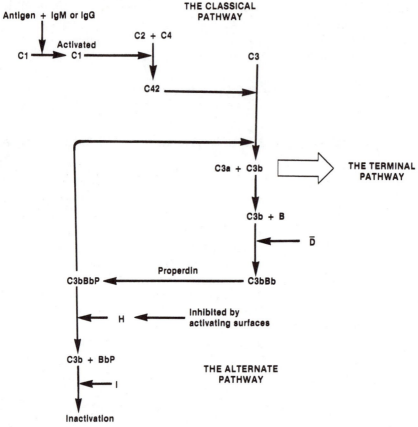

FIGURE 14-4. The "classical" and "alternate" pathways for the activation of C3. (From Tizard, I. Veterinary Immunology, 2nd ed. W. B. Saunders, Philadelphia, 1982. With permission.)

C4   The fourth component of complement is a three-chain glycoprotein, containing an α chain MW 93,000, a β chain MW 78,000 and a γ chain of 33,000 MW (Fig. 14–5). Active C1s acts on the α chain of C4 to cleave off a small fragment from the N terminus called C4a, and to leave the major fragment C4b. C4b is very unstable in the free form, and, unless it binds rapidly to an immunoglobulin Fab region, it will be broken down by C4b inactivator to an inactive product C4bi. C4 can bind to complement receptors on neutrophils, platelets and lymphocytes (CR1).

C4 Variants

Two antigenic variants of C4 are commonly found bound to cell membranes. In humans, these are known as C4A (Rogers antigen) and and C4B (Chido antigen). They are coded for by loci F and S respectively located within the major histocompatibility complex (see Chap. 3). In mice, a nonhemolytic variant of the C4 molecule is

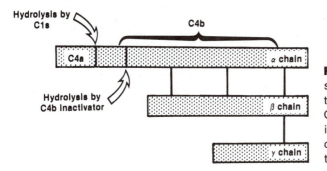

FIGURE 14–5. The structure of C4. C1s activates the molecule by cleaving off C4a leaving C4b. C4b inactivator inactivates C4b by cleaving another peptide off the α chain.

Slp (sex-linked protein). This is structurally and antigenically similar to C4, but each of its three peptide chains has a slightly different molecular weight than true C4.

C2 C2 is a glycoprotein with a molecular weight of 117,000. Activated C1s splits the C2 into C2a and C2b. The C2a binds to C4b or C4bi to generate a complex, C4b2a, but this complex breaks down spontaneously as the C2a decays to C2ai. The remaining C4b can form more of this complex if more C2a is provided. C4b can also interact with C1 to permit more efficient activation of C2. C4b2a has several different functions. First, and most important it can cleave C3. The complex C4b2a is therefore called classical C3 convertase. Second, C4b2a can bind to C3b to form C4b2a3b, which acts on C5 and is called C5 convertase.

The Third Component of Complement

By far the most important of the complement components is C3. C3 is a β globulin with a molecular weight of 190,000 composed of two chains, an α chain of 120,000 daltons and a β chain of 70,000 daltons linked by two disulfide bonds (Fig. 14–6). C3 is synthesized by liver cells and by macrophages and is the complement component of highest concentration in serum. In order for the complement cascade to proceed, C3 must be activated by proteolytic cleavage. C4b2a, the classical C3 convertase acts on N terminus of the α chain of C3 to split off a small, 6000 to 8000-dalton fragment. The small fragment is called C3a and the remainder of the molecule is called C3b.

The Alternative Pathway of C3 Convertase Production

While C3 may be activated by the classical pathway as described above, it may also be activated through the **alternative pathway.** Native C3 breaks down slowly but spontaneously in plasma, and as a result C3b is continuously generated in normal serum. C3b has the unique property of participating in its own hydrolysis as a component of the alternative pathway C3 convertase.

Factor B B is a 100,000-dalton globulin that binds to C3b through a magnesium-dependent bond. This complex, C3bB, has very weak C3-convertase activity. However, if factor B is cleaved by the serum enzyme known as factor D into Ba and an 80,000-MW fragment called Bb, then the complex C3bBb develops very potent C3-convertase activity.

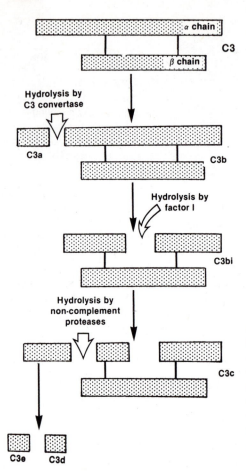

FIGURE 14-6. The activation and breakdown of C3. C3a released by the activity of classical or alternate C3 convertase, has anaphylatoxic activity. C3b is the biologically active form of C3 that initiates the terminal portion of the complement pathway. C3b is inactivated by factor I. (Modified from Harrison, R. A., and Lachmann, P. J. Mol. Immunol. *17:* 227, 1980. With permission.)

B is cleaved by the serum enzyme known as factor D into Ba and an 80,000-MW fragment called Bb, then the complex C3bBb develops very potent C3-convertase activity.

Factor D   Factor D is an α globulin, MW 23,500, which functions as a serine esterase to cleave factor B into Ba and Bb. Factor D, however, only acts on B after it is bound to C3b. As a result its overall activity is regulated by the supply of C3b.

The alternate C3 convertase, C3bBb, is capable of splitting C3 and so generating more C3b. Clearly, this positive loop could proceed in a runaway fashion unless rigorously controlled. This control function is undertaken by factors H and I, which degrade C3bBb, and by properdin (factor P), which stabilizes it. The net rate at which C3b,Bb becomes available depends upon the balance between the activities of these factors.

Factor P   Properdin. Properdin is a γ globulin, MW 220,000, which can bind to C3b reversibly. It exists in two conformational forms, one of which, the activated form, binds more firmly. Properdin stabilizes the alternate convertase C3bBb by slowing the spontaneous dissociation of Bb.

Factors H and I   The factors that normally retard the production of active C3bBb are known as factors H and I. Factor H (once known as β1H) is a β globulin, MW 150,000. It accelerates the dissociation of Bb from C3b. C3b can accept another Bb molecule unless inactivated by factor I. Factor I (once known as C3b inactivator) is a two-chain β globulin that cleaves the α chain of C3b to convert it to an inactive form C3bi. Factor I cannot act on C3b, however, when it is bound to Bb. Thus, in order to destroy C3bBb, factor H must first separate the two components.

In a normal, stable situation, factors H and I can destroy C3bBb as fast as it is generated and, as a result, this pathway for C3-convertase activation remains essentially inactive.

However, factor-H activity is itself regulated by the presence of surfaces containing sialic acid. Sialic acid enhances the affinity of factor H for C3b up to a hundredfold. In the presence of surfaces deficient in sialic acid, such as bacterial cell walls for example, factor-H activity is depressed. As a result, the production of C3bBb greatly exceeds its destruction and it proceeds to activate C3 in large quantities (Fig. 14-7). The surfaces that inhibit factor H and thus activate the alternate pathway include some virus-infected cells, some tumor cells, cell walls from many bacteria, aggregated immunoglobulins, foreign particles, such as asbestos, and cells that have had their sialic acid artificially removed by means of sialidases (neuraminidases). Antibody may act to permit activation of the alternate pathway on cell membranes by masking sialic-acid residues.

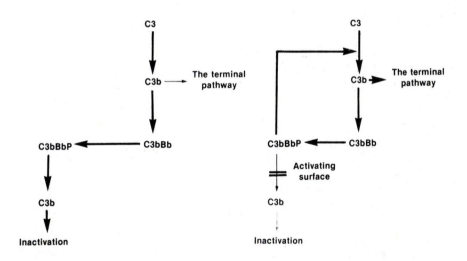

FIGURE 14-7.   The activation of the alternate complement pathway in the presence of activating surfaces results in the generation of large quantities of C3 convertase (C3bBbP) that would normally be destroyed. (From Tizard, I. Veterinary Immunology, 2nd ed. W. B. Saunders, Philadelphia, 1982. With permission.)

Other Methods of Generating C3b

C3b may be generated through the activities of many proteolytic enzymes. For example, the enzymes from activated phagocytic cells or by thrombin on platelets. As a result, C3b may be generated in sites of inflammation or in areas of thrombosis.

The Terminal Complement Pathway

Both C4b2a, the classical C3 convertase and C3bBb, the alternate C3 convertase, act on C3 to cleave off C3a and generate C3b. C3b acts as the initiator of the terminal complement pathway by binding to either C4b2a or to C3bBb to generate an enzyme known as C5 convertase (Fig. 14–8).

C5 is a two-chain β globulin, MW 206,000 (Fig. 14–9). The α chain, MW 141,000 and the β chain MW 83,000 are bound by disulfide bridges. C5 convertase, from either the classical or alternate pathways, splits the chain to remove a peptide known as C5a, which has a molecular weight of 11,000, and the residue is termed C5b. This C5b binds to C6 to form a complex C5b6. In the unbound state C5b decays rapidly. C6 is a β globulin, 95,000 MW, consisting of a single polypeptide chain. It is not cleaved on binding to C5b. C7, a 120,000 MW β globulin, can bind to the C5b6 complex either in solution or bound to cell membranes. C5b67 can bind to unsensitized cell membranes and provoke the destruction of innocent bystander cells through a mechanism known as reactive lysis. Fluid phase C5b67 rapidly decays to C5i67, a complex which is cytolytically inert but which has chemotactic activity.

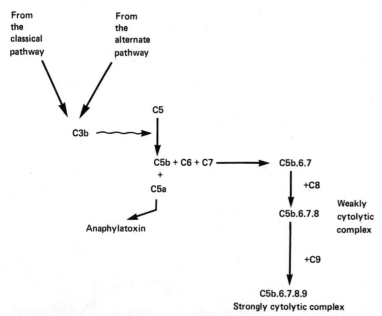

FIGURE 14–8. The terminal complement pathway. For details, see the text. (From Tizard, I. Veterinary Immunology, 2nd ed. W. B. Saunders, Philadelphia, 1982. With permission.)

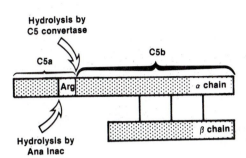

Hydrolysis by
C5 convertase

C5a

C5b

Arg

α chain

β chain

Hydrolysis by
Ana Inac

FIGURE 14–9. The structure, activation, and breakdown of C5. The molecule is activated by C5 convertase. C5b participates in the terminal pathway. C5a is rapidly destroyed in serum by anaphylatoxin inactivator (Ana Inac). This is a carboxypeptidase that, by removing the terminal arginine, leaves a peptide (C5a des arg), which is devoid of anaphylatoxic activity (i.e., it does not contract smooth muscle) but is a very potent neutrophil chemotactic agent.

Membrane-bound C5b67 binds C8 (C8 is a three-chain α globulin, MW 163,000). The entire C5b678 complex acts as an initiator to induce the polymerization of C9. Thus 12 to 15 C9 molecules come together to form a tubular structure consisting of poly C9 (mono C9 is a single-chain α globulin, MW 71,000). Tubular poly C9 forms a large doughnut-shaped structure that can insert itself into a cell membrane (Fig. 14–10). As a result, the central "hole" of the poly C9 forms a transmembrane channel in the membrane and osmotic lysis of the target cell occurs.

Regulation of the Complement System

The biological consequences of complement activation are so significant and potentially dangerous that the system must be very carefully regulated. This regulation is accomplished through the activities of control proteins (Fig. 14-11). We have already discussed how the alternate pathway is regulated through the activities of controlling proteins H and I.

C1 Inactivator   C1 inactivator (C1INH) is a 105,000 Mr αglycoprotein that controls the assembly of C4b2a (classical C3 convertase) by binding to, and blocking the activities

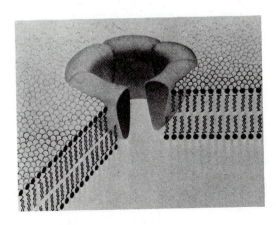

FIGURE 14–10. A hypothetical model of a cell-membrane lesion created by the action of complement. The walls of the lesion appear to consist of poly C9 (From The complement system, by M. Mayer. Copyright © 1973 by Scientific American, Inc. All rights reserved.)

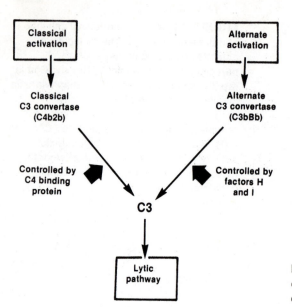

FIGURE 14–11. The basic control mechanisms of the complement cascade.

of active C1r and C1s. Normally, C1s acts on C2 to cleave off C2b. After further degradation by plasmin, C2b develops kininlike activity. In individuals who suffer from a congenital deficiency of C1INH, excessive amounts of this C2 kinin are produced. Since the C2 kinin increases vascular permeability, affected individuals suffer from attacks of widespread edema, which, if it involves the larynx, may cause the victim to suffocate. The disease caused by C1INH deficiency is known as hereditary angioedema.

C4-bp   C4 binding protein (C4-bp) is a heat-stable β globulin that binds to classical C3 convertase (C4b2a), accelerates the decay/dissociation of C2a, and destroys its activity. It may act in a similar manner to factor H of the alternate pathway insofar as it acts with Factor I to cleave the α chain of C4b into two inactive fragments, C4d and C4c.

S Protein   S protein is an α glycoprotein with a molecular weight of 88,000. It appears to bind to C5b67 and, by preventing the attachment of this complex to membranes, inhibits bystander lysis. Low-density lipoproteins have a similar activity.

Immunoconglutinins

The activation of complement components, either by enzymic activity or through conformational changes results in the formation of autoantibodies against newly formed antigenic determinants. These autoantibodies are known as **immunoconglutinins** (abbreviated to IK). An immunoconglutinin called C3 nephritic factor, (it was found in the serum of patients with renal disease) is directed against the alternate C3 convertase (C3bBb). When C3 nephritic factor binds to C3bBb, it not only stabilizes the complex but in binding to its antigens can also activate complement by the classical pathway. Other immunoconglutinins may be directed against determinants on C3b, C2 and C4. In cattle, buffalo, and other bovidae, there is a serum protein, called **conglutinin** that can also bind to fixed C3b. Although it is not an immunoglobulin, it, like the immunoconglutinins can clump (strictly speaking, conglutinate) C3b-coated particles. The biological significance of conglutinin is unknown.

The Biological Consequence of Complement Activation

The complement system plays a major role in host defense both through destruction of invading microorganisms and through mediation of inflammatory reactions. In addition, the complement system may contribute to tissue injury as a result of excessive inflammatory responses (Fig. 14–12).

Cell Adherence Many cells possess receptors for complement components. The most important of these receptors, called CR1, is a 205,000-dalton glycoprotein found on neutrophils, macrophages, and B lymphocytes. The receptor may be shed and reabsorbed to cells fairly freely. CR1 is able to bind C3b strongly and C4b weakly. Particles coated with C3b bind to cells through these receptors in a phenomenon called immune adherence.

A second group of complement receptors are known as CR2. CR2 receptors are found on some B cells and neutrophils. They bind the breakdown products of C3 namely

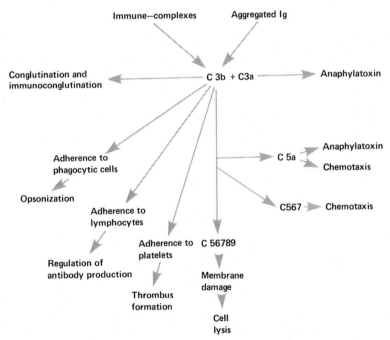

FIGURE 14–12. Some of the many biological consequences of complement activation. (From Tizard, I. Veterinary Immunology, 2nd ed. W. B. Saunders, Philadelphia, 1982. With permission.)

C3d and C3bi. Monocytes, B cells, some null cells, and neutrophils have a C1q receptor while B cells have a receptor for factor H.

Complement-Mediated Opsonization   Phagocytic cells possess both Fc and CR1 receptors. As a result, both antibody and complement-coated particles bind to these cells and can therefore be phagocytosed. If, for some reason, these particles cannot be ingested, then neutrophils may be induced to secrete their lysosomal enzymes. These enzymes in turn will cause inflammation and tissue damage and may activate C3 or C5.

Complement-Mediated Secretion   CR1 receptors are found on nonprimate platelets. Adherence of C3b-coated particles to these platelets results in the secretion of the vasoactive factors histamine and serotonin, and effectively promotes local inflammation.

Complement-Mediated Immune Regulation.   CR1 receptors are found on some B cells but not on T cells. The function of these receptors is unclear but they are probably involved in the regulation of the B-cell response. Thus complement depletion delays the antibody response to thymus-dependent antigens and prevents the switch from IgM production to production of other immunoglobulin classes. The binding of C3b to B lymphocytes stimulates them to secrete a chemotactic lymphokine and it also regulates the splenic antibody response through an effect on antigen localization.

     The binding of C3 to receptors appears to exert a regulatory function on the development of immunological memory. Depletion of C3 abrogates memory-cell and germinal-center production—probably because of alterations in the localization of antigen.

Complement-Mediated Cytolysis   If the complement sequence proceeds to completion, the membrane-attack complex is formed. This complex can be seen by electron microscopy to be ring shaped with a central electron-dense area surrounded by a lighter ring of poly C9 (Fig. 14–10). This ring structure is incorporated into the lipid membrane of cells and, as a result, a channel is formed through which the cell is lysed. It is not clear whether the channel is through the center of the complex or around its periphery. Nevertheless, the lysis of cells by complement is compatible with the formation of "holes" in the cell membranes.

     For Gram-negative bacteria, a single "hit" by a complement membrane-attack complex is insufficient for bactericidal activity, since this only disrupts the outer bacterial cell membrane. In order to complete the lytic process by rupturing the inner cell membrane, the enzyme lysozyme is required. Thus bacterial destruction by complement is a "two-hit" process.

Complement-Mediated Chemotaxis   During the process of activation of the complement cascades, a number of chemotactic factors are generated. These include C5a, C5a67, C3e and Bb (Table 14–2). There appear to be subtle differences in the nature of their targets. Thus C5a67 is chemotactic for neutrophils and eosinophils only, while C5a attracts not only neutrophils and eosinophils but also macrophages and basophils. When C5a attracts neutrophils, it stimulates their metabolism especially their respiratory burst, aggregates them, and causes them to release thromboplastins. C5a in vivo is rapidly broken down by a carboxypeptidase that removes the terminal arginine and forms C5a des arg, which is equally potent but only in the presence of whole serum.

TABLE 14–2 Complement Derived Chemotactic Factors

Factor	Target
C3a	(Eosinophils)?
C5a	Neutrophils, eosinophils, macrophages
C5a des arg in presence of serum	Neutrophils, eosinophils, macrophages
C567	Neutrophils, eosinophils
Bb	Neutrophils
C3e	Leukocytosis promotion

C3e derived from the α chain of C3c (Fig. 14–6) will cause a leukocytosis on intravenous administration and appears to have the ability to mobilize leukocytes from bone marrow.

Complement-Mediated Inflammation   C3a and C5a also function as **anaphylatoxins,** that is, they cause smooth muscle such as that found in the intestine wall to contract. This reaction is independent of histamine but may be due to leukotrienes since it is inhibited by lipoxygenase inhibitors. These two factors also provoke degranulation of skin mast cells at exquisitely low concentrations (10^{-12} and 10^{-15}M) and also act on platelets to promote their release of histamine and serotonin. The name **anaphylatoxin** was introduced to describe the toxic activities of immune complexes containing these peptides. If these peptides are treated with carboxypeptidases or a naturally occurring serum inhibitor (anaphylatoxin inactivator) to remove the terminal arginine, their toxic activities are inhibited although they retain the ability to block the activities of the intact peptides, and treated C5a (C5a des arg) retains its chemotactic activity (Fig. 14-13).

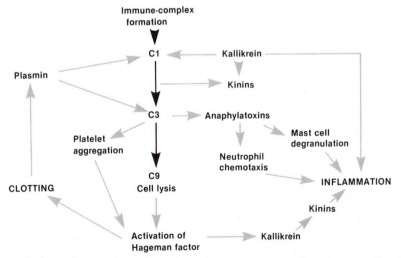

FIGURE 14–13.   Some of the more important interactions between the clotting, complement, and inflammatory systems. (From Tizard, I. Veterinary Immunology, 2nd ed. W. B. Saunders, Philadelphia, 1982. With permission.)

Complement Genes

C4, C2, and factor B are coded for by Class III genes located within the MHC. C3 is coded by a gene locus on the same chromosome as the MHC but is located some distance away.

As described in Chapter 3, in mice, the C4 gene locus is located adjacent to the gene locus for the related protein Slp. In man, there appear to be two C4 loci and within each locus are multiple alleles. Chido and Rogers "blood group" antigens are variants of C4 derived from each of these loci, FA and SB. In guinea pigs there is a single C4 locus. C4 is synthesized as a single chain precursor molecule (pro-C4) which is converted to C4 by the action of plasmin.

C3 and C5 are also processed in a similar manner—the pro-C3 or C5 is cleaved by a plasmin-like enzyme to generate the multichain complement component.

The gene for factor B, known as Bf, is located close to the C2 gene but is under independent control.

Complement Deficiencies

In general, congenital deficiencies of complement components result in an increased susceptibility to infections. In humans, the most severe conditions occur in individuals deficient in C3. They suffer from recurrent bacterial infections, especially pyococcal infections in a manner similar to agammaglobulinemic individuals (Chap. 18). In contrast to the severe effects of a C3 deficiency, congenital deficiencies of other complement components are not necessarily lethal. Thus individuals with C6 or C7 deficiencies have been described who are quite healthy. The lack of discernible effect of these deficiencies suggests that the terminal portion of the complement pathway leading to lysis is not biologically essential. Notwithstanding this, individuals deficient in C5 tend to suffer from recurrent neisserial meningitis as do properdin-deficient individuals. In C5-deficient mice, it is possible to show that phagoctytosis of *Neisseria gonorrhoeae* is delayed.

Deficiencies of C2, C1r or C4 are commonly associated with the presence of the autoimmune disorder systemic lupus erythematosus (SLE) (Chap. 21). Since SLE may, in some cases, be mediated by a virus, the occurrence of this condition in conjunction with C2 or C4 deficiency may reflect a defect in antiviral resistance.

Deficiencies of the complement control proteins have also been described. A deficiency of the C1 inactivator leads, as has already been described, to hereditary angioedema as a result of the overproduction of C2 kinin. A congenital deficiency of factor H leads to hypocomplementemia as a result of uncontrolled activation of the alternate pathway and the patients have suffered from a hemolytic-uremic syndrome. A factor I deficiency has a similar effect and presents a clinical picture similar to that of a C3 deficiency—severe recurrent infections (Table 14-3).

Interrelationships between the Complement and Clotting Systems

The interaction between antigen and antibody and the activation of the complement system may influence the clotting process in several ways (Fig. 14–13). Immune complexes, particularly if deposited on blood-vessel walls, may trigger thrombus formation through acti-

TABLE 14–3   Complement Deficiency States

Deficient Component	Clinical Manifestations
C1q	Hypogammaglobulinemia
C1r	Systemic lupus
C4	Systemic lupus
C2	Systemic lupus or healthy
C3	Severe immunodeficiency usually neisserial infections
C5	Severe immunodeficiency
C6	Healthy or neisserial infections
C7	Healthy
C1 inhibitor	Hereditary angioedema
I	Severe immunodeficiency
H	Hemolytic uremic syndrome
P	Neisserial infections

vation of Hageman factor. Second, C1 inhibitor can act to inhibit not only the activities of C1 but also of thrombin and factors XI and XII, as well as plasmin and kallikrein. Third, C3b, as mentioned earlier, can cause platelet aggregation. This aggregation can lead to the release of adenosine diphosphate, which, in turn, mediates further platelet aggregation, the release of vasoactive factors, particularly histamine and serotonin, and the release of platelet procoagulants, which accelerate the clotting process. As a consequence, extensive immune-complex formation within the blood-vascular system may give rise to a disseminated intra-vascular coagulation (DIC), in which there is generalized activation of the clotting system, and fibrin is deposited within small blood vessels. Finally, a direct role for complement in the clotting process is implied by the observation that, in rabbits congenitally deficient in C6, there is a defect in whole-blood clotting time that may be corrected by the addition of physiological amounts of purified C6. The significance of this phenomenon is not clear at this time.

The Fibrinolytic System

The fibrinolytic system, as its name implies, acts to control the clotting process by digestion of fibrin. It consists of a series of linked enzyme reactions that eventually generate the fibrinolytic enzyme plasmin from its precursor plasminogen. Being a proteolytic enzyme, plasmin can activate both C1 and C3 and is, in turn, inhibited by C1 inactivator. Because plasminogen activators are found closely associated with neutrophil surfaces, plasmin may be generated and complement subsequently activated at sites of neutrophil accumulation. This activation of complement contributes significantly to the inflammatory lesions that occur when immune complexes are deposited in tissues (Chap. 22).

The Complement Fixation Test

The activation of the complement system by immune complexes results in the generation of factors capable of disrupting cell membranes. If the immune complexes are generated on erythrocyte surfaces, then the erythrocyte membranes are lysed, and hemolysis occurs. It is possible to use this reaction to measure serum antibody levels. The most important test of this type is the hemolytic complement fixation test (CFT). The CFT is one of the most widely applicable of all immunological techniques. Once the required reagents are prepared and standardized, the CFT may be used to detect many immune interactions. The end point is very easily read and, unlike the hemagglutination tests, does not depend upon the settling of the erythrocytes and is less affected by prozones. In addition, this test does not depend upon the availability of purified suspensions of antigens and is therefore commonly used in the diagnosis of viral diseases. The most important disadvantage of this test is its complexity, particularly with regard to the standardization and preparation of the reagents required.

The hemolytic CFT is performed in two parts (Fig. 14–14). First, antigen and the serum under test (deprived of its complement by heating at 56°C) are incubated in the presence of normal guinea-pig serum, which provides a source of complement. (Guinea-

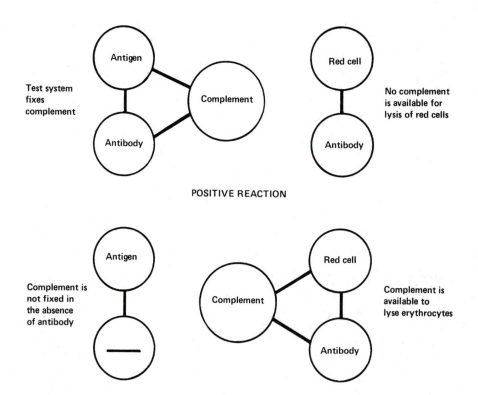

FIGURE 14–14. The principle of the complement fixation test. Complement, if fixed by antigen and antibody, is unavailable to lyse the indicator system. In the absence of antibody, the complement will remain unfixed and available for lysis of the indicator system. (After Roitt, I. Essential Immunology. Blackwell Scientific Publications, Oxford, 1971. From Tizard, I. Veterinary Immunology, 2nd ed. W. B. Saunders, Philadelphia, 1982. With permission.)

pig serum is most commonly used because its complement has a high hemolytic activity—that is, it lyses erythrocytes well.) After allowing the antigen–antibody–complement mixture to react for a short period, the amount of free complement remaining is measured by adding an "indicator system" consisting of antibody-coated sheep erythrocytes. Lysis of these erythrocytes, seen as the development of a transparent red solution, is a negative result, since it indicates that complement was not fixed and that antibody was, therefore, absent from the serum under test. Absence of lysis (seen as a cloudy red cell suspension) is a positive result. It is usual to titrate the serum being tested so that, if antibodies are present in that serum then, as it is diluted the reaction in each tube will change from no-lysis (i.e., positive) to lysis (i.e., negative). The titer may be considered to be the highest dilution of serum in which no more than 50 percent of the red cells are lysed.

Before a hemolytic CFT is performed, all reagents, to be used, antigen, complement, sheep erythrocytes, and antibody against these erythrocytes (hemolysin) must be carefully standardized. For example, addition of the correct amount of complement is critical, since too little complement results in incomplete lysis, while excessive complement is not completely fixed by immune complexes and therefore will lead to false-negative results. Excessive antigen interferes with complement fixation, while insufficient antigen may fail to fix complement in demonstrable amounts. The hemolysin should be heated at 56°C for 30 min in order to destroy its content of complement.

Anticomplementary Effects   One problem commonly encountered when performing CFT's is the presence of anticomplementary activity in the serum under test. That is, the test serum appears to fix complement in the absence of antigen. There are several possible reasons for this behavior. For example, any immune complexes present will effectively bind some complement. Similarly, the presence of bacterial contaminants in serum may activate complement through the alternate pathway.

Cytotoxicity Tests   Complement may cause membrane damage, not only to erythrocytes but also to nucleated cells and to protozoa. Antibodies against cell surface antigens thus may be measured by reacting target cells with antibody in the presence of complement and estimating the resulting cell death. A simple method of doing this is to add a dye such as trypan blue or eosin-Y to the cell suspension. Living cells do not take up these dyes, while dead ones stain intensely. This form of test is employed in the identification of histocompatibility antigens (Chap. 19).

Sources of Additional Information

Chan, A. C., et al. Identification and partial characterization of the secreted form of the fourth component of human complement: Evidence that it is different from the major plasma form. Proc. Natl. Acad. Sci. USA., *80*:268–272, 1983.

Chenoweth, D. E., and Hugli, T. E. Demonstration of a specific C5a receptor on intact human polymorphonuclear leukocytes. Proc. Natl. Acad. Sci. USA, *75*:3943–3947, 1978.

Colten, M. R., Alper, D. A., Rosen, F. S. Genetics and biosynthesis of complement proteins. N. Engl. J. Med., *304*:653–656, 1981.

Fearon, D. T., and Austin, K. F. Current concepts in immunology. The alternative pathway of complement. A system for host resistance to microbial infection. N. Engl. J. Med. *303*:259–263, 1980.

Kolb, W. P., and Muller-Eberhard, H. J. The membrane attack mechanisms of complement. Isolation and subunit composition of the C5b-9 complex. J. Exp. Med., *141*:724–735, 1975.

Mayer, M. M. The complement system. Sci. Am., *229*:54–70, 1973.

Osler, A. G. Complement Mechanisms and Functions. Foundations of Immunology series. Prentice-Hall, Englewood Cliffs, N.J., 1976.

Pangburn, M. K., et al. Activation of the alternative complement pathway: recognition of surface structures on activators by bound C3b. J. Immunol., *124*:977–982, 1980.

Podack, E. R., et al. Membrane attack complex of complement: A structural analysis. J. Exp. Med., *151*:301–313, 1980.

Polley, M. J., and Nachman, R. The human complement system in thrombin-mediated platelet function. J. Exp. Med., *147*:1713–1721, 1978.

Porter, R. R., and Reid, K. B. M. The biochemistry of complement. Nature, *275*:699–704, 1978.

Roos, M. H., Atkinson, J. P., and Shreffler, D. C. Molecular characterization of the Ss and Slp (C4) proteins of the mouse H-2 complex: Subunit composition, chain size polymorphism and an intracellular (Pro-Ss) precursor. J. Immunol., *121*:1106–1115, 1978.

15

Immunity at Body Surfaces

Although mammals possess an extensive array of defense mechanisms within tissues, it is at the body surface that invading microorganisms are first encountered and largely repelled or destroyed. The protective systems at body surfaces achieve this by establishing, through physical and chemical mechanisms, local environmental conditions suitable for only the most adapted microorganisms. These surfaces are populated by an extensive microbial flora that, because it is well adapted, is also of low pathogenicity and effectively prevents the establishment of other, more poorly adapted and potentially pathogenic organisms. This environmental defense system is supplemented by immunological mechanisms in areas where the physical barriers to invasion are relatively weak.

Nonimmunological Surface-Protective Mechanisms (Table 15-1)

That most obvious of the body surfaces, the skin, serves a number of functions, one of which is to present a barrier to invading microorganisms. The skin carries a dense and stable resident bacterial flora whose composition is regulated by a number of factors, including continuing desquamation, desiccation, and a relatively low pH that is due, in part, to the presence of fatty acids in sebum. If any of these environmental factors is altered, then the composition of the skin flora is disturbed, its protective properties are reduced, and invasion may occur in consequence. Thus, skin infections tend to occur in areas such as the axilla or groin where both pH and humidity are relatively high. Similarly, individuals forced to stand in water or mud for prolonged periods show an increased frequency of foot infections as the skin becomes sodden, its structure breaks down, and its resident flora changes in response to alterations in the local environment.

The importance of the resident flora is seen to much greater effect in the digestive tract, where it is essential not only for the control of potential pathogens but also for the digestion of some foods, such as cellulose in the diet of herbivores. In addition, the natural

TABLE 15-1   Some Nonimmunological Protective Mechanisms that Assist in Preventing Microbial Invasion at Body Surfaces

Type	Examples
Physical mechanisms	Dessication
	pH extremes
	Desquamation
	Mucus barrier
	Fluid flow (e.g., saliva, urine, milk, vomiting, diarrhea)
Chemical factors	Lysozyme
	Fatty acids
	Gastric acid
	Proteolytic enzymes
Biological factors	Competition with normal flora
	Antibiosis
	Generation of anaerobic or acidic conditions

development of the immune system depends upon the continuous antigenic stimulation provided by intestinal flora. Because of the absence of a bacterial flora, germ-free animals have poorly developed secondary lymphoid organs.

If the natural flora of the intestine is eliminated or its composition drastically altered (by aggressive antibiotic treatment, for example), then dietary disturbances result and the overgrowth of potential pathogens may occur. The flora of the digestive tract normally acts competitively against potential invaders through a number of mechanisms that supplement the other physical defenses of this system. Thus, in the mouth, the flushing activity of saliva is complemented by the generation of peroxides from streptococci. In the stomach of some animals, the gastric pH may be sufficiently low to have some bactericidal and viricidal effect, although this effect varies greatly between species and between meals, and the pH in the center of a mass of ingested food may not necessarily drop to low levels. Some foods, such as milk, are known to be potent buffers.

Farther down the intestine, the resident bacterial flora tends to ensure that the pH is kept relatively low and the contents anaerobic. The intestinal flora is also influenced indirectly by the diet; for instance, the intestine of milk-fed animals tends to be colonized largely by lactobacilli, which produce large quantities of bacteriostatic lactic and butyric acids. These acids inhibit colonization by potential pathogens, such as *Escherichia coli,* so that animals suckled naturally tend to have fewer digestive upsets than animals weaned early in life. In the large intestine, the bacterial flora is composed largely of strict anaerobes.

Lysozyme (Chap. 17), the antibacterial and antiviral enzyme, is synthesized in the gastric mucosa and in macrophages within the intestinal mucosa. As a consequence, it is found in relatively large quantities in the intestinal fluid. The role of phagocytic cells in the intestine is not clear, but macrophages can migrate through the intestinal wall and may be active for a short time within the lumen.

In the urinary system, the flushing action and low pH of urine generally provide adequate protection; however, when urinary stasis occurs, urethritis resulting from the unhindered ascent of pathogenic bacteria is not uncommon. In adult women, the vagina is lined by a squamous epithelium composed of cells rich in glycogen. When these cells desquamate, they provide a substrate for lactobacilli that, in turn, generate large quantities of lactic acid, which protects the vagina against invasion. Glycogen storage in the vaginal epithelial cells is stimulated by estrogens and thus occurs only in sexually mature individuals. Because of this, vaginal infections tend to be commonest prior to puberty and after the menopause.

The protective mechanisms of the mammary gland are, presumably, not of the most effective kind, at least in that biological anomaly the modern dairy cow. The flushing action of the milk serves to prevent invasion by some potential pathogens, while milk itself contains bacterial inhibitors. A general term for these antibacterial substances in milk is **lactenins.** Lactenins include complement, lysozyme, the iron-binding protein lactoferrin, and the enzyme lactoperoxidase. Lactoferrin competes with bacteria for iron and therefore renders it unavailable for their growth. It also enhances the neutrophil respiratory burst. Milk contains high concentrations of lactoperoxidase and thiocyanate (SCN^-) ions. In the presence of exogenous hydrogen peroxide, the lactoperoxidase can oxidize the SCN^- to bacteriostatic products such as sulfur dicyanide. The hydrogen peroxide may be produced by bacteria, such as streptococci or, alternatively, by the oxidation of ascorbic acid. Some strains of streptococci are resistant to this bacteriostatic pathway, since they possess an

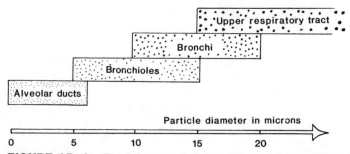

FIGURE 15–1. The influence of size on the site of deposition of particles within the respiratory tract: Particles greater that 10 μm in diameter will be trapped in the upper respiratory tract. Only particles less than 5 to 6 μm diameter will react in the alveolar ducts.

enzyme that reduces the SCN^-. IgA appears to enhance the activity of lactoperoxidase. The phagocytic cells released into the mammary gland in response to irritation may also contribute to antimicrobial resistance not only through their phagocytic efforts but also by providing additional lactoferrin and lysosomal peroxidases.

The respiratory tract differs from the other body surfaces in that it is in intimate connection with the interior of the body and it is required by its very nature to allow unhindered access of air to the alveoli. The system obviously requires a filter. In fact, air entering the respiratory tract is largely deprived of any suspended particles by turbulence that directs particulate matter onto its mucus-covered walls, where it adheres. The turbulence is brought about by the conformation of the turbinate bones, the trachea, and the bronchi. This "turbulence filter" serves to remove particles as small as 5μm in size before they reach the alveoli (Fig. 15–1).

The walls of the upper respiratory tract are covered by a layer of mucus produced by goblet cellls and provided with "antiseptic" properties through its content of lysozyme and IgA. This mucus layer is in continuous flow, being carried from the bronchioles up the bronchi and trachea by ciliary action or backward through the nasal cavity to the pharynx. Here the "dirty" mucus is swallowed and presumably digested in the intestinal tract. Particles smaller than 5μm that can by-pass this "mucociliary escalator" and reach the alveoli are phagocytosed by alveolar macrophages. Once these cells have successfully ingested particles, they migrate to the mucus "escalator" and, in this way, are also carried to the pharynx and eliminated (Table 15–1).

Immunological Surface-Protective Mechanisms

Immunoglobulins A and E   In addition to the environmental and chemical factors that protect body surfaces, two immunoglobulin classes are found in relatively high concentration in secretions such as saliva, intestinal fluid, nasal and tracheal secretions, tears, milk and colostrum, and urine and the secretions of the urogenital tract (Table 15–2). Immu-

TABLE 15-2   IgA in Human Body Secretions

	Concentration (mg/100 ml)
Serum	100–300 (15% A2, 85% A1)
Bile	50–80
Parotid saliva	5–28
Colostrum	150
Intestinal fluid	14–75
Respiratory secretions	50–110
Prostatic fluid	25
Urine	0.01–0.10
Vaginal fluid	65
Tears	60–120
Milk	≃1600

noglobulin E tends to be largely associated with immunity to parasites and Type I hypersensitivities (see Chap. 17 and 20). Immunoglobulin A, however, appears to have evolved specifically for the purpose of protecting body surfaces.

The IgA monomer is a 6.8S molecule with a molecular weight of about 160,000 having a typical four-chain, Y-shaped structure and a somewhat elevated carbohydrate content relative to the other immunoglobulin classes. It tends to polymerize and is, therefore, usually found as a 9.3S dimer with the subunits bound together through a J chain. IgA has several extra cysteine residues in its chains. As a result, the short interchain disulfide bonds make the chains very compact and shield vulnerable peptide bonds from proteolytic enzymes. IgA dimers bind a protein (with a molecular weight of 71,000 synthesized by intestinal epithelial cells and hepatocytes, termed secretory component) to produce secretory IgA (SIgA). SIgA is a 10.8S molecule with a molecular weight of about 400,000 (Fig. 6–15), which renders IgA even more resistant to proteolysis by digestive enzymes.

Although it is apparent that IgA exerts a significant protective effect on mucosal surfaces, its mode of action is not completely clear. IgA, for instance, is not bactericidal, does not bind to macrophages or enhance phagocytosis, and fixes complement only by the alternate pathway. It can, however, neutralize viruses, as well as some viral and bacterial enzymes, and it may function in some ADCC systems. Its most important mode of action is to prevent the adherence of bacteria and viruses to epithelial surfaces. The importance of this adherence may be seen, for example, in diseases of the intestinal tract caused by strains of *E. coli* possessing the K88 antigen. The K88 antigen is a piluslike structure by which these organisms bind to intestinal epithelial cells (Fig. 15–2), so preventing their expulsion and promoting proliferation and enterotoxin production.

How to Show that IgA is Secreted in Bile.

In order to demonstrate the fate of serum IgA, it was necessary to inject animals with purified homologous IgA labelled with [125]I. The animals (rats in this case) were given this labelled immunoglobulin intravenously, and blood and bile samples were taken at intervals.

The radioactivity in each of these fluids was then counted.

TABLE 15–3   Amounts of Radioactive IgA Secreted in Serum and Bile

Time After Injection	cpm in Serum/ml	cpm in Bile/ml
15 min	8.2×10^5	
1 hr	4.2×10^5	4.2×10^6
2 hr	3.3×10^5	5.4×10^6
3 hr	2.8×10^5	1.6×10^6
3 hr	2.2×10^5	0.4×10^6

> Thus, 2 hr after injection, the level of IgA in bile was up to 12 times higher than that in serum. If the bile duct was ligated, then the IgA radioactivity in serum fell very slowly, at a rate comparable to that of the other immunoglobulin classes. This presumably reflects normal protein catabolism.
>
> *Orlans, E., et al. Rapid active transport of immunoglobulin A from blood to bile. J. Exp. Med., 147:588–592, 1978.*

Antibodies made specifically against K88 antigen can inhibit bacterial adherence and hence protect animals against disease caused by these strains of *E. coli.* Prolonged exposure of these bacteria to IgA may interfere with the expression of K88.

IgA is synthesized by plasma cells in the gut-associated lymphoid tissue (GALT) in response to local antigenic stimulation (Fig. 15–3). Much of this IgA diffuses directly into the intestinal lumen. As it diffuses, its J chain combines with secretory component synthesized by intestinal epithelial cells. The IgA is taken into the epithelial cells by endocytosis, transported across them by the microtubule system, and is discharged from the apical sur-

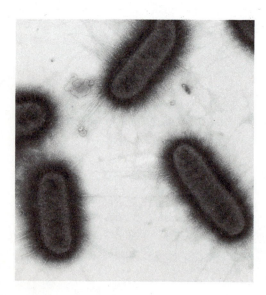

FIGURE 15–2. *E. coli* covered by a dense mat of K88 attachment pili (original magnification x35,000). (Courtesy of Dr. C. L. Gyles.)

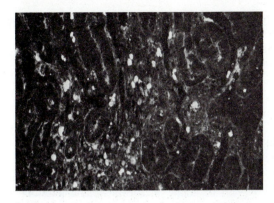

FIGURE 15–3. An immunofluorescence photomicrograph showing IgA-positive cells in the villi and submucosa of the rabbit small intestine. (Courtesy of Dr. D. Befus.)

face directly into the intestinal lumen. A significant proportion of the IgA, however, also diffuses into the portal circulation and is thus carried to the liver. Hepatocytes also synthesize secretory component and incorporate it into the membrane, where it acts as an IgA receptor. The blood-borne IgA thus binds to hepatocytes, is taken up by endocytosis, and is carried across the hepatocyte cytoplasm to be released into the bile canaliculi. Bile is, therefore, rich in IgA, and is a major route by which IgA reaches the intestinal lumen (Fig. 15–4). It is probably also a route by which antigens bound to circulating IgA can be removed from the body.

The plasma cells in the GALT arise from precursor B cells. These B cells, upon encountering antigen, respond in a manner similar to that of lymphocytes elsewhere in the

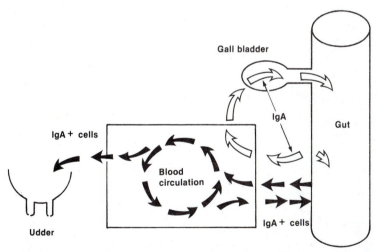

FIGURE 15–4. IgA (white arrows) is produced in the intestinal wall; some enters the gut directly, but most enters the portal circulation and is removed by the liver, entering the intestine through the bile. IgA-producing cells (black arrows) leave the intestinal wall and circulate for a short period before either returning to the intestine or migrating to other body surfaces, such as the mammary gland.

body—that is, they divide and some differentiate into plasma cells. Some of these responding B cells also migrate into intestinal lymphatics, from which they reach the thoracic duct and the blood circulation. These recirculating IgA^+B cells have an affinity for body surfaces in general. As a result, they colonize the intestinal tract, the respiratory tract, the urogenital tract, and the mammary gland. This means that priming at one site will permit antibodies to be synthesized and secondary responses to occur at sites remote from the priming site.

The movement of IgA-secreting B cells from the intestine to the mammary gland is of major importance, since it provides a route by which intestinal immunity can be transferred to the newborn through milk. Oral administration of antigen to a pregnant animal will result in the appearance of IgA antibodies in its milk. In this way, the intestine of the newborn animal will be flooded by antibodies directed against intestinal pathogens. T cells originating within the Peyer's patches also tend to home specifically to the intestinal mucosa.

Immunity in the Gastrointestinal Tract

The gastrointestinal tract is probably the major site of antigenic stimulation in animals. The intestine contains, in total, more lymphoid tissue than the spleen. Antigenic particles, such as bacteria, can penetrate the intestinal mucosa relatively easily and, in this way, gain access to the lacteals and portal vessels. These organisms are subsequently trapped in the mesenteric lymph nodes and liver. Other antigens may enter the body via the surface lymphoid tissues. For instance, the tonsils are particularly vulnerable to invasion by microorganisms.

Tonsils possess a peculiar structural weakness in that their squamous epithelial covering is particularly thin at the bottom of the tonsillar crypts (Fig. 15–5). Viruses especially

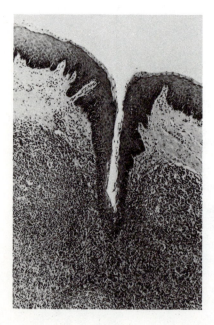

FIGURE 15–5. A section of tonsil showing a tonsilar crypt: Note how thin the epithelium is at the base of the crypt. An easy invasion route for many organisms (original magnification x150). (Specimen kindly provided by Dr. S. Yamashiro. From Tizard, I. Veterinary Immunology, 2nd ed. W. B. Saunders, Philadelphia, 1982. With permission.)

may enter the body by this route and multiply locally in the tonsil prior to the development of a viremia. Peyer's patches are covered with a specialized epithelium consisting of M cells. These M cells are capable of taking up antigen very efficiently. For example, they can engulf a whole bacterium and persent it to the lymphocytes in the Peyer's patches. The tonsils and Peyer's patches consist of relatively organized lymphoid tissues, possessing all the components required to mount an immune response—namely, T cells, helper cells, B cells, and macrophages. Nevertheless, most IgA is formed in diffuse lymphoid nodules and in isolated plasma cells found in the walls of the intestine, in salivary glands, and in the gall bladder (Fig. 15–3). If bacteria succeed in penetrating the intestinal wall, then, in the ensuing inflammatory response, capillary permeability will increase, and IgG will be free to diffuse from the bloodstream to the area of invasion. Thus, IgG may also act to protect body surfaces, but usually only secondarily to an inflammatory reaction.

It is difficult to confer prolonged protection against intestinal infection by using killed organisms as a vaccine. Oral vaccination, however, may be of some use if the vaccine contains live organisms capable of colonizing the gastrointestinal tract. For example, volunteers given live cholera organisms remain resistant for at least 5 or 6 yr.

Cell-mediated immune responses can also occur in the wall of the intestine. Lymphocytes with NK activity and capable of antibody-dependent cellular cytotoxicity (ADCC) for virus-infected cells may be readily found among the intestinal epithelial cells (Fig. 15–6). There has been a report that the protozoan parasite *Giardia lamblia* can be attacked by cytotoxic lymphocytes within the intestinal lumen.

Immunity in the Mammary Gland

The mammary gland is protected in nonspecific fashion by the physical barrier of the teat canal, by the flushing action of the milk, and by the presence of lactenins, of which the lactoperoxidase-thiocyanate system, lactoferrin, and lysozyme are probably the most important. In addition, milk contains IgA and IgG1 in low concentrations. In simple-stomached animals, IgA predominates, whereas in ruminants, the reverse is the case.

IgA is usually synthesized locally in the mammary gland. Many of these IgA-producing cells are derived from lymphoblasts originating in Peyer's patches and mesenteric

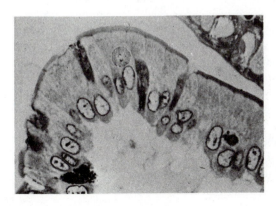

FIGURE 15–6. An intraepithelial lymphocyte: These small lymphocytes are probably important in mounting a cell-mediated immune response within the intestinal wall. (Courtesy of Dr. D. Befus.)

lymph nodes in late pregnancy and during lactation. Once these cells colonize the gland, they provide a local source of antibodies.

Human colostrum is commonly rich in macrophages and lymphocytes. These macrophages can process antigen, and their supernatants can enhance IgA production from blood lymphocytes. Milk lymphocytes are primarily T cells. They may survive for some time in the intestine of a suckling animal, but their significance is unclear.

Immunity in the Urogenital Tract

Antibodies of several classes, but particularly IgA, are found in cervicovaginal mucus, and a local immune response may be directed against organisms that cause infections of the cervix or vagina. The presence of agglutinating antibodies in vaginal mucus has been used as a diagnostic test for several infectious diseases of animals, such as trichomoniasis and brucellosis. (The local immune response to trichomoniasis is largely mediated by IgE; see Chap. 17.)

IgA is present in small amounts in normal urine, produced, presumably, by lymphoid tissues in the walls of the urinary tract. If, however, a kidney infection occurs, then IgG may also be found in relatively large amounts because of the breakdown in the glomerular barrier and defects in tubular reabsorption. Urinary IgA and IgG prevent colonization of the urinary tract by preventing bacterial adherence to epithelial cells.

Immunity in the Respiratory Tract

In addition to the tonsils, the respiratory tract possesses a considerable amount of lymphoid tissue in the form of nodules in the walls of the bronchi as well as lymphocytes distributed diffusely throughout the lung and the walls of the airways. The immunoglobulin synthesized in these tissues is mainly secretory IgA, particularly in the upper regions of the respiratory tract. In the bronchioles and alveoli, however, the secretions contain a relatively large amount of IgG, the concentration of which is intermediate between the levels in the trachea and in serum. IgE is also synthesized in significant amounts in the lymphoid tissues of the upper respiratory tract. As on other body surfaces, IgA in the respiratory tract is thought to protect by preventing adherence of antigenic particles, including microorganisms, whereas IgG is probably of major importance only when acute inflammation and transudation of serum protein occur. This situation will arise, for example, following a Type I hypersensitivity reaction mediated by locally produced IgE, and it is tempting to suggest that the combination of IgA and IgE synthesis at mucosal surfaces is, therefore, not entirely fortuitous. It is possible that these immunoglobulins work in concert, so that IgA produces a surface immunity serving to prevent antigen adherence and penetration. If, in spite of the presence of IgA, antigen gains access to the tissues, then the subsequent IgE-mediated hypersensitivity reaction may serve to increase vascular permeability and make available large quantities of potent IgG in the resulting fluid exudate.

Large numbers of cells may be washed out of the lungs by lavage with saline. These include alveolar macrophages and lymphocytes. The lymphocytes are largely T cells. It is possible to demonstrate the production of macrophage migration inhibition factor by these cells under experimental situations and to show alveolar macrophage activation following infection with *Listeria monocytogenes*. It is likely, therefore, that cell-mediated immune reactions may be readily invoked among the cells that exist within the lower respiratory tract.

Sources of Additional Information

Bienenstock, J., and Befus, A. D. Mucosal immunology. Immunology, *41*:249–270, 1980.

Brandtzaeg, P. Transport models for secretory IgA and secretory IgM. Clin. Exp. Immunol., *44*:221–232, 1981.

Crago, S. S., et al. Secretory component on epithelial cells is a surface receptor for polymeric immunoglobulin. J. Exp. Med., *147*:1832–1837, 1978.

Guy-Grand, D., Griscelli, C., and Vassalli, P. The mouse gut T lymphocyte: a novel type of cell. J. Exp. Med., *148*:1661–1677, 1978.

Husband, A. J., and Gowans, J. L. The origin and antigen-dependent distribution of IgA-containing cells in the intestine. J. Exp. Med., *148*:1146–1160, 1978.

Kaltreider, H. B. Expression of immune mechanisms in the lung. Am. Rev. Resp. Dis., *113*:347–397, 1976.

Lamm, M. E. Cellular aspects of immunoglobulin A. Adv. Immunol., *22*:223–290, 1976.

McDermott, M. R., Befus, A. D., and Bienenstock, J. The structural basis for immunity in the respiratory tract. Int. Rev. Exp. Path., *23*:47–112, 1982.

Orlans, E., et al. Rapid active transport of immunoglobulin A from blood to bile. J. Exp. Med., *147*:588–592, 1978.

Schrader, J. W., Scollary, R., and F. Battye. Intramucosal lymphocytes of the gut: Lyt-2 and Thy-1 phenotype of the granulated cells and evidence for the presence of both T cells and mast cell precursors. J. Immunol., *130*:558–564, 1983.

Tomasi, T. B., et al. Mucosal immunity: the origin and migration pattern of cells in the secretory system. J. Allerg. Clin. Immunol., *65*:12–19, 1980.

Tomasi, T. B., Jr. The immune system in secretions. Prentice Hall, Englewood Cliffs, N.J., 1976.

Walker, W. A., and Isselbacher, K. J. Intestinal antibodies. N. Engl. J. Med. *297*:767–773, 1977.

Woloschak, G. E., and Tomasi, T. B. The immunology and molecular biology of the gut-associated lymphoid tissue. CRC Crit. Rev. Immunol. *4*:1–18, 1983.

16

Vaccines and Vaccination

The observation that individuals who recovered from some infectious diseases were resistant to subsequent reinfection long preceded the development of the science of immunology and our understanding of the immune response. Indeed, it was the attempts made to reproduce this phenomenon in a controlled fashion by Jenner and Pasteur that provided the impetus for the early development of immunology. Their efforts to produce immunity by artificial exposure to infectious agents were so successful that many diseases, for long major scourges of mankind, were rapidly controlled. Vaccines were developed against smallpox, rabies, tetanus, anthrax, cholera, and diphtheria, and this success has been responsible in part for the recent phenomenal increase in the world's population. Fortunately, in many areas, these successes in the development of human vaccines have been matched by similar developments in the production of vaccines against animal diseases, thus expanding the food supply and at least slowing the widening of the gap between food supply and demand. In general, immunization procedures involve giving antigen derived from an infectious agent to an individual so that an immune response is mounted and resistance to that infectious agent is therefore stimulated. This is known as active immunization. Alternatively, preformed antibodies may be administered to a susceptible recipient in order to confer a transient but immediate state of immunity—a process called passive immunization.

Three criteria must first be satisfied in determining whether vaccination is either possible or desirable in controlling a specific disease. The first is the absolute identification of the causal organism. While this appears to be a very obvious requirement, it has not always been followed in practice, at least in some diseases of domestic animals.

Second, it must be established that an immune response can, in fact, protect against the disease in question—one reason why smallpox vaccine must never be used to treat recurrent herpes infections or warts. Other examples of nonprotective immune responses are seen in the virus disease of horses, equine infectious anemia, and in the parvovirus disease of mink, Aleutian disease, in which the immune response itself is responsible for many of the disease processes and vaccination therefore increases its severity.

Finally, vaccination is not without some disadvantages. Before using any vaccine, one must be absolutely certain that the risks involved do not exceed those due to the chance of contracting the disease itself. Smallpox has been eradicated globally since Oct. 26, 1977. Since smallpox vaccination may cause encephalitis, disseminated vaccinia, or eczema with a significant mortality, there is now no possible reason whatsoever to give smallpox vaccine to normal individuals.

More recently, there has been a considerable debate on the risks of *Bordetella pertussis* vaccination relative to the hazards of whooping cough. Vaccination reduces the number of cases about seventyfold, while reducing deaths fourfold. On the other hand, vaccination induces about twice as many cases of encephalitis as does the natural disease (5.0 cases/million of postvaccinal encephalitis as compared with 2.5 cases/million postinfection encephalitis). Clearly, the relative benefits of this vaccination must be carefully analyzed.

Types of Immunization Procedures

Passive immunization and active immunization are the two methods by which an individual can be rendered resistant to an infectious agent. Passive immunization produces a temporary resistance by transferring antibodies from a resistant to a susceptible individual. These passively transferred antibodies give immediate protection, but, since they are gradually catabolized, this protection wanes, and the recipient eventually becomes susceptible to infection once again (Fig. 16–1).

Active immunization has several advantages over passive immunization. This technique involves administering antigen to individuals so that they respond by mounting a protective immune response. Reimmunization or exposure to the infectious agent will result in a secondary immune response. The major disadvantage of this form of response is that the protection conferred is not immediate. Its advantage is that it is long-lasting and capable of restimulation.

Passive Immunization

Passive immunization requires that antibodies be produced in a donor by active immunization and that these antibodies, after purification, be given to susceptible recipients in order to confer immediate protection. These antibodies may be raised in animals of any species and against a wide variety of pathogens. For example, they can be produced in man against measles or hepatitis, in horses against tetanus, and in dogs against canine distemper.

One of the most important passive immunization procedures has been the protection of man and animals against the toxigenic organism *Clostridium tetani* by means of antisera raised in horses. Antibodies made in this way are known as antitoxins and were produced in young horses by a series of immunizing inoculations. The toxins of the Clostridia are proteins, and they can be rendered nontoxic by denaturation with formaldehyde. Formaldehyde-treated toxins are known as toxoids. Initially, the horses were inoculated with tox-

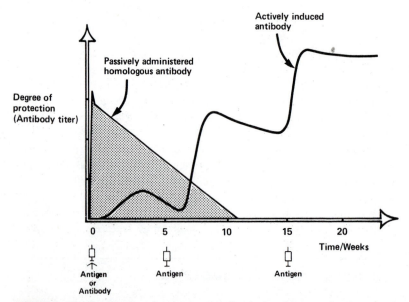

FIGURE 16–1. The levels of serum antibody (and hence the degree of protection) conferred by active and passive methods of immunization. (From Tizard, I. Veterinary Immunology, 2nd ed. W. B. Saunders, Philadelphia, 1982. With permission.)

oids, but once antibodies were produced, subsequent injections contained purified toxin. The responses of the horses were monitored—once their antibody levels were sufficiently high, the horses were bled. Bleeding was undertaken at regular intervals until the antibody levels dropped when the horses were again boosted with antigens. Plasma was separated from the horse blood and treated with ammonium sulfate to concentrate and purify the globulin fraction. This purified antibody preparation was then dialyzed, filtered, titrated, and dispensed.

This equine antiserum conferred prompt immunity to tetanus, but was not devoid of side effects. Horse tetanus antitoxin may indeed be given safely to horses, in which it is not regarded as foreign, and will persist for a relatively long period of time, being removed only by catabolism. If, however, this antiserum is given to an animal of another species, such as a human, then it is regarded as foreign, an immune response is mounted against it, and it is rapidly eliminated (Table 16–1). While it is not possible to completely destroy all the immunogenicity of the horse antibodies, it is usual to treat equine antitoxins with pepsin so as to destroy the immunoglobulin-Fc region and leave intact only the portion of the molecule required for toxin neutralization, the $F(ab')_2$ fragment.

If the amount of circulating horse immunoglobulin is relatively large when the recipient begins to produce antibodies, immune complexes form within the bloodstream. These may provoke a Type III hypersensitivity reaction known as serum sickness (Chap. 22). If repeated doses of horse antitoxin are given to an individual, a Type I hypersensitivity reaction, such as anaphylaxis, may occur (Chap. 20). Finally, the presence of high levels of circulating antibody may interfere with active immunization against the same antigen (Chap. 13). This is a phenomenon similar to that seen in newborn animals passively protected by maternal antibodies and reflects the negative feedback exerted by immunoglobulins on the B cell response.

In order to check the potency of preparations of antitoxin, comparison must be made with an international biological standard. In the case of tetanus antitoxin, this is done by comparing the dose necessary to protect guinea pigs against a fixed dose of tetanus toxin, with the dose of the standard preparation of antitoxin required to do the same. Alternatively, the potency of an antitoxin can be measured by estimating its ability to flocculate a fixed amount of toxin as compared with the standard antitoxin. This technique measures the ability of the antitoxin to combine with toxin and has some advantages, since toxins are relatively unstable and their intrinsic toxicity may fluctuate while their antigenicity remains constant. The international standard antiserum for tetanus toxin is a quantity held at the State Serum-Institute in Copenhagen. An international unit (IU) of tetanus antitoxin is the specific neutralizing activity contained in 0.03384 mg of the international standard.

About 250 units of antitoxin are normally given to humans to confer immediate protection against tetanus, although the exact amount should vary with the severity of tissue damage, the degree of wound contamination, and the time elapsed since injury. About

TABLE 16–1 The Adverse Consequences of Passive Immunization

Short-lived immunity
Serum sickness
Suppression of active immunization
Anaphylaxis

10,000 units may be given to individuals with clinical tetanus in an attempt to bind free toxin and hasten recovery, although this procedure is not very effective.

Because of the problems encountered when equine antiserum is used in humans, it is preferable to use antiserum of human origin wherever possible. This human immune serum globulin is commonly obtained from convalescent donors. It is usually purified and concentrated. Its potency, however, may be rather variable. Other common passive immunizing agents used in humans include antisera against measles, hepatitis A and B, rubella, varicella, rabies, vaccinia (smallpox), diptheria, tetanus, and botulism (Table 16–2).

Measles immune serum globulin (ISG) is commonly given to susceptible contacts of infected individuals in order to prevent the disease or, alternatively, to immunodeficient individuals who may not be able to mount an active immune response. Hepatitis-A ISG can be used for postexposure prophylaxis to individuals who run the risk of exposure to this disease either through their occupation or area of residence. Hepatitis-B ISG is used for immediate protection of individuals exposed to this disease through accidental skin puncture with a contaminated needle or exposure to infected blood or body fluids. Rubella ISG may be given to susceptible pregnant women who have been exposed to rubella but whose pregnancy is not terminated.

Varicella immune globulin is of use in immunosuppressed children—e.g., leukemia patients—exposed to chicken pox. Rabies immune globulin either of human or equine origin is used in conjunction with postexposure prophylaxis of rabies. It is given in a divided dose, half intramuscularly and the remainder injected around the bite wound in an effort to establish an antibody barrier to the spread of the rabies virus.

Active Immunization

The most important advantages of active immunization as compared with passive protection are the prolonged duration of protection and the recall and boosting of this protective response by repeated injections of antigen.

The ideal vaccine to be used for active immunization should be cheap, stable, and adaptable to mass vaccination. It should give prolonged strong immunity with an absence of adverse side effects and ideally stimulate an immune response distinguishable from that due to natural infection so that vaccination does not interfere with diagnosis.

TABLE 16–2 Passive Immunizing Agents Used in Humans

Disease	Origin	Use
Measles	Human	Postexposure
Hepatitis A	Human	Postexposure, Preexposure
Hepatitis B	Human	Postexposure
Rubella	Human	Postexposure
Varicella	Human	Prophylaxis in immunosuppressed individuals
Botulism	Equine	Postexposure and treatment
Diphtheria	Equine	Postexposure
Rabies	Human or equine	Postexposure
Tetanus	Human or equine	Postexposure and treatment
Vaccinia	Human	Treatment of complications of vaccination

It is most important that vaccines be free of adverse side effects. This clearly precludes the use of virulent living organisms. Remember, however, that this was the method first used by the Chinese in vaccinating against smallpox (Chap. 1). The Chinese reduced the hazards of vaccination by selecting the smallpox scabs from the mildest cases available. Nevertheless, the procedure was still hazardous until Jenner reported on the use of the relatively avirulent cowpox. Unfortunately, not all infectious agents have a readily available avirulent counterpart. For this reason, if living organisms must be used in a vaccine, they have to be treated in such a way that they lose their disease-producing ability. The term used for this loss of virulence is **attenuation.**

The commonly used methods of attenuation involve adapting organisms to unusual environmental conditions so that they lose the ability to replicate extensively in their usual host. For example, the Bacille Calmette-Guerin (BCG) strain of *Mycobacterium bovis* was rendered avirulent by growing it for 13 years on a bile-saturated medium. At the end of that time, the organisms had adapted well to growing in bile, but had lost the ability to grow and cause disease in humans. BCG is used as a vaccine against tuberculosis. A similar situation occurred in Pasteur's original fowl-cholera experiments (Chap. 1), in which the organism was grown under conditions where there was a shortage of nutrients and, as a result, lost its ability to cause disease in chickens.

While bacteria may be attenuated by growth in abnormal culture conditions, a similar process can be undertaken with viruses. Prolonged tissue culture, especially in cells of a species that the virus does not normally infect, has the effect of reducing the virulence of viruses. Thus, attenuated living poliovirus vaccine contains viruses grown in monkey-tissue culture. Rubella virus vaccine may contain virus prepared in duck-embryo cells.

As an alternative to growth in tissue culture, some viruses may be attenuated by growth in eggs. These include the 17D strain of yellow fever and strains of canine distemper virus used for vaccination of dogs. One interesting method of attenuation is to adapt the virus to growth at slightly lower temperatures than normal. Thus, the vaccine against the herpes virus responsible for infectious bovine rhinotracheitis uses a temperature-sensitive mutant. This vaccine is given intranasally to cattle so that the temperature-sensitive organism can replicate within the relatively cool nasal mucosa. It cannot spread within the body, however, and so cause disease, because the body temperature is too high.

Attenuation of organisms for use in vaccines has both advantages and disadvantages. In general, vaccines containing living organisms are very effective and give prolonged strong immunity. Because in effect, they cause transient infection of the vaccinee, only a few inoculating doses are required and adjuvant need not be employed—as a result, there is less chance of provoking adverse hypersensitivity reactions. In addition, live virus vaccines may provoke a rapid protective response through stimulation of interferon production.

On the other hand, live vaccines may be difficult and expensive to produce. There exists the possibility that they may contain dangerous extraneous organisms and, more important, cause disease as a result of either residual virulence (i.e., they may not be fully attentuated) or of reversion to a more virulent form.

In order to avoid these disadvantages, it is commonly necessary to use organisms that have been killed or inactivated. In such cases, it is desirable that the "dead" organisms be as antigenically similar to the living organisms as possible. Therefore, a crude method of killing microorganisms, such as heating, which causes extensive protein denaturation, tends to be unsatisfactory.

If chemical inactivation is to be used, it is essential that the chemicals produce little change in the antigens responsible for protective immunity. One commonly used inactivating compound is formaldehyde, which acts on amino and amide groups of proteins and on free amino groups in purines and pyrimidines to form cross-links and thus confer structural rigidity. Alkylating agents that cross-link nucleic acid chains are quite suitable for killing organisms, since, by leaving the surface proteins of organisms unmodified, they do not interfere with antigenicity. Examples of such alkylating agents include ethylene oxide, ethyleneimine, acetylethyleneimine, and B. propiolactone.

The advantages and disadvantages of vaccines containing living or "dead" organisms may be seen in the vaccines used against poliomyelitis (Table 16–3).

Live oral poliovirus vaccines contain a mixture of three strains of attentuated poliovirus (Types 1, 2, and 3) grown in monkey kidney epithelial cells. The vaccine is administered orally as a liquid generally dropped onto a sugar cube. As a result, the vaccine strains colonize the intestine and provoke an immune response similar to that induced by natural infection by poliovirus. This response includes the production of secretory antibodies in the intestine as well as serum antibodies. Consequently, the vaccine produces a very long-lasting humoral and intestinal immunity, thus reducing the need for repeated boosters. The administration of the vaccine is very simple and does not require trained personnel, while the vaccine itself is relatively cheap and can be grown on human cells, thus reducing the need to use increasingly rare and precious monkeys. On the other hand, since oral poliovaccination results in infection of recipients, the vaccine virus may spread to household contacts and nonvaccinees. If the vaccinee is already carrying a population of other enteroviruses, a common situation in underdeveloped tropical countries, then viral interference may prevent colonization by the polio vaccine virus.

As with many live-virus vaccines, there is a very slight risk that the vaccine virus may cause disease. It has been estimated that the rate of paralytic disease in vaccine recipients

TABLE 16–3   The Relative Merits of Living and Inactivated Poliovirus Vaccines

Advantages of Inactivated Vaccine	Advantages of Live Vaccine
Produces humoral immunity	Humoral and intestinal immunity
May be incorporated into other vaccines	Rapid onset of protection No chance that surviving traces of virulent virus will cause infection.
Will not revert to virulent form	Easy to administer
May be used in immunodeficient individuals	Blocks intestinal spread
May be used in tropical countries	Cheaper than inactivated
Will not spread	More people get the full course since few boosters are required

is about 1 case in 4 million doses of vaccine distributed, although in contacts of vaccine recipients, there is about 1 case of paralytic poliomyelitis in 2 million doses of vaccine distributed. This oral poliovirus vaccine is, of course, contraindicated in immunodeficient recipients.

The advantages of killed poliovirus vaccines effectively reflect the disadvantages of oral poliovirus vaccines. Thus, killed polio vaccine can be readily incorporated with other injectable vaccines as part of a single vaccination program. This method is, of course, very safe in that there is no chance of reversion to a virulent form provided it is properly inactivated. It also can be used in tropical areas where other enteroviruses interfere with the live vaccine. It is perfectly safe for immunodeficient individuals.

On the other hand, in order to get a good protective response, multiple booster injections are required and individuals must return for boosters at regular intervals. Killed poliovirus vaccine will not prevent intestinal colonization by wild-type virus, since it will not provoke local immunity. Finally, since it must be injected, it must be very pure and, because it is grown in monkey cells, it is costly.

As stated previously, one notable feature of the use of oral polio vaccine is that the vaccine virus may spread to and infect individuals other than the vaccinee. In some respects this may be considered to be an advantage since these contacts are protected in turn and the overall protected status of the population is thereby enhanced. On the other hand, the seeding of human population with poliovirus vaccine in this way can provide a potential opportunity for the vaccine virus to revert to the wild type and occasionally, therefore, cause paralytic poliomyelitis.

Thus, both types of vaccine have risks and benefits. The final choice as to which one to use must be made only in conjunction with an assessment of local conditions and requirements.

Subunit Vaccines

In the search for effective vaccines, much attention has been given to the elimination of unwanted antigenic material. Viruses grown in tissue culture or bacteria grown in culture fluid commonly contain culture-fluid components. These must be removed and, indeed, the inevitable end point of this purification process is the isolation of the individual antigens within an organism that can provoke a protective immune response (Table 16-4).

In the case of bacteria, this procedure is usually relatively simple. The most obvious examples are the vaccines against diphtheria and tetanus, which utilize not the whole bacterium but a purified preparation of its exotoxin detoxified by treatment with formaldehyde. These bacterial toxoids have proved to be excellent and effective immunizing agents.

Vaccines against bacterial meningitis contain purified bacterial cell-wall polysaccharides against two types of *Neisseria meningitidis*—groups A and C. Antipneumococcal vaccine usually contains a mixture of purified polysaccharides from each of 14 different types of *Streptococcus pneumoniae* (Types 1, 2, 3, 4, 6A, 7F, 8, 9N, 12F, 14, 18C, 19F, 23F, and 25). These are known to cause 68% of pneumococcal pneumonia in the United States. The vaccine also prevents a further 17% of cases through antigenic cross-reactivity. Some strains of *E. coli* that cause enteric disease of animals attach to the intestinal wall by means of specialized attachment pili. Vaccines enriched with these attachment pili are able to reduce the severity of disease caused by pilus-bearing strains. Over the past 15 years, many

TABLE 16–4   Some Subunit Vaccines Used in Man and Animals

Vaccine	Subunit
Bacterial	
Tetanus	
Botulism	Toxin
Diphtheria	
S. pneumoniae	Capsular polysaccharide
Meningococci	Capsular polysaccharide
E. coli	Adherence pili
Viruses	
Rabies	Capsid proteins
Foot-and-mouth virus	
Influenza	
Hepatitis B	Synthetic capsid antigenic determinants
Foot-and-mouth virus	

studies have been conducted to investigate the protective effects of ribosomal preparations from bacteria. While the results have been very encouraging, none has been incorporated into a commercially available vaccine.

In contrast to the relative ease with which purified bacterial antigens may be obtained, viral subunits are difficult and expensive to produce and usually are not available in sufficient quantity for vaccination purposes.

In order to obtain purified viral antigen, recourse must, therefore, be made to DNA recombination technology. The first successful example of a vaccine produced in this way is directed against foot-and-mouth-disease virus. In this disease, the virus is extremely simple, the protective antigen (VP 3) is well recognized, and the viral genes that code for this antigen have been mapped (Fig. 16–2). The RNA genome of the foot-and-mouth disease virus has been isolated and duplicated into DNA by means of the enzyme reverse transcriptase. This DNA is then carefully cut by restriction endonucleases so that it only contains the gene for VP 3. The DNA is then inserted into an *E. coli* plasmid, the plasmid inserted into *E. coli,* and the *E. coli* grown. These bacteria commence to synthesize large quantities of VP 3 that may be harvested, purified, and incorporated into a vaccine. This technique is an effective method of isolating, in an economical fashion, sufficient quantities of viral antigen for use in a vaccine and may be very widely employed in future.

An alternative and much superior method of producing a subunit vaccine is to synthesize the protective antigen completely. This synthesis has been accomplished experimentally for hepatitis B, MS2 phage, diphtheria toxin, foot-and-mouth-disease virus, and influenza A. By knowing the complete amino-acid sequence of the major antigenic proteins of these organisms, it is possible to identify the sequences that are hydrophilic and thus most likely to be located on the surface of the molecule. It may be predicted that these sequences will function as antigenic determinants. When peptides containing these synthetic determinants are used to immunize animals, they provoke protective immunity. This technique clearly has a number of significant advantages over gene-splicing techniques, being, for example, much safer although rather more expensive.

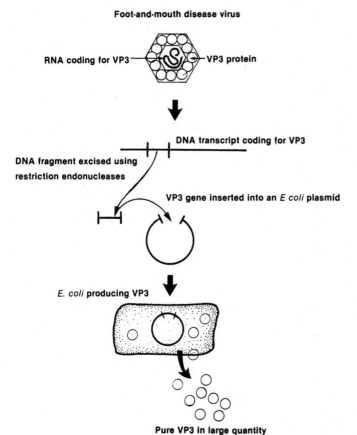

Foot-and-mouth disease virus

RNA coding for VP3 — VP3 protein

DNA transcript coding for VP3

DNA fragment excised using
restriction endonucleases

VP3 gene inserted into an *E coli* plasmid

E. coli producing VP3

Pure VP3 in large quantity

FIGURE 16–2. The production of large quantities of VP3 antigen from the foot-and-mouth disease virus by the use of gene-splicing techniques. The purified VP3 derived from bulk culture of *E. coli* may be used in a foot-and-mouth-disease vaccine.

The Use of Vaccines

Route of Administration

Most human and animal vaccines are designed to be administered by intramuscular or subcutaneous injection. Injections, however, are relatively time-consuming and painful and clearly bear a risk of carrying unwanted organisms into an individual. Thus, when very large numbers of people or animals must be vaccinated under less-than-ideal conditions, other methods of vaccination are employed. The use of a high-pressure jet injector can serve as a painless, sterile method of administering antigen.

Some antigens may be given orally—for example, poliomyelitis vaccine in humans. In the poultry industry, it is common to administer vaccines to very large flocks by incorporating the vaccine either in the feed or in the drinking water. An alternative method of mass vaccination used in veterinary medicine is to expose animals to a vaccine aerosol so that they will inhale the antigen. This technique is particularly useful for vaccines directed against diseases of the respiratory tract, since it provokes the production of local antibodies.

Adjuvants

In human vaccines, the only widely employed adjuvants are aluminum salts, especially aluminium phosphate (Table 16–5). In domestic animals, a wider variety of adjuvants are employed. The major restriction on adjuvants is that they should neither be toxic nor should they adversely affect the quality of the meat from an animal. Saponin, used in anthrax vaccine, is an exception to this rule, since it is required to cause local tissue damage and anaerobic conditions so that the anthrax spores in the vaccine may germinate.

Vaccination Schedules

It is not difficult to establish a simple immunization schedule to be followed as children grow up (Table 16–6). It may be modified as appropriate if vaccination is begun at a later age than normal. In addition, certain legal requirements such as the requirement that children must be vaccinated against measles before admission to school, will also influence the timing of vaccination schedules.

Since newborn animals are passively protected by maternal antibodies, it is sometimes difficult to successfully vaccinate them in early life. Thus, if measles vaccine is given to children before 12 months of age, it is necessary to give a second dose at about 15 months in order to ensure adequate protection. In dogs and cats, vaccines given before 10 weeks must be repeated at about 15 weeks while in cattle, sheep, pigs, and horses, any vaccine

TABLE 16–5   Active Immunizing Agents Used in Man

Disease	Vaccine Type	Adjuvant
Tuberculosis	Modified live (BCG)	None
Cholera	Bacterin	None
Diphtheria	Toxoid	Aluminium phosphate
Influenza	Inactivated vaccine	None
Measles	Modified live	None
Meningococcus	Polysaccharide	None
Mumps	Modified live	None
Pertussis	Bacterin	Aluminium phosphate
Plague	Bacterin	None
Pneumococcus	Polysaccharide	None
Poliomyelitis	Inactivated or modified live	None
Rabies	Inactivated	None
Rubella	Modified live	None
Staphylococcus	Toxoid	None
Tetanus	Toxoid	Aluminium phosphate
Typhoid	Bacterin	None
Typhus	Inactivated	None
Yellow fever	Modified live	None

TABLE 16-6 An Example of a Routine Immunization Schedule for Normal Infants and Children

Recommended Age	Vaccine*
2 months	DTP 1 OPV 1
4 months	DTP 2 OPV 2
6 months	DTP 3
15 months	MMR
18 months	DTP 4 OPV 3
4–6 yr	DTP 5 OPV 4
14–16 yr and repeated every 10 yr thereafter	DT

*DTP—Diphtheria toxoid, tetanus toxoid, and pertussis vaccine

OPV—Oral poliomyelitis vaccine containing types 1, 2, 3

MMR—Live measles mumps, and rubella in a single vaccine.

given before six months must be repeated. In domestic animals, if protection is required early in life, it may be possible to vaccinate the pregnant mother so that peak antibody levels may be achieved at the time of colostrum formation.

The interval between booster doses of vaccine varies, but, as a general rule, inactivated vaccines generally produce a weak immunity that requires frequent boosters, perhaps as often as every six months as in the case of cholera vaccine. On the other hand, live vaccines produce a much more persistent immunity—for example BCG vaccine does not require boosting, and yellow-fever vaccine requires a booster dose only every ten years.

Contraindications of Vaccination

The most important contraindications to vaccination involve the administration of live vaccines to immunodeficient or pregnant humans. Thus, it is critical that no live vaccine be given to patients with immunodeficiency diseases, patients with malignancies that will adversely affect immunity, such as leukemias and lymphomas, and patients undergoing immunosuppressive therapy.

While inactivated vaccines and toxoids may be given to pregnant women, live viral vaccines must not be given because of the potential risk to the developing fetus, particularly not measles and rubella vaccines. On the other hand, under conditions where the risk of disease is very high, as in yellow fever or poliomyelitis, the theoretical risk may be less important and the vaccine given to pregnant women.

Failures in Vaccination

The immune response, like other biological phenomena, never confers absolute protection and is never equal in all numbers of a vaccinated population. For example, since the immune response is influenced by a large number of factors, the range of immune responses in a large random population tends to follow a normal distribution (Figs. 16–3 and 16–4).

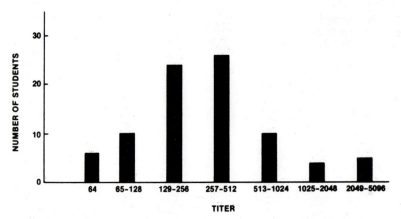

FIGURE 16-3. The distribution of antibody titers to rabies in 120 recently vaccinated students. A small number produce a fairly poor response and, hence, will be poorly protected. Similarly, a few will generate a very good response (titers > 2049) and will be well protected.

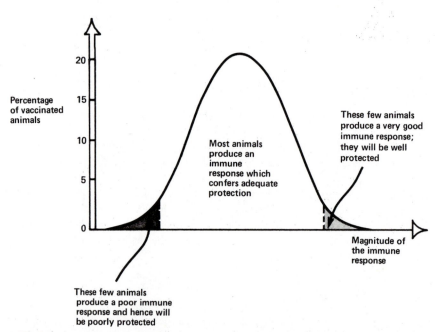

FIGURE 16-4. The hypothetical normal distribution of immune responses in a population of vaccinated individuals. (From Tizard, I. Veterinary Immunology, 2nd ed. W. B. Saunders, Philadelphia, 1982. With permission.)

This means that, while most individuals respond to a vaccine by mounting an average immune response, a small proportion will mount a very poor immune response. This group may not be protected against disease in spite of vaccination. It is, therefore, highly improbable that 100% of a random population will be protected by vaccination. The size of this unreactive portion of the population will vary with the type of vaccine employed and the number of booster doses given. Its significance will also vary. Thus, for any individual, the lack of protection is, of course, serious. It may well be, however, that, from a public health viewpoint, less than 100% protection may be quite satisfactory if it prevents the spread of disease within the population. This phenomenon is known as herd immunity and its effect is due to the reduced probability of a susceptible individual encountering an infected one.

A second type of apparent vaccine failure can occur when the immune response is depressed. As mentioned earlier, this effect may be due to clinical immunosuppression, or it may be due to a high stress situation. Thus extremes of cold and heat or malnourishment may all inhibit the immune response.

The third major group of vaccine failures may be due to the possibility that the individual was incubating the disease prior to vaccination, or to the death of a supposedly live vaccine as a result of inadequate storage or the excessive use of alcohol while swabbing the skin, a procedure that may inactivate a virus vaccine (Table 16–7).

Adverse Consequences of Vaccination

Residual virulence, toxicity, and allergic reactions are perhaps the three most important groups of problems associated with the use of vaccines (Table 16–8). Thus, a mild measles rash may be seen in some children vaccinated against measles. Vaccines containing whole killed Gram-negative bacteria, such as the cholera and typhoid vaccines, may be intrinsically toxic owing to the presence of endotoxins. These endotoxins may cause soreness, fever, malaise, and headache. Influenza vaccines also commonly cause fever, malaise, and myalgia (muscle pain). In an attempt to reduce these symptoms, it is possible to treat the influenza virus preparation with detergents that cause its disruption and reduce the prevalence of side effects. Unfortunately, this preparation is slightly less immunogenic than the untreated vaccine. Some of the older rabies vaccines, especially those produced in duck embryos, commonly caused severe systemic toxic reactions. The newer rabies vaccines that utilize hamster kidney cells or the vaccines grown in human diploid fibroblast cultures are much less toxic.

Like any antigen, vaccine preparations have the ability to provoke hypersensitivity reactions. Thus, a Type I immediate hypersensitivity can occur not only in response to the

TABLE 16–7   Reasons for Vaccine Failure

Ineffective vaccine	Death of supposedly living vaccine
	Wrong strain of organism employed
	Inadequate vaccine
Failure in the immune response	Genetically unresponsive individual
	Immunosuppressed individual
	Passively immunized individual
Apparent vaccine failure	Individual incubating the disease

TABLE 16–8 Some of the Adverse Consequences of Active Immunization

Mechanism	Effect
Toxicity	Fever
	Pain
	Leukopenia
Residual virulence	Mild disease
Type I hypersensitivity	Anaphylaxis
	Urticaria
Type III hypersensitivity	Purpura
	Serum sickness
Type IV hypersensitivity	Granuloma formation
Autoimmunity	Guillain-Barré syndrome
	Encephalitis

organisms but also to some of the contaminating antigens, such as egg proteins in measles, mumps, influenza, rabies or yellow-fever vaccines. Some vaccines may contain trace amounts of antibiotics, for example, neomycin, and should not be given to patients with a history of allergy to this drug. As with other types of hypersensitivity, this type of reaction is more commonly associated with multiple injections of antigen and is, therefore, associated with the use of dead vaccines.

Epinephrine (Chap. 20) should always be immediately available when vaccines are injected in order to treat the occasional case of anaphylaxis that may occur.

Type III and Type IV hypersensitivity reactions (Chap. 22 and 23) are potential problems that may appear, for example, as local Arthus reaction developing 2 to 8 hours after injection. This reaction seems to be a particular problem following pneumococcal vaccination.

Under some circumstances, autoimmune disorders may be provoked by vaccination. For example, an allergic encephalitis may be provoked by the use of vaccines, such as the rabies vaccines, which contain central-nervous tissue. An idiopathic polyneuritis (Guillain-Barré syndrome) has been associated with the use of certain virus vaccines (most notably swine influenza). This is a self-limiting paralytic syndrome that occurred in about ten persons per/million vaccinated with swine flu in 1976. Of those affected, 5 to 10% have some residual weakness, and about 5 percent may die.

Mixing of Vaccines

It is obviously advantageous if two or more vaccines can be given to an individual simultaneously, but there are certain problems associated with this method. First, adverse reactions may be additive. Alternatively, completion or interference between antigens may prevent optimal responses from occurring to all the components in the mixture. For this reason, only commercially prepared mixtures should be employed. It is, of course, essential that live and inactivated vaccines should not be mixed in the same syringe, since the preservative in the inactivated vaccine may effectively inactivate the live vaccine. Similarly, live virus vaccines should not be administered within six weeks of a patient receiving immune globulins. Commonly employed vaccine mixtures used in humans include diphtheria, pertussis, and tetanus (DPT), and measles, mumps, rubella. In animals, very complex mixtures can be used, containing up to six different immunizing organisms.

Sources of Additional Information

Clancy, R. L., et al. Specific immune response in the respiratory tract after administration of an oral polyvalent bacterial vaccine. Inf. Immunol. *39:*491–496, 1983.

Dick, G. Immunization. Update Books, London/New Jersey, 1978.

Hennessen, W., and Huygelen, C., eds. Immunization benefits versus risk factors. Dev. Biol. Stand., *43:*1–476, 1979.

Hilleman, M. R., et al. Polyvalent pneumococcal polysaccharide vaccines. Bull. WHO *56:*371–375, 1978.

Horstmann, D. M. Control of poliomyelitis: a continuing paradox. J. Inf. Dis., *146:*540–549, 1982.

Lerner, R. A. Synthetic vaccines. Sci. Am., *248:*66–74, 1983.

Symposium. Advances in the application of attenuated and killed vaccines. Am. J. Clin. Pathol. *70:*113–196, 1978.

17

Immunity to Infection

As pointed out at the beginning of this book, the animal body must defend itself from two major groups of pathogens. The first group are the pathogens that arise outside the body. These are, of course, the bacteria, viruses, fungi, protozoa, and helminths, which can invade the body and cause disease. The second group are the abnormal cells that arise within the body—these include virus-infected and chemically modified cells as well as cancer cells.

While this is very arbitrary classification, it provides a simple basis for the major division of the immune system into the antibody-mediated and cell-mediated branches. Thus, antibodies are primarily involved in immunity to free infectious agents, while the cell-mediated immune responses are directed against cell-associated antigens.

Mechanisms of Antibacterial Resistance

While immunologists tend to be preoccupied with the specific cell- and antibody-mediated immune responses, it must be pointed out that these represent only a portion of the defenses available to the animal body. Three general types of protection can, in fact, be identified. First, there is resistance as a result of species insusceptibility. Examples of this include *Neisseria gonorrhoea,* which will grow well only in man despite its relatively simple in vitro growth requirements, or *B. abortus,* an important mammalian pathogen, which is unable to infect chickens. The second type of protection is due to the presence of nonimmunological inhibitory substances, and the third type is mediated by the specific immune responses. The specific immune responses are probably the most important of these protective mechanisms, as is demonstrated by the inevitably fatal consequences of a failure to develop a functioning immune system (Chap. 18).

General Factors Influencing Resistance

The most important of the general factors that influence disease resistance are genetic. Under natural conditions, disease is but one of the selective pressures to act on a population. The spread of disease through such a population may therefore eliminate all susceptible animals but leave a resistant residue to multiply and make use of the newly available resources, such as food. The genetic factors that influence resistance in this way are many and complex. Some of the most important may include immune-response genes and genes that influence macrophage activity.

A second group of nonspecific factors that influence disease resistance are hormonal. Age-related resistance is, in many cases, under hormonal influence. Thus thyroxine, low doses of steriods, and estrogens may stimulate the immune response, while high doses of steroids, testosterone, and progesterone are immunosuppressive. In heavily stressed individuals, increased steroid production may be immunosuppressive and so help to precipitate disease.

The last group of the major nonspecific factors that influence disease resistance are nutritional. Severe malnutrition, specifically protein deficiency, may impair immunoglobulin production (perhaps through a stress mechanism). The negative protein balance incurred in heavily parasitized animals may also have an adverse effect on the immune response. It is of interest to note, however, that mild protein–calorie deficiency may enhance immune responsiveness. The stressful effect of surgery may also be magnified by the increase in protein catabolism, which occurs following surgical intervention and results in a temporary immunosuppression.

Specific Chemical Factors Contributing to Resistance

Convincing evidence for the ability of animal tissues to discourage bacterial invasion is readily available when we consider the relative infrequency of bacterial infections as a consequence of minor skin wounds. Some of this resistance is due to the presence of potent antibacterial factors in tissues (Table 17–1), perhaps the most important of which is lysozyme, a bactericidal enzyme first recognized by Sir Alexander Fleming, the discoverer of penicillin. Lysozyme is found in tissues and in all body fluids with the exception of cerebrospinal fluid, sweat, and urine. It is found in particularly high concentrations in tears and egg white. Lysozyme splits the acylaminopolysaccharides of the cell walls of some Gram-positive bacteria so killing them, and it is also capable of participating in the destruction of some Gram-negative organisms in conjunction with complement (Fig. 17–1). While many of the bacteria killed by lysozyme are considered to be nonpathogenic, it might reasonably be pointed out that this susceptibility could account for their lack of pathogenicity. Lysozyme is found in very high concentrations in the lysosomes of neutrophils, and so tends to accumulate in areas of acute inflammation, including sites of bacterial invasion. The pH optimum for lysozyme activity, although somewhat low (pH3 to pH6), is easily achieved in these areas as well as within phagosomes, and, as a consequence, it is here that its antibacterial activity is largely exerted. Finally, lysozyme may act as a potent opsonin, facilitating phagocytosis in the absence of specific antibodies and under conditions in which its enzymic activity may be ineffective.

The observation that kidneys remain relatively unaffected in tuberculosis led to the isolation of two tetra-amines called spermine and spermidine, which, in conjunction with

TABLE 17–1   Some Nonimmunological Protective Factors Found in Body Tissues and Fluids

Group	Name	Major Sources	Activity Against
Enzymes	Lysozyme	Serum; leukocytes	Gram-positive and -negative bacteria; some viruses
Basic peptides and proteins	β-Lysin	Platelets	Gram-positive bacteria
	Phagocytin	Neutrophils	
	Leukin	Neutrophils	
	Plakin	Platelets	
Iron binding proteins	Tranferrrin	Serum	Gram-positive and -negative bacteria
	Lactoferrin	Leukocytes; milk	
Basic amines	Spermine; spermidine	Pancreas; kidney; prostate	Gram-positive bacteria
Complement components	—	Serum	Bacteria; viruses; protozoa
Peroxide splitting mechanisms	Myeloperoxidase; xanthine oxidase	Neutrophils; milk	Bacteria; viruses; protozoa
Interferon	—	Most cells but not neutrophils	Viruses; some intracellular protozoa

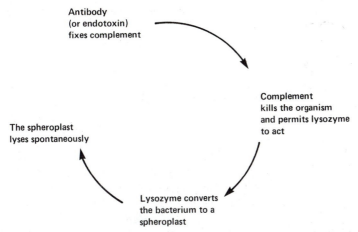

FIGURE 17–1. The interaction between complement and lysozyme that causes lysis of Gram-negative bacteria. (From Tizard, I. Veterinary Immunology, 2nd ed. W. B. Saunders, Philadelphia, 1982. With permission.)

a serum α globulin, form a bactericidal complex active against acid-fast organisms, cocci, and *Bacillus anthracis*.

Free fatty acids are also inhibitory to bacterial growth under some circumstances. In general, unsaturated fatty acids, such as oleic acid, tend to be bactericidal for Gram-positive organisms, while saturated fatty acids are fungicidal. Because of this, scalp ringworm of children, which is somewhat refractory to conventional medical treatment, may resolve spontaneously at puberty when the amount of saturated fatty acids in sebum increases.

A number of peptides and proteins rich in basic amino acids (lysine and arginine) and with potent antibacterial properties, have been isolated from mammalian cells and tissues. They are commonly derived from proteins digested as a result of the release of proteolytic enzymes from neutrophils or platelets. β lysin, a polypeptide active against *Bacillus anthracis* and the clostridia, is released from platelets as a result of their interaction with immune complexes.

One of the most important factors that influence the success or failure of bacterial invasion is the level of iron in body fluids. Most bacteria such as *Staphylococcus aureus*, *E. coli*, *Pasteurella multocida* and *Mycobacterium tuberculosis* require iron for growth. Within the body, however, iron is largely associated with the iron-binding proteins transferrin, lactoferrin, haptoglobin, and ferritin. In addition, serum iron levels tend to drop following bacterial invasion as a result of cessation of intestinal iron absorption and increased production of haptoglobin by the liver. The result of this action is to effectively hinder bacterial invasion. A similar situation occurs in the mammary gland when, in response to bacterial invasion, neutrophils release their stores of lactoferrin and, in this way, enhance the bactericidal power of milk. In spite of the sequestration of iron, some bacteria, such as *Mycobacterium tuberculosis* and *E. coli* succeed in invading the body because they can release potent iron chelating compounds called "siderophores" (mycobactin and enterochelin respectively). These siderophores have such a high affinity for iron that they can withdraw it from the serum proteins and render it available to the bacteria. In conditions in which serum iron levels are elevated, such as the hemolytic anemias, animals may become extremely susceptible to bacterial infection.

Peroxide-generating mechanisms, which are important in neutrophils and in milk, have been discussed elsewhere (Chap. 4 and Chap. 15).

Specific Resistance to Bacterial Disease Mediated by the Immune System

There are four basic mechanisms by which the specific immune responses combat bacterial infections (Table 17–2). These are (1) the neutralization of toxins or enzymes by antibody; (2) the killing of bacteria by antibodies, complement, and lysozyme; (3) the opsonization of bacteria by antibody (and complement), which results in phagocytosis and destruction of bacteria; and (4) the phagocytosis and intracellular destruction of bacteria by activated macrophages. The relative importance of each of these processes depends upon the organisms involved and the mechanisms by which they cause disease.

Immunity to Exotoxigenic Organisms

In diseases caused by exotoxigenic organisms such as the clostridia or *B. anthracis,* the function of the immune response must be not only to eliminate the invading organisms, but also to neutralize any toxin produced by them. Unfortunately, destruction of these bacteria may be quite difficult, especially if they are embedded in a mass of necrotic (dead) tissue. Nevertheless, antibodies can readily neutralize bacterial exotoxins. It is thought that neutralization occurs as a result of blocking of the combination between the toxin and its receptor on a host cell. IgG is the immunoglobulin almost totally responsible for toxin neutralization since IgM usually has insufficient avidity. The neutralization process, therefore, involves competition between receptor and antibody for the toxin molecule, and it is apparent that once the toxin has combined with the receptor, antibody will be relatively ineffective in reversing this combination. This result is observed in practice when the dose of antitoxin required to produce clinical improvement in a disease such as tetanus is greatly in excess of that required to prevent the development of clinical disease.

Immunity to Systemically Invasive Organisms

Protection against invasive bacteria is generally mediated by antibodies directed against their surface antigens. Antibodies against antigens in the interior of these organisms, such as ribonucleoprotein or enzymes,

TABLE 17–2   A Classification of the Immunologoical Mechanisms of Antibacterial Immunity

Components of the Immune Systems Employed	Bacterial Antigen	Result
Antibody with complement (and lysozyme)	Bacterial surface antigens	1. Bacteriolysis 2. Phagocytosis
Antibody (alone)	Protein toxins or enzymes	Toxin or enzyme neutralization
Activated macrophages	Possibly bacterial ribonucleoprotein	Intracellular destruction of organism

are consequently of only limited usefulness in protection (although bacterial ribonucleo-protein may have a significant role to play in the development of cell-mediated immunity).

Antibody directed against capsular (K) antigens may serve to neutralize the anti-phagocytic properties of the capsule, so opsonizing the organisms and permitting bacterial destruction by phagocytic cells to take place. In organisms lacking capsules, antibodies directed against somatic (O) antigens may serve a similar function. The precise fate of many organisms is dependent upon the immunoglobulin class involved and whether complement is activated. Thus, IgG is commonly a much more effective opsonin than IgM in the absence of complement. IgM, however, is much more effective at activating complement than IgG and thus is the most effective opsonin in the presence of complement.

While some bacteria are phagocytosed and destroyed by neutrophils or macrophages, others may be killed while they are still free in the circulation. The bactericidal activity of serum is mediated by antibodies, complement, and lysozyme. Together, antibodies and complement can cause the development of cell-wall lesions similar to those seen by electron microscopy of complement-lysed red cells. By itself, however, this lesion seems to be insufficient to kill many Gram-negative bacteria. Moreover, the action of complement on bacteria appears to reveal a substrate for lysozyme, and this enzyme, therefore, acts on the bacterial cell membrane following complement activity and so produces bacteriolysis (Fig. 17–1). Gram-negative organisms may activate the alternate complement pathway as a result of inhibition of factor-H activity, or alternatively, in some cases, may directly activate the classical pathway as a result of the interaction between lipid A and C1q. Complement may, therefore, act in the absence of antibody.

On a molar basis, IgM is about 500 to 1000 times more efficient than IgG in opsonization in the presence of complement and about 100 times more potent than IgG in sensitizing bacteria for complement-mediated lysis. Therefore, during a primary immune response, the quantitative deficiency of the IgM response is compensated for by its quality, so ensuring early and efficient protection.

Immunity to Facultative Intracellular Parasites Certain organisms of major importance, particularly *Brucella, Mycobacteria, Listeria, Legionella,* some *Corynebacteria,* and the *Salmonellae,* are engulfed by macrophages but are resistant to subsequent intracellular destruction. These organisms (which are, therefore, "facultative" intracellular parasites) can replicate within macrophages in an environment free of antibody, and as a consequence, the normal humoral immune response is relatively ineffective (Fig. 17–2). In addition, protective immunity to these organisms cannot be satisfactorily induced by the use of vaccines composed of killed bacteria. Passively transferred antiserum will not confer protection, although passively transferred lymphocytes will (Table 17–3).

It appears, therefore, that protection against this type of bacterium is cell-mediated. While macrophages from unimmunized animals are normally incapable of destroying these organisms, this capacity is acquired by the macrophages of infected animals about ten days after onset of infection. The changes that occur in these activated macrophages include an increase in cell size, in metabolic activity, and in the size and number of their lysosomes (Fig. 12–6). These changes are reflected in a marked increase in the bactericidal capacity of the cells (see Fig. 12–5). The changes themselves are a reflection of a form of "acquired cell-mediated immunity," which is mediated through lymphokines released by sensitized T cells on exposure to bacterial antigens, possibly their ribonucleoprotein (Fig. 17–3). The

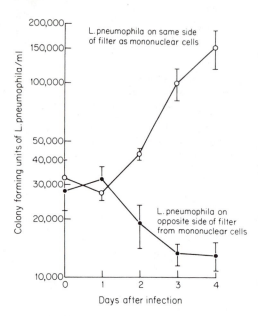

FIGURE 17-2. *Legionella pneumophilia* multiplies only when in direct contact with monocytes. The cultures were set up in paired culture separated by 0.05-μm pore filters. These filters permitted molecules but not the bacteria to pass. (Reproduced from *The Journal of Clinical Investigation,* 1980 Vol. 66, p. 441 by copyright permission of The American Society for Clinical Investigation. Courtesy of Dr. M. A. Horwitz.

How it was Shown that Lymphocytes were Needed for Immunity to Intracellular Bacteria

Mice were infected with a sublethal dose of *Listeria monocytogenes.* Once they developed immunity, they were killed and their serum and spleens removed. Normal syngeneic mice were then inoculated with either normal or immune living mouse spleen cells, normal or immune frozen (and thus dead) spleen cells, or normal or immune mouse serum, and challenged with virulent *L. monocytogenes* at the same time.

The results were as follows.

TABLE 17-3   Response to *L. monocytogenes*

Treatment	Deaths/Challenged
Control	9/10
Live normal cells (4 mouse equivalents)	6/10
Live immune cells (4 mouse equivalents)	0/10
Frozen immune cells (4 mouse equivalents)	10/10
Frozen normal cells (4 mouse equivalents)	9/10
Immune serum (0.2 ml)	19/19
Normal serum (0.2 ml)	19/20

Thus this form of immunity was only transferred by living spleen cells from immune animals.

Miki, K., and MacKaness, G. B. The passive transfer of acquired resistance to Listeria monocytogenes. *J. Exp. Med., 120: 93–103, 1964.*

response of these macrophages tends to be relatively nonspecific, particularly in *Listeria* infections, and these "activated" cells are therefore capable of destroying a wide range of normally resistant bacteria. Thus an animal recovering from an infection with *Listeria monocytogenes* shows increased resistance to infection by *Mycobacterium tuberculosis*. The development of these activated macrophages often coincides with the appearance of delayed (Type IV) hypersensitivity to intradermally administered antigen.

Modification of Bacterial Disease by the Immune Response

The development of an antibacterial immune response will, of course, have a profound influence on the course of infection. At its best this will result in a cure. In the absence of a curative response, however, the disease may be profoundly modified. Perhaps the most dramatic example of modification is observed in leprosy. Leprosy is classified as either tuberculoid or lepromatous (Table 17–4). Tuberculoid leprosy found in about 80% of infected individuals is associated with relatively high resistance on the part of the infected individual as a result of cell-mediated immune response to the leprosy bacillus. Thus, patients with tuberculoid leprosy have few organisms in their tissues and thus few lesions. The lesions are infiltrated with mononuclear cells and the patients give a positive delayed hypersensi-

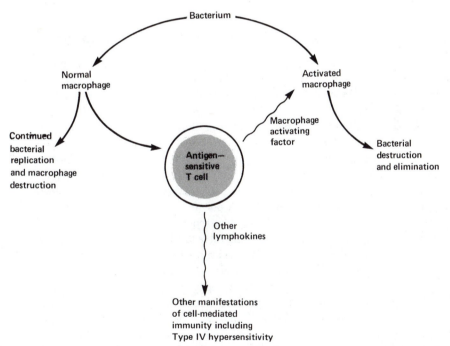

FIGURE 17–3. The principle of acquired cellular immunity to facultative intracellular parasites: Macrophages activated by T cells acquire the capacity to destroy otherwise resistant bacteria. (From Tizard, I. Veterinary Immunology, 2nd ed. W. B. Saunders, Philadelphia, 1982. With permission.)

TABLE 17-4 A Comparison of Tuberculoid and Lepromatous Leprosy

	Tuberculoid	Lepromatous
Resistance	High	Low
Presence of *M. leprae* in tissues	±	+ + + +
Lymphocyte infiltration in lesions	+ + +	−
Antibodies to *M. leprae*	≈ 20%	95%
Immune-complex lesions	−	+ + + +
Auto-antibodies	≈ 10%	≈ 40%
Lepromin test	+ + +	−

tivity reaction to an intradermal bacterial extract (called lepromin). Most of these patients do not have detectable antibodies to *Mycobacterium leprae*.

In contrast, lepromatous leprosy found in about 20% of the cases is associated with low resistance to the disease. These patients do not mount a detectable cell-mediated response but make high levels of antibodies to *M. leprae*. They may also develop immune-complex lesions (Type III hypersensitivity) and autoantibodies to normal tissues. The lesions in these patients are extensive, and are densely infiltrated with organisms. The prognosis of lepromatous leprosy is, as a result, much poorer than for tuberculoid leprosy.

Methods Employed by Bacteria in Evading the Immune Responses

Bacteria, like most parasites, are not well served either by the death of their chosen host or by their immune elimination. Mechanisms have thus evolved by which the consequences of the immune responses may be evaded. We have already discussed such features as the use of antiphagocytic capsules and facultative intracellular parasitism, both of which tend to delay bacterial destruction. Some organisms such as *E. coli, S. aureus, M. tuberculosis,* and *Pseudomonas aeruginosa* secrete factors that can depress phagocytosis by neutrophils. The most extreme form of this is shown by *Pasteurella haemolytica,* which secretes factors that kill ruminant alveolar macrophages but not macrophages from swine, horses, or humans. *P. hemolytica* is an important cause of pneumonia in cattle and sheep.

Other organisms can inhibit the bactericidal activities of cells in a more subtle fashion. For example, the carotenoid pigments responsible for the color of *S. aureus* can quench singlet oxygen and so enable it to survive the respiratory burst. *P. multocida* is also capable of inhibiting the respiratory burst, whereas strains of *E. coli* and salmonellae may carry plasmids that confer resistance to complement-mediated lysis. Other protective devices employed by pathogenic bacteria include the production of proteolytic enzymes specific for IgA produced by *Neisseria gonorrhoeae, S. pneumoniae, N. meningitidis, Hemophilus influenza,* and *Strep. sanguis.*

Campylobacter fetus, an organism that normally colonizes the male and female genital tracts in cattle, shows cyclical antigenic variation. The successful destruction of a major portion of this bacterial population by a local immune response leaves a residual population of organisms that possess antigenic determinants differing from those of the original population. This residual population may multiply and be largely eliminated in turn by a second immune response, leaving a residual population of a third antigenic type. This process may be repeated for a prolonged period, and because of the poor memory in the IgA-producing system (Chap. 15), the organisms may reutilize antigens without stimulating a strong secondary immune response. Organisms that release immunosuppressive factors include *Vibrio cholera, Treponema pallidum* and *Mycobacterium tuberculosis. Bordetella pertussis* releases a highly active adenylate cyclase within phagocytic cells. As a result, it provokes a rise in intracellular cyclic AMP and a severe depression of phagocytosis.

Mechanisms of Antiviral Resistance

Nonimmunological Defense Mechanisms

Just as nonimmunological factors influence susceptibility to bacterial disease, so they modify and control the outcome of many viral infections. Lysozyme, for example, is capable of destroying several viruses, as are many of the intestinal enzymes. Bile is a powerful neutralizer of some viruses, so much so that Robert Koch, the great German microbiologist, first successfully vaccinated cattle against rinderpest with the bile of animals dying from that disease.

Interference and Interferons

Probably the most important of the nonimmunologic antiviral defense mechanisms is interference. Interference is the name given to the inhibition of viral replication by the presence of other viruses. One cause of this inhibition is the production of interferons. Interferons are released from virus-infected cells within a few hours after viral invasion, and high concentrations of interferon may be achieved within a few days in vivo, at a time when the primary immune response is still relatively ineffective (Fig. 17–4). For example, following exposure to influenza virus, peak serum interferon levels may be reached one to two days later and then decline, although they are still detectable at seven days. In contrast, antibodies are usually not detectable in serum until five to six days after virus administration.

Interferons, as described previously, are a class of glycoproteins with molecular weights that vary according to the method used to induce them but that generally lie between 20,000 and 34,000. Three major classes are recognized in humans and mice (Table 17–5): interferon α (IFN α), a family of at least eight different molecules derived from virus-infected leukocytes; interferon β (IFN β) derived from virus-infected fibroblasts; and interferon γ (IFN γ), a lymphokine derived from antigen-stimulated T cells. IFN-α and IFN-β are stable at pH2, whereas IFN-γ is labile at low pH. All are heat-stable and only weakly antigenic.

Antiviral Activities of Interferon

Interferons act on target cells to induce an antiviral state (Fig. 17–5). They first bind to receptors on the target-cell membrane. Interferons are probably not taken into the target, since they retain their activity when bound to agarose beads. They then stimulate the for-

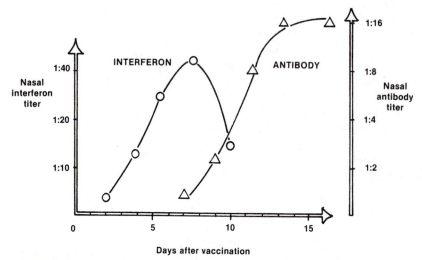

FIGURE 17-4. The sequential production of interferon and antibody following intranasal vaccination of calves with infectious bovine rhinotracheitis vaccine. (From data kindly provided by Dr. M. Savan.)

mation of two new enzymes. One enzyme is 2′5′-oligoadenylate synthetase, which acts on ATP to generate 2′5′A, a complex adenyl phosphate polymer; 2′5′A in turn activates a cellular endoribonuclease that inhibits viral RNA production.

The other enzyme, a protein kinase, is activated by double-stranded RNA. It then acts to inhibit viral protein synthesis by inhibiting the activities of an initiating factor.

It is probable that different interferons act at different steps in the virus-replication cycle, and the mechanism may vary between different viruses. For example, some interferons seem to block the release of murine leukemia viruses from cells.

Virus-induced interferons are relatively species-specific; for example, bovine interferon appears to be most effective when acting on bovine cells, human interferon on human cells, and so on. They are not, however, virus-specific, and interferon induced by one virus may be equally effective when acting against other, unrelated viruses. The ability of cells to produce interferon varies. T cells appear to represent the major source of interferon in many virus diseases (Chap. 12), whereas other cells, such as those from the kidney, are relatively poor interferon producers, and neutrophils, since they do not synthesize protein, produce no interferon.

Although live or inactivated viruses are normally considered to be the most important stimulators of interferon production, interferons may also be induced by other stimuli. For

TABLE 17-5   The Classification of Interferons

Source	Name	Target	Effect
Leukocytes	IFN-α	Virus-infected cells	Blocking of viral replication
Fibroblasts	IFN-β	Suppressor cells	Immunosuppression
T, B, or NK cells	IFN-γ	T and NK cells	Enhanced cytotoxicity

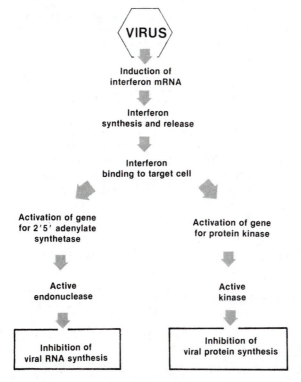

FIGURE 17–5. The two major antiviral activities of interferon.

example, bacterial endotoxins provoke the release of interferon from target cells within a few minutes of exposure. This interferon differs both in size and in heat stability from that produced by virus-infected cells and is probably released preformed from stores within cells. Other substances that can induce interferon production include plant extracts, such as phytohemagglutinin, and some synthetic polymers that act by mimicking the action of viral RNA. One of the most potent of these synthetic polymers (poly I:C) is a copolymer of inosinic and cytidilic acids. Poly I:C may, if given at the right time, increase survival in experimental virus infections.

A second and probably much more important role for the interferons is the regulation of immune reactivity (Chap. 13). Interferons can enhance both suppressor and cytotoxic cell activity (see Table 13–5). The result of stimulating cytotoxic cells, especially NK cells, is enhancement of antitumor and anti-virus-infected-cell immunity.

How to Detect Interferon

The most usual assays for interferon involve measurement of its antiviral effects. As can be imagined, a large number of in vitro assay systems have been developed for this purpose. In general, for human-interferon assays, a standard virus preparation—bovine vesicular stomatitis virus (VSV), Indiana strain—is grown in human fibroblast cultures.

Normally, a set of fibroblast cultures is established under standard conditions.

The putative interferon-containing samples are added to these cultures at various dilutions and incubated for 18 to 24 hours. The fibroblast monolayers are then washed and a standard quantity of VSV is added to each culture. Normally, the VSV is allowed to adsorb to the cells for 45 minutes. Excess virus is then removed and the monolayer overlaid with melted agar. After 48 hours' incubation, the monolayers are stained and virus plaques are seen as cleared areas in the monolayer. If interferon was present in the samples, then it will reduce the number of plaques formed. A greater than 50 percent reduction in virus plaques is considered significant. However, in order to confirm that the antiviral activity is indeed interferon, it is necessary to ensure that the activity belongs to a protein by showing that it is destroyed by trypsin. It should not be sedimented by 100,000 g in the ultracentrifuge. (Remember, other viruses could block plaque formation by interference.) It should block the activities of other viruses, but it should be species-specific. Its sensitivity to low pH and heat will enable it to be classified as a particular type of interferon.

The Destruction of Viruses and Virus-Infected Cells by Antibody

The capsids of viruses contain antigenic glycoproteins, and it is against these and the envelope that antiviral immune responses are largely mounted (Table 17–6).

Antibodies may either destroy free viruses, or prevent virus infection of cells, or destroy virus-infected cells by a number of different mechanisms.

Since viruses first must bind to target cells in order to infect them, antibodies may neutralize viruses by blocking their attachment to cell receptors. The efficiency of this form of virus neutralization varies with the virus. Thus the T-even phages, (T2, T4, and so on) which have only one critical attachment site, can be neutralized by blocking that site with a single immunoglobulin molecule. On the other hand, orthomyxoviruses, such as influenza, have multiple binding sites. Neutralization of influenza will, therefore, occur only

TABLE 17–6   Antibody-mediated Anti-viral Activity

Components Employed	Target	Result
Antibodies	Virus surface antigen	Blocking of viral adsorption or penetration; phagocytosis
Complement	Virus surface antigens	Virolysis by the alternate pathway
Antibodies and Complement	Virus surface antigen	Virolysis, phagocytosis, blocking of viral adsorption or penetration
	Cell-bound viral antigen	Cytolysis of infected cells; blocking of viral shedding
Antibodies and cytotoxic cells	Cell-bound viral antigen	Cytolysis of infected cells; blocking of viral shedding

when all of these are blocked and will thus require much higher immunoglobulin levels. Very small virus particles may behave as if their entire surface is critical.

The combination of antibody with virus is not viricidal in itself, since splitting of virus–antibody complexes can lead to the release of fully infectious virus. Nevertheless, antiviral antibodies may act as opsonins, promoting the phagocytosis of virus particles by macrophages; clump virus particles, so reducing the number of infectious units available for cell invasion; or initiate complement-mediated virus neutralization.

Complement plays a critical role in protection against viruses. The complement cascade may be activated by antibody bound to virus surfaces, by activation through the alternate pathway, or by direct activation of C1q by viral glycoproteins. For viruses, which have a membranelike envelope, the complement pathway may go to completion and thus cause virolysis. Other viruses, however, may be neutralized by the complement components up to C3b. C3b probably neutralizes the virus by blocking critical sites the same way antibodies do.

Antibodies and complement are active, not only against free virions, but also against viral antigens expressed on the surface of infected cells. These cells may be destroyed by antibody-mediated opsonization or by complement-mediated lysis. Antibody binding to the surface of a virus-infected cell does not always destroy it. Thus, it may strip off viral antigens or, alternatively, suppress their production. As a result, infected cells may cease to carry viral antigen on their surfaces and become persistently infected. Cells infected with herpes simplex virus may develop Fc receptors. These receptors may protect infected cells against immune lysis.

Antibody-dependent cellular cytotoxicity (ADCC) is probably of major importance as a mechanism of destruction of virus-infected cells (Fig. 17–6). In this process, cytotoxic cells with Fc receptors bind and lyse antibody-coated target cells. ADCC is a very efficient procedure since it is mediated by concentrations of antibody several hundredfold less than those required to produce complement-dependent lysis of the same cells. The lesions that

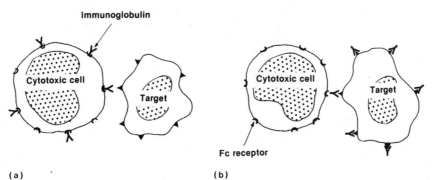

(a)   (b)

FIGURE 17-6. Two ways in which antibody-dependent cellular cytotoxicity may be initiated. The second method **(B)** is clearly related to opsonization since the target cell is coated with immunoglobulin. It may be that cytotoxicity may occur when phagocytosis is frustrated either by the physical state of a target cell—if, for example, it is firmly attached to a surface—or by the inability of the cytotoxic cell to undertake phagocytosis—for example, if it is a K cell.

develop on ADCC targets are similar to, but larger than complement lesions and complement does potentiate ADCC. The cells that have been implicated in ADCC include macrophages, polymorphonuclear cells (neutrophils and eosinophils), and a subset of null lymphocytes that carry Fc receptors and are called K (for *killer*) cells. These K cells are almost certainly identical to NK cells.

The immunoglobulins involved in virus neutralization include IgG and IgM in serum and IgA in secretions. It is possible that IgE also plays a protective role, since humans with a selective IgE deficiency have an increased susceptibility to respiratory infections.

The Destruction of Viruses and Virus-Infected Cells by Cell-Mediated Immune Mechanisms

Although serum antibodies and complement are capable of neutralizing free virus and of destroying virus-infected cells, it is the cell-mediated immune mechanisms that are most important in controlling virus diseases (Table 17–7). This is readily seen in immunodeficient humans (Chap. 18). Those who are defective in their ability to mount an antibody-mediated response (Bruton-type agammaglobulinemia), suffer severely from recurrent bacterial infections but tend to respond normally to smallpox vaccination and to recover from mumps, measles, chicken pox, poliomyelitis, and influenza. In contrast, humans who have a congenital deficiency in their cell-mediated immune response are commonly resistant to bacterial infection, but highly susceptible to virus diseases. Thus, they may die from generalized vaccinia if vaccinated against smallpox. Notwithstanding this, it is probable that normally, antibodies and cell-mediated mechanisms act cooperatively, so that antibodies eliminate circulating virus, while the cell-mediated immune responses eliminate infected cells. An example of this cooperative approach is seen in rabbit fibroma infections in which antibody eliminates circulating virus while the cell-mediated immune response causes tumor regression.

Virus-infected cells develop new antigens on their surface membranes. These new antigens may arise as a result of viruses budding from the cell surface or as a result of the cell synthesizing virus-coded protein. For example, oncogenic viruses may provoke infected cells to produce tumor-specific antigens and depress production of nontumor antigens. It was pointed out above that cells infected with herpes simplex virus generate Fc receptors. Virus-infected cells therefore may be recognized as foreign and thus provoke immunological

TABLE 17–7   Cell-Mediated Antiviral Activity

Components Employed	Target	Result
Antibodies and cytotoxic cells	Cell-bound viral antigen	Cytolysis of infected cells; blocking of viral shedding
Activated macrophages	Cell-bound viral antigen	Macrophage-mediated phagocytosis or cytolysis
Cytotoxic lymphocytes	Cell-bound viral antigen	Cytolysis of infected cells
NK cells	Cell-bound viral antigen	Cytolysis of infected cells

attack. Although antibody and complement, or antibody and K cells can play a role in this process, cytotoxic T cells are probably the major contributors to the destruction of these cells.

When the process of destruction of virus-infected cells by cytotoxic T cells is investigated, it has been found that, in most cases, both the target and the cytotoxic T cell must be histocompatible. Thus, in 1974, Zinkernagel and Doherty showed that cytotoxic lymphocytes from mice immune to lymphocytic choriomeningitis virus (LCM) only lyse LCM-infected target cells if they share H-2 antigens with the cytotoxic cells (Table 12–3). The loci that regulate this map in the Class I regions (K or D) of the MHC. Thus, the cytotoxic T cells must interact not only with viral antigens but also in some way with Class I antigens. The precise mechanisms of this recognition process are unclear. Some investigators have suggested that the cytotoxic cells recognize Class I antigens modified by the virus. Others maintain that the T cells recognize two distinct antigens, the virus-coded antigens and the Class I antigens, while a third hypothesis suggests that T cells recognize a Class I antigen–virus complex.

When studying specific T-cell-mediated cytotoxicity for tumor cells and virus-infected cells, it was noticed that lymphocytes from normal unsensitized donors exerted a considerable degree of cytotoxicity on their own. This spontaneous cell-mediated cytotoxicity has been ascribed to the existence of natural killer (NK) cells and may be of major importance in antiviral immunity. It is markedly stimulated by interferon and, as a result, NK activity is rapidly enhanced soon after onset of virus infection. It therefore serves to provide protection prior to the development of specific cell-mediated cytotoxicity.

NK cells are found in peripheral lymphoid tissues such as the spleen, lymph nodes and peripheral blood, although they originate in the bone marrow. They are nonadherent, nonphagocytic cells. Most have low avidity Fc γ receptors but some have Fc μR. They are Ia$^+$, CR1$^+$, Lyt1$^+$23$^+$ TL$^-$ in mice but may possess very low levels of Thy-1 on their surfaces. NK cells are probably a heterogenous population, since they differ in their relative effectiveness in destroying different target-cell populations. Morphologically, they have been identified as large granular lymphocytes in peripheral blood.

It has gradually become apparent that NK cells are very similar if not identical to, the K cells implicated in ADCC (p. 300). The cells have a similar tissue distribution and strain distribution. Both are relatively radiation-resistant and cyclophosphamide-susceptible. Interferon may also enhance K-cell activity, and both cell types have Fc receptors.

When a lymphocyte suspension is mixed with virus-infected cells, NK-cell-enhancing activity may be detected in the supernatant fluid. This activity is mediated by both interferon and interleukin 2. Unlike T cells, NK cells are not MHC-restricted in their activity and can also act across species barriers, possibly because NK cells recognize a few, common, antigenic determinants. Virus-infected cells are much more sensitive to natural cell-mediated cytotoxicity than their normal counterparts, but it is still unclear whether the NK cells recognize virus-coded antigens or some alternative target structure.

Macrophages also exert a significant antiviral activity. Viruses are readily taken up by macrophages and are usually destroyed. If the viruses are noncytopathic but are able to grow within macrophages, then a persistent infection will result. Under these circumstances, the macrophages must be activated in order to eliminate the virus. This activation is readily accomplished by interferon. An example of this process is seen in birds immunized against fowl pox. The macrophages of these birds show an enhanced antiviral effect against Newcastle-disease virus and acquire the ability to prevent intracellular multiplication of *Salmonella gallinarum,* a feature that is not a property of normal macrophages.

Evasion of the Immune Response by Viruses

The relationship between host and virus must be established on the basis of mutual accommodation so that its long-term continuation is ensured. Failure to establish it results in elimination of either host or virus, an undesirable consequence for both parties. One aspect of this adaptation involves the avoidance by the virus of the attentions of the immune system.

This evasion may be accomplished by several mechanisms, one of the simplest of which is antigenic variation. A good example is seen among the influenza viruses. The influenza viruses possess a number of different surface antigens, of which the hemagglutinins and neuraminidases are most important. There are 13 different hemagglutinins and 9 neuraminidases among the type-A influenza viruses, and they are identified according to a nomenclature system recommended by the World Health Organization (Table 17–8). Thus, the hemagglutinin of the swine influenza virus is classified as H1 and its neuraminidase as N1. Influenza viruses in a human population show an antigenic drift as mutation and selection gradually change the amino-acid sequences of the hemagglutinins and neuraminidases in a seemingly random fashion. As a result, there is great antigenic variation within each subtype. This drift permits the virus to persist in a population for many years. In addition, influenza viruses sporadically exhibit a major antigenic shift, in which a new strain develops whose hemagglutinins show no apparent relationships to the hemagglutinins of previously known strains. Such a major change cannot be produced by mutation and is probably due to recombination between two virus strains. It is the development of these influenza viruses with a completely new antigenic structure that accounts for the periodic

TABLE 17–8   Examples of Influenza A Viruses and their Antigenic Structures

Species	Virus Strain	Antigenic Structure*
Human	A/Hong Kong/8/68† (Hong Kong Flu)	H3N2
	A/Japan/305/57 (Asian Flu)	H2N2
	A/Brazil/11/78	H1N1
	A/Bangkok/1/79	H3N2
	A/New Jersey/76 (Swine Flu)	H1N1
Equine	A/Equine/Prague/1/56	H7N7
	A/Equine/Miami/1/63	H3N8
Swine	A/Swine/Iowa/15/30	H1N1
Avian	A/Fowl Plague/Dutch/27	H7N7
	A/Duck/England/56	H11N7
	A/Turkey/Ontario/6118/68	H8N4

*There are many other antigens known among the human and avian influenza viruses.

†The first number is the isolate number; the second is the year of isolation.

pandemics of this disease in humans. In horses and pigs, in contrast, the rapid turnover of the population ensures the persistence of influenza without the necessity for antigenic drift. As a result, the antigenic structure of equine and swine influenza viruses has remained relatively stable since they were first described.

A second form of virus adaptation is seen in equine infectious anemia (EIA), Aleutian disease (AD) of mink, and African swine fever. Although infected animals mount an immune response to these agents, the antibodies formed are incapable of virus neutralization. Thus, virus-antibody complexes from AD-infected mink or EIA-infected horses are fully infectious. The precise reason for the inability of antibody to neutralize these viruses is not clear, although it is assumed that antibody must bind to a "noncritical" site on the virus. It has also been suggested that some form of antigenic variation may occur.

An alternative evasive process has been observed in measles-infected cells in humans and in LCM-infected cells in mice. Antibody against measles virus will normally kill measles-infected cells. If, however, there is insufficient antibody present to be immediately lethal, then an infected cell may respond by removing the measles antigens from its surface. Once these antigens are lost, the infected cells are refractory to cytolysis, although presumably, the virus is itself unable to spread. Removal of the measles antibody permits re-expression of measles antigen.

Of particular interest to immunologists are the virus diseases in which profound immunosuppression occurs (Table 17–9). In many cases, the immunosuppression may be due to virus-induced destruction of lymphoid tissues. In some of these, only the primary lymphoid organs are involved. For example, mice may be infected by a herpes virus that causes massive necrosis of the thymic cortex. This "viral thymectomy" will naturally result in the occurrence of immunological defects. In poultry, the virus of infectious bursal disease destroys the cells of the bursa of Fabricius. This virus is not completely specific for the bursa, since it may also damage the spleen and thymus. These organs, however, usually recover while the bursa atrophies. The consequences of this infection, as might be predicted, are most evident in young birds infected immediately after hatching since they are unable to make normal levels of antibody. If infection by the bursal disease virus is delayed for several weeks after hatching, then antibody production tends to be relatively normal.

TABLE 17–9   Some Viruses that Affect Lymphoid Tissues

Viruses that destroy lymphoid tissues
  Herpes simplex
  Dengue
  Measles
  Canine distemper
  Bovine virus diarrhea
Viruses that stimulate lymphoid tissues
  Aleutian disease
  Epstein-Barr Virus
Viruses that cause lymphoid neoplasia
  Mareks disease
  Feline leukemia
  Bovine leukemia
  Murine leukemias

Some viruses affect secondary lymphoid organs. For example, the virus of canine distemper has a predilection for lymphocytes, which it rapidly destroys. The destruction of lymphoid tissues in this disease accounts in large part for its clinical features. If germ-free dogs are infected by virulent distemper virus, they suffer from only a relatively mild disease, presumably because secondary infection cannot occur. Perhaps the most dramatic of these conditions is Acquired Immune Deficiency Syndrome (AIDS) of man. Although the cause of this disease remains unknown, preliminary evidence suggests that it may be associated with infection with human T cell leukemia virus (Chap. 18).

A more complex interaction between lymphocytes and virus is seen in infectious mononucleosis (Fig. 17–7). The causal agent, Epstein-Barr virus (EBV), infects only B cells, most of which possess specific receptors for the virus. The virus provokes these B cells to proliferate in nonspecific fashion. These abnormal B cells, however, are recognized as

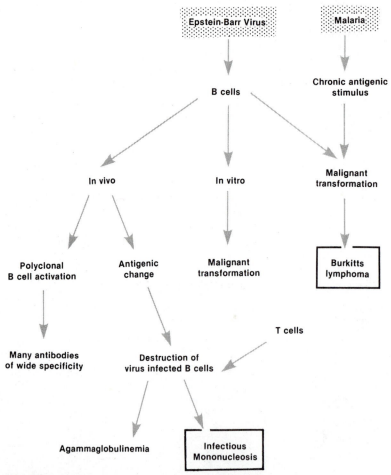

FIGURE 17–7. A schematic view of the relationships between the diseases associated with Epstein-Barr virus.

foreign by the T-cell system. As a result, cytotoxic T-cell production is provoked, and the T cells proceed to attack and destroy the virus-infected cells. It is these cytotoxic T cells that are the atypical mononuclear cells found in the blood of patients with infectious mononucleosis.

Sometimes, the T cells fail to prevent the abnormal B-cell proliferation induced by EBV. In this case, two alternative syndromes may develop—fatal infectious mononucleosis or an uncontrolled leukemia-like syndrome.

Burkitt's lymphoma is a tumor of B cells. It is generally restricted to certain areas of the tropics since it is commonly associated with concurrent malaria and EBV infections. EBV may also be implicated in the pathogenesis of lymphomas that develop in patients treated with the immunosuppressive drug, cyclosporin A (see p. 341).

The polyclonal B-cell activation seen in infectious mononucleosis results in the production of many different antibodies. Antibodies to sheep, bovine, and human red blood cells, lymphocytes, DNA, bovine serum, albumin, thyroglobulin, Newcastle-disease virus, and human IgG have all been described. One antibody consistently produced is directed against N-glutamyl glucosamine. This antigen, also called Paul Bunnell antigen, is found on bovine erythrocytes, mouse T cells, and on the spleen and T cells of some humans. Its detection has long provided a method of diagnosis of infectious mononucleosis.

Other mechanisms of virus-induced immunosuppression include the release of soluble immunosuppressive proteins, for example, interferon or a 15,000-dalton glycoprotein from feline leukemia virus, which prevents lymphocyte blastogenesis. Viral neuraminidases may alter lymphocyte membranes and hence interfere with lymphocyte recirculation. They may also render cells susceptible to lysis by complement through the alternate pathway (Chap. 14).

Immunologically Mediated Enhancement of Viral Disease

There exist a number of fairly well-defined situations in which the immune responses directed against viruses enhance, rather than prevent, the expression of clinical disease. A good example is lymphocytic choriomeningitis (LCM). In this disease, vertical transmission of the virus from female mice to their offspring causes relatively asymptomatic infection because of neonatal tolerance. Horizontal transmission between immunologically competent individuals, on the other hand, can lead to severe immunologically mediated disease as cytotoxic lymphocytes attack virus-infected cells within the brain. Immunosuppressive treatment given before the clinical signs appear will, therefore, prevent the appearance of LCM.

In contrast to the immune response against bacteria, antiviral immunity is, in many cases, very long-lasting. The reasons are not completely clear, but they appear to be related to virus persistence within cells, perhaps in a slowly replicating or a nonreplicating form as typified by the herpes viruses. The persistent virus may periodically boost the immune response of the infected animal and, in this way, generate prolonged immunity to superinfection. This type of infection can only be countered by an immune response directed against infected cells, and even this may be ineffective if the virus does not influence the antigenic structures on the cell surface. The immune responses in these cases, although not capable of eliminating virus, may prevent the development of clinical disease and therefore serve a protective role. Immunosuppression of persistently infected animals may permit disease to occur. The association between stress and the development of some virus diseases is well recognized (for example, cold sores caused by Herpes simplex virus), and it is likely that the increased levels of steroid production occurring in stressful situations may be sufficiently immunosuppressive to permit activation of latent viruses or infection by exogenous ones.

Mechanisms of Resistance to Protozoa

Nonimmunological Defense Mechanisms

Although the nonimmunological mechanisms of resistance to protozoa have not been fully clarified, they appear, in general, to be qualitatively similar to those that operate in bacterial and viral diseases. Species and genetic influences are perhaps of most significance; for example, *Trypanosoma lewisi* is found only in the rat and *Trypanosoma musculi* in the mouse, where neither causes disease.

Presumably, these species differences are but a development of somewhat more subtle influences. Perhaps the best analyzed case of genetically determined resistance to protozoan disease is sickle cell anemia in humans. Individuals who inherit the sickle cell trait possess hemoglobin S (HbS) in which a residue of valine has replaced a residue of glutamic acid present in normal hemoglobin. The changes in the shape of the hemoglobin molecule induced by this substitution cause deoxygenated hemoglobin molecules to aggregate, thus distorting the shape of the erythrocytes and resulting in increased erythrocyte fragility and clearance. Individuals who are homozygous for the sickle cell gene die when young from the results of severe anemia. Heterozygous individuals are also anemic, but, in west central Africa, the fact that red blood cells containing hemoglobin S are not parasitized by *Plasmodium falciparum* ensures that these individuals are resistant to malaria. As a consequence, more of these heterozygotes tend to survive to reproductive age than normal persons. The mutation is, therefore, maintained in the human population at a relatively high level.

Immunological Defense Mechanisms

The obvious inadequacies of the immune responses to many parasites led early investigators to conclude that successful parasites were, in general, poorly immunogenic. This is not the case; most parasites are fully antigenic, but in their adaptation to a parasitic existence they have developed mechanisms through which they may survive in the presence of an immune response. Therefore, like other antigenic particles, protozoa can stimulate both humoral and cell-mediated immune responses. In general, antibodies serve to control the level of parasites that exist free in the bloodstream and tissue fluids, whereas cell-mediated immune responses are directed largely against intracellular parasites (Fig. 17–8).

Serum antibodies directed against protozoan surface antigens may opsonize, agglutinate, or immobilize them. Antibodies together with complement and cytotoxic cells may kill them, and some antibodies (called ablastins) may act to inhibit protozoan enzymes in such a way that their replication is prevented.

For many years, it was thought that a common feature of protozoan infection was

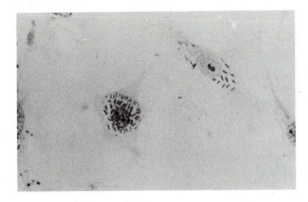

FIGURE 17–8. Mouse macrophages growing in tissue culture and infected with tachyzoites of *Toxoplasma gondii*. *T. gondii* is a facultative intracellular parasite. (Courtesy of Dr. C. H. Lai. From Tizard I. Veterinary Immunology, 2nd ed. W. B. Saunders, Philadelphia, 1982. With permission.)

premunition. **Premunition** is the term used to describe resistance that is effective only if the parasite persists in the host and wanes rapidly when all parasites are eliminated. This is probably not an absolute phenomenon but is of importance in resistance to certain blood protozoa.

Evasion of the Immune Response by Protozoa

Most important protozoan parasites have evolved mechanisms for evading the consequences of their hosts' immune responses. In general, these mechanisms resemble those evolved by other types of organisms. For example, many protozoa are immunosuppressive.

Parasite-induced immunosuppression may be of great assistance to the parasite. For example, *Babesia bovis* is immunosuppressive for cattle. As a result, its host vector, the tick *Boophilus microplus,* is more able to survive on an infected animal. Consequently, infected cattle have more ticks than noninfected animals and the efficiency of transmission of *B. bovis* is greatly enhanced. It must also be pointed out, however, that parasite-induced immunosuppression commonly leads to the death of host animals as a result of secondary infection, so it is not necessarily always beneficial to the parasite.

In addition to immunosuppression, protozoa have evolved two other extremely effective immunoevasive techniques. One involves becoming either hypo- or nonantigenic, and the other involves acquiring a capacity for the rapid and repeated alteration of surface antigens. An example of a hypoantigenic organism is the cyst stage of *T. gondii,* which appears not to stimulate a host response. As an alternative to the evolution of nonimmunogenic stages, some protozoa can become functionally nonantigenic by masking themselves with host antigens. Examples of these include *Trypanosoma theileri* in cattle and *Trypanosoma lewisi* in rat. These are both nonpathogenic trypanosomes that can survive in the bloodstream of infected animals because they become covered with a layer of host serum proteins and so are not regarded as foreign.

Although the absence of antigenicity may be considered the ultimate stage in the evasive process, many protozoa, especially the trypanosomes, have evolved the techniques of antigenic variation to a high degree of sophistication. If humans are infected with the pathogenic trypanosomes *T. rhodesiense* or *T. gambiense* and the parasitemia is checked at regular intervals, it is found that the numbers of circulating organisms fluctuate greatly,

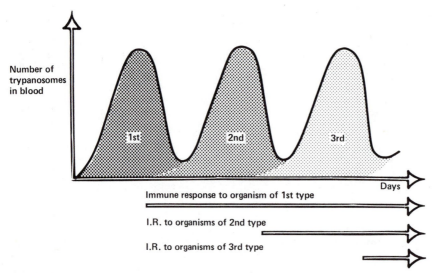

FIGURE 17–9. A schematic diagram depicting how antigenic variation may account for the cyclic parasitemia observed in trypanosomiasis: Each peak represents the growth of a new antigenic variant. (From Tizard, I. Veterinary Immunology, 2nd ed. W. B. Saunders, Philadelphia, 1982. With permission.)

periods of high parasitemia alternating regularly with periods of low or undetectable parasitemia (Fig. 17–9). Serum taken from infected individuals will react with trypanosomes isolated prior to the time of bleeding, but not with those taken subsequently. Each peak period of high parasitemia corresponds to the development of a population of trypanosomes of a new antigenic type. The elimination of a population of one antigenic type leads to a fall in blood parasite levels. From the survivors, however, a proportion of parasites develop new surface antigens and a fresh population arises to produce yet another period of high parasitemia. This cyclical fluctuation in parasite levels with each peak reflecting the appearance of a new antigenic variant population can continue for a long time.

The sequence of antigens produced appears to be almost entirely random and is not provoked by antibody. Trypanosomes grown in tissue culture also show spontaneous antigenic variation. By means of electron microscopy, it can be shown that the variant antigen forms a thick coat over the surface of the trypanosome. When antigenic change occurs, the proteins in the old coat are shed and replaced by an antigenically different protein. Analysis of the genetics of this process indicates that the trypanosomes possess a large number of genes for coat protein and that antigenic variation occurs as a result of random gene rearrangement and selection.

Trypanosomiasis is not the only protozoan infection in which antigenic variation is seen. Minor antigenic variations have been recorded in babesiosis, in which relapse strains appear to be antigenically different from the original strains. Antigenic variation is also seen in malaria, although the range of antigens and the differences between them are relatively small.

Vaccination against Malaria

Malaria is arguably the most important disease in the world today, and it would be a tremendous advance if we could vaccinate humans again it. This has become particularly important since many insecticides used for mosquito control have become unavailable or ineffective.

The form of the parasite injected by a mosquito is called a sporozoite. Sporozoite vaccines may well work; however, a large number of sporozoites are inoculated and all must be destroyed in order to prevent infection. Since sporozoites are only present in the bloodstream for about 30 minutes, this may be insufficient time for their total destruction.

An alternative type of vaccine that may be developed is directed against the bloodstream form of the organism called merozoites. Antibodies against merozoites may be effective but only when invoked using a powerful adjuvant. No such adjuvant is available at the present time.

At present it seems probable that a sporozoite vaccine may be developed first, especially since the genes for the protective antigen have been cloned and the antigen synthesized in bacterial cultures.

Since parasitic protozoa seek to evade the immune responses, it is not surprising that they also invade immunosuppressed individuals. Organisms that are normally maintained in a relatively quiescent state by the immune response, such as the cyst forms of *T. gondii,* are capable of changing to more active form and producing severe disease in immunosuppressed animals. For this reason, acute toxoplasmosis is commonly seen in patients immunosuppressed for transplantation purposes or for cancer therapy.

Mechanisms of Resistance to Helminths

The immune system has not been conspicuously successful in producing absolute resistance to helminth (parasitic worm) infections in mammals. In a sense, it has been detrimental, since the IgE-mediated immune reactions appear to have evolved largely for the control of these parasites. In western society, where parasites are largely controlled by hygienic measures, the problem of allergies is probably of much greater social significance than parasitism. On a worldwide basis, however, and in relation to domestic animals, helminth parasites remain of major signficance.

It is not surprising that the immune system is relatively inefficient in controlling helminth parasites. After all, these organisms have adapted to an obligatory parasitic existence, and, presumably, this adaptation has involved dealing with the immune system and either overcoming or evading it. Helminths are, therefore, not maladapted pathogenic organisms but fully adapted obligate parasites whose very survival depends on reaching some form of accommodation with the host. Consequently, if an organism of this type causes disease, it is likely to be expressed either very mildly or subclinically. Only when helminth parasites invade a host to which they are not fully adapted, or in unusually large numbers, does acute disease occur.

Nonimmunological Defense Mechanisms

The factors that influence the course of helminth infections are many and complex. They include not only the influences of host-derived factors but also of factors derived from other helminths within the same host. For example, both intraspecies and interspecies competition are known to occur. In the former case, it is evident, particularly with respect to tapeworm infections, that the presence of adult worms in the intestine delays the further development of larval stages in the tissues. In interspecies competition, competition between helminths for mutual habitats and nutrients serves to control the numbers and composition of an animal's helminth population.

The age and sex of the host influences worm burdens through hormonal processes. In animals whose sexual cycle is seasonal, parasites tend to synchronize their reproductive cycle with that of the host. For instance, female sheep show a "spring rise" in fecal nematode ova, which coincides with lambing and the onset of lactation. Similarly, the development of helminth larvae ingested by cattle in autumn tends to be inhibited until spring. Perhaps the most evolved organisms in this respect are the nematodes of the genus *Toxocara,* the larvae of which may migrate from an infected bitch to the liver of the fetal puppy, resulting in a congenital infection. Once born, the infected pups can reinfect their mother by the more conventional fecal-oral route.

Immunological Defense Mechanisms

Humoral Mechanisms   Helminths, in general, can be found in two situations in the body: in tissues as larval forms or within the gastrointestinal or respiratory tracts as adults. Obviously, the form of the immune response that is most effective against these stages differs considerably.

Although conventional antibodies of the IgM, IgG, and IgA classes are produced in response to helminth antigens, an increasing body of evidence suggests that the most significant immunoglobulin class involved in resistance to helminths is IgE. For example, IgE levels are usually extremely elevated in parasitized individuals; many helminth infestations are associated with the characteristic signs of Type I hypersensitivity, including eosinophilia, edema, asthma, and urticarial dermatitis; and many helminth infections, such as ascariasis, are accompanied by a positive passive cutaneous anaphylaxis (PCA) reaction to worm antigens (Chap. 20). Many helminth antigens preferentially stimulate IgE production, so investigators who handle helminths regularly may become sensitized to worm antigens. These individuals then suffer from asthmatic attacks or cutaneous wheal-and-flare reactions (urticaria) on exposure to worms. In addition to being potent stimulators of IgE production against themselves, helminth antigens are also capable of acting as adjuvants, specific for IgE production against other, nonhelminth antigens.

Although IgE production and the allergies that result from it are considered by some to be only a nuisance, they appear to be of considerable benefit in controlling worm burdens. One of the best examples is the "self-cure" reaction seen in sheep infected with gastrointestinal nematodes, particularly *Hemonchus contortus.* These worms, which are embedded in the intestinal and abomasal mucosa, secrete antigens during their third ecdysis that act as allergens. As a result, the development of a worm burden provokes a local acute Type I hypersensitiviy reaction in the parasitized regions of the intestine. The combination of helminth antigens with mast-cell-bound IgE leads to mast-cell degranulation and the release of vasoactive amines. These compounds stimulate smooth-muscle contraction and increase vascular permeability. Thus, in the self-cure reaction, violent contractions of the intestinal musculature and an increase in the permeability of intestinal capillaries occur, allowing an efflux of fluid into the intestinal lumen. This combination results in dislodgment and expulsion of the major portion of the animal's gastrointestinal worm burden (Fig. 17–10). In sheep that have just undergone self-cure, their PCA antibody titer is high (Chap. 20) and experimental administration of helminth antigens will result in acute anaphylaxis, confirming the role of Type I hypersensitivity in this phenomenon. A similar reaction is seen in fascioliasis in calves, in which peak PCA titers coincide with expulsion of the parasite.

IgE has other roles to play in the reduction of helminth burdens in animals. For example, macrophages may bind to helminth larvae such as schistosomulae (immature forms of schistosomes) through an IgE-mediated pathway and cause their destruction. By mediating mast-cell degranulation, IgE stimulates release of ECF-A (eosinophil chemotactic factor of anaphylaxis). This material mobilizes the body's eosinophil pool and provokes the release of large numbers of eosinophils into the circulation. It is for this reason that an eosinophilia is so characteristic of helminth infections (Fig. 5–6). Eosinophils serve at least two roles. First, they contain enzymes capable of neutralizing the vasoactive agents released from mast cells (Chap. 20). Second, in conjunction with antibodies and complement, eosinophils are capable of killing some helminth larvae and hence serve a protective function. Eosinophils attach to helminths by means of IgG and IgE. They then degranulate, releasing their granule contents onto the helminth cuticle (Fig. 17–11). The major basic protein of

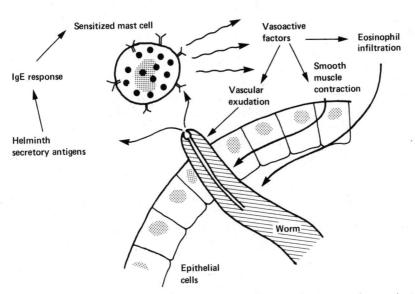

FIGURE 17–10. The probable mechanism of the self-cure reaction against intestinal helminths. (From Tizard, I. Veterinary Immunology, 2nd ed. W. B. Saunders, Philadelphia, 1982. With permission.)

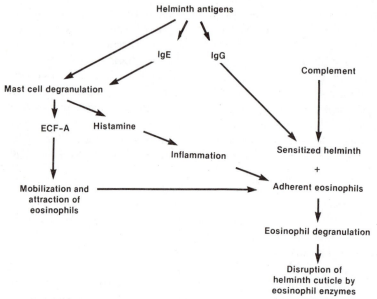

FIGURE 17–11. Some of the mechanisms by which mast cells, IgE, IgG, and eosinophils may interact to destroy helminths: Recent evidence suggests that eosinophils may also attach to helminths through IgE. (From Tizard, I. Veterinary Immunology, 2nd ed. W. B. Saunders, Philadelphia, 1982. With permission.)

the granules can cause direct damage to the cuticle and also promotes the adherence of additional eosinophils. The cytotoxic effects of eosinophil major basic protein are enhanced by mast-cell-derived factors, such as histamine, as well as by complement.

While the IgE–eosinophil-mediated antihelminth response is perhaps the most sigsignificant mechanism of resistance to helminths, antibodies of other immunoglobulin classes also play a protective role. The mechanisms involved include complement-mediated cuticular damage (Fig. 17–12), antibody-mediated neutralization of the proteolytic enzymes used by larvae to penetrate tissues, blocking of the anal and oral pores of these larvae by immune complexes as antibodies combine with their excretory and secretory products (Fig. 17–13), and prevention of ecdysis and inhibition of larval development by antibodies directed against exsheathing antigens.

Cell-Mediated Immunity Many helminths, particularly those that undergo tissue migration, may be considered as functional xenografts. It is somewhat remarkable, therefore, that they are not precipitously rejected by the cell-mediated immune system. Their survival is a reflection of the success of their adaptation to existence within mammalian tissues. Nevertheless, there is evidence to suggest that sensitized T lymphocytes and activated macrophages may successfully attack helminths that are either deeply embedded in the intestinal mucosa or undergoing prolonged tissue stages.

Sensitized T lymphocytes depress the activities of helminths by two mechanisms. First, the development of an inflammatory response of the delayed-hypersensitivity type tends to attract mononuclear cells to the site of larval invasion and renders the local envi-

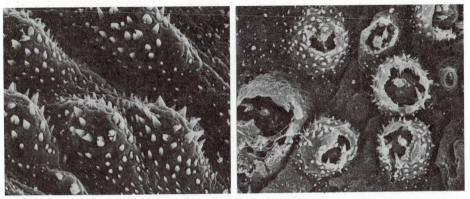

FIGURE 17–12. Scanning electron micrographs of the surface of an adult male *Schistosoma mansoni:* **A)** intact tubercles after incubation in normal mouse serum and complement in vitro; **B)** tubercle damage after incubation in immune mouse serum and complement in vitro (original magnification x3000). (Courtesy of Dr. K. Rasmussen.)

ronment unsuitable for growth or migration. Second, cytotoxic lymphocytes may be capable of causing larval destruction. Thus, it has been shown that the treatment of experimental animals with BCG vaccine, a treatment that stimulates the T-cell system, inhibits the metastases of hydatid cysts *(Echinococcus granulosus)* and, in these treated animals, the space that surrounds the cysts may be filled with large lymphocytes. It is also not uncommon to observe large lymphocytes adhering firmly to migrating nematode larvae in vivo.

Evasion of the Immune Response by Helminths

Although the preceding discussion has noted a number of mechanisms whereby animals resist helminth infection, it is obvious, even to a casual observer, that these responses are not fully effective. The success of this adaptation is seen at its most marked extent in tapeworm infections where cysticerci appear to be able to survive indefinitely in muscle despite

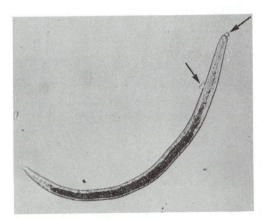

FIGURE 17–13. A *Toxocara canis* larva after incubation in specific antiserum: The immune precipitates at the oral and excretory pores are indicated by arrows. (Courtesy of Dr. D. H. DeSavigny.

the host's response. Several mechanisms may be considered to play a role in this adaptation. These include mimicry of host antigens, absorption of host antigens, antigenic variation, blocking of antibodies, and tolerance (Table 17-10).

The first of these mechanisms introduces the concept that helminths may synthesize histocompatibility or blood-group antigens to match those of their host. It is clear that a helminth cannot synthesize all antigens it could possibly require, since such synthesis would demand the existence of a genetic system similar in complexity to the antibody-producing system. Nevertheless, partial mimicry of host antigens is indeed possible, so that, for example, sheep respond to fewer antigens of *H. contortus* than do rabbits. This fact suggests that *H. contortus* possesses a closer antigenic similarity to sheep, its natural host, than to rabbits, which it does not normally infect. It has also been shown that many trematodes and cestodes are capable of synthesizing blood-group antigens, which, if they happen to be identical to those of the host, also serve to reduce the effective antigenicity of the worm.

Second, there is a considerable amount of evidence to suggest that tissue helminths may be protected from the consequences of their hosts' immune response by the adsorption of host antigens onto their surface. An example of this is the adult *Schistosoma mansoni*, a trematode that lives in the mesenteric blood vessels of humans and that is capable of adsorbing host erythrocyte and histocompatibility antigens to its surface. Cysticerci can also adsorb histocompatibility antigens in this way.

A third mechanism of evasion of the immune response involves antigenic variation. Although helminths have not evolved a system as efficient as that seen in trypanosomiasis, gradual antigenic variation is recognized. Thus, the cuticular antigens of *T. spiralis* larvae show extensive changes following each molt. Even during their growth phase, they show quantitative changes in the expression of surface protein antigens.

Another response that may contribute to the survival of parasitic helminths is immunosuppression. For example, sheep infected with *H. contortus* may become specifically suppressed so that they are unreactive to *H. contortus* even though they remain responsive to unrelated antigens. The mechanisms involved in this response are unknown. They may involve induction of specific suppressor cells, as has been demonstrated in filariasis, or, alternatively, they may result from the production of blocking antibody in a manner anal-

TABLE 17-10   Methods Employed by Helminths in Order to Evade the Host's Immune Response

Hiding of helminth antigens
   Protective coating with antibody, complement, host histocompatibility
   antigens, serum proteins, or blood-group antigens.
Loss of helminth antigens
   Antigenic variation
   Shedding of helminth surface antigens
Release of soluble factors that
   Inhibit complement activity
   Inhibit mast-cell degranulation
   Inhibit lymphocyte proliferation
Selective stimulation of production of
   Suppressor cells
   Blocking antibodies

ogous to that seen in pregnancy and in some neoplastic conditions (Chap. 19). In other helminth infections, such as trichinosis, infected animals are nonspecifically immunosuppressed. This immunosuppression is reflected in a lowered resistance to other infections, a poor response to vaccination, and a prolongation of skin graft survival.

Sources of Additional Information

Allison, A. C., et al. Virus-associated immunopathology: animal models and implications for human disease. Bull WHO, *47:* 257–274, 1972.

Bloom, B. R. Games parasites play: how parasites evade immune surveillance. Nature, *279:* 21–26, 1979.

Capron, A., Dessaint, J. P., and Capron, M. Immunoregulation of parasite infections. J. Allerg. Clin. Immunol., *66:* 9–196, 1979.

Eckles, D. D., et al. SB-restricted presentation of influenza and herpes simplex virus antigens to human T-lymphocyte clones. Nature, *301:* 716–718, 1983.

Gresser, I. On the varied biological effects of interferon. Cell. Immunol. *34:* 406–415, 1977.

Miki, K., and MacKaness, G. B. The passive transfer of acquired resistance to *Listeria monocytogenes.* J. Exp. Med., *120:* 93–103, 1964.

Mims, C. A. The Pathogenesis of Infectious Disease. Grune and Stratton, New York, 1976.

Mitchell, G. F. Effector cells, molecules and mechanisms in host-protective immunity to parasites. Immunology, *38:* 209–223, 1979.

Mitchell, G. F. Responses to infection with metazoan and protozoan parasites in mice. Adv. Immunol. *28:* 451–511, 1979.

Morrison, D. C., and Ryan, J. L. Bacterial endotoxins and host immune responses. Adv. Immunol. *28:* 293–450, 1979.

Notkins, A. L. Viral Immunology and Immunopathology. Academic Press, New York, 1975.

Porterfield, J. S. Antibody-mediated enhancement of rabies virus. Nature, *290:* 542, 1981.

Schwab, J. H. Immunosuppression by bacteria. *In* Hobart, M. R., and Neter, E., eds. The Immune System and Infectious Diseases. S. Karger, Basel, 1975, pp. 64–65.

18

Defects in the Immune System

Inherited defects in the immune system generally impair the ability of an individual to mount either a cell-mediated or an antibody-mediated immune response, or alternatively, impair the ability of phagocytic cells to process antigen or control the invasion of infectious agents. The consequences of these inherited deficiencies have served as excellent indicators of the site of the genetic lesion and have confirmed the basic arrangement of the immune system.

In general, immunodeficiencies are recognized clinically by symptoms that suggest a defect in either protection against infection—as reflected by recurrent severe, intractible infections—or a defect in surveillance, as reflected by neoplasia. Clinically, it is essential that such cases be very carefully investigated to ensure that any immunodeficiency detected is not secondary to a nongenetic cause. Repeated infections may be due, for example, to malnutrition or some aspects of life style. Secondary immunodeficiencies are associated with many virus infections such as rubella, cytomegalovirus, feline leukemia, or canine distemper (Chap. 17). Thymic atrophy and lymphopenia are common manifestations of many virus diseases. Many environmental toxins, such as polychlorinated biphenyls, polybrominated biphenyls, dioxanes, cigarette smoke, iodine, lead, cadmium, methyl mercury, and DDT have a suppressive effect on the immune system, as do deficiencies of copper, zinc, vitamin E, and selenium.

Immunoglobulin synthesis is very much reduced in animals suffering from absolute protein deficiencies. Thus, immunosuppression develops in animals with protein loss due to renal failure (nephrotic syndrome), in malnourished individuals, in heavily parasitized or tumor-bearing animals, and following severe burns or trauma.

Acquired Immune Deficiency Syndrome (AIDS)

Beginning in 1979, physicians began to notice a remarkable incidence of two unusual conditions among active homosexuals. These conditions were a rare lymphoid tumor known as Kaposi's sarcoma and a severe pneumonia caused by an opportunistic pathogen, *Pneumocystis carinii*. Upon investigation, affected individuals were found to be profoundly immunosuppressed as a result of an almost total loss of T cells.

As the number of cases of AIDS grew it began to be observed among other segments of the population. Intravenous drug abusers who tend to share syringes and needles and individuals suffering from hemophilia A were among the affected groups. Hemophiliacs require frequent transfusions of pooled plasma; this plasma is obtained from a large number of donors, many of whom are derelict. These observations suggest that AIDS may be transmitted by an infectious agent present in plasma. However, AIDS has also been described in the heterosexual partners of affected individuals and in male Haitians living within the United States or Canada.

This latter group of victims presents a dilemma since there is no obvious source of infection. One possible factor that may contribute to the syndrome is human T-cell leukemia virus (HTLV). This virus, which is normally associated with a rare form of T-cell leukemia, is found in a high percentage of AIDS patients. HTLV is endemic in the West Indies, including Haiti.

Although there is no evidence that HTLV "causes" AIDS, there are several animal models in which a retrovirus can cause either a T-cell tumor or a T-cell loss.

Close examination of the AIDS syndrome indicates that it may be one of three types: a severe T cellular immunodeficiency associated with opportunistic infections; a chronic benign lymphadenopathy; or Kaposi's sarcoma. In all cases, the major T-cell loss is associated with $T4^+$ cells. These are the T cells with helper function. $T8^+$ suppressor cells are usually at normal levels.

The size of the AIDS epidemic is reaching alarming proportions. The mortality has already reached 75% and will climb higher since no one has yet recovered from the disease and the number of cases has been doubling every six months since 1979.

Congenital Immunodeficiencies

As a general rule, a defect in the production of lymphoid stem cells will be reflected in a deficiency of both the antibody-mediated and the cell-mediated immune responses. A defect that occurs only in the T-cell development pathway will be reflected by an inability to mount a cell-mediated immune response, although antibody production may be relatively normal. Similarly, a lesion restricted to the B-cell system will be reflected by an absence of antibody-mediated immune responses (Fig. 18–1) (Table 18–1).

Stem-Cell Deficiency Diseases

The most severe congenital immunodeficiency state recognized in humans results from a defect in the development of primordial bone marrow stem cells as a result of which neither

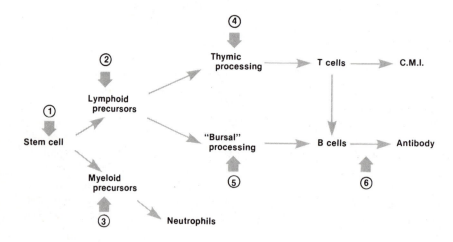

1 Reticular dysgenesis
2 Severe combined immunodeficiency
3 Neutrophil defects
4 Thymic aplasia
5 Agammaglobulinemia
6 Deficiencies in individual immunoglobulins

FIGURE 18–1. The points in the immune system at which development blocks may lead to immune deficiencies. (From Tizard, I. Veterinary Immunology, 2nd ed. W. B. Saunders, Philadelphia, 1982. With permission.)

TABLE 18-1   The Major Congenital Immunodeficiency Syndromes in Man

Syndrome	Target	Mode of inheritance
Reticular dysgenesis	Stem cells	Unknown
SCID (DiGeorge Syndrome)	T cells	Variable
SCID due to ADA deficiency	T cells	Autosomal recessive
Thymus hypoplasia (Nezelof's syndrome)	T cells (B cells)	Variable
Nucleoside phosphorylase deficiency	T cells	Autosomal recessive
Congenital hypogammaglobulinemia (Bruton type)	B cells	X-linked
Common variable immunodeficiency	B cells	Autosomal recessive
IgA deficiency	Excessive suppressor cells	Variable
IgM deficiency	?	Unknown
IgG subclass deficiency	?	X-linked
Wiscott-Aldrich syndrome	T cells	X-linked
Ataxia-telangiectasia	T cells (B cells)	Autosomal recessive

myeloid (neutrophils, etc.) nor lymphoid cells (T and B lymphocytes) develop. This condition, known as reticular dysgenesis, results in the very early death of affected individuals as a result of recurrent intractible infections.

Only slightly less severe are the combined immune deficiencies in which lymphoid stem cells fail to develop. As a result, neither the T- nor B-cell systems develop to maturity, and no immune responses can be mounted. These congenital combined immune deficiencies are a heterogeneous group of disorders, with a variety of lesions, modes in inheritance, and degrees of immunologic dysfunction. They generally present as severe recurrent infections during the first weeks of life. Affected children commonly develop oral candidiasis, pneumonias caused by low-grade pathogens such as *Pneumocystis carinii*, and chronic diarrhea. Unless successfully treated, these children will die within the first two years of life. Combined immunodeficiencies may be diagnosed by an absence of lymphocytes from peripheral blood, reduced or absent serum immunoglobulin levels, and an inability to mount either cell-mediated and antibody-mediated immune responses. On autopsy, both the primary and secondary lymphoid organs are devoid of lymphocytes.

Combined immunodeficiency (CID) may be an X-linked recessive, autosomal recessive, or a sporadic disease. One of the most interesting autosomal recessive forms of CID is due to an inherited deficiency of the enzyme adenosine deaminase (ADA).

ADA converts the nucleosides deoxyadenosine and adenosine to deoxyinosine and inosine, respectively (Fig. 18-2). In ADA-deficient patients, deoxyadenosine is not destroyed but accumulates in the bloodstream. It is then taken up by T cells and phosphorylated. As a result, deoxyadenosine phosphate accumulates within T cells, where it inhibits the enzyme ribonucleotide reductase and thus blocks DNA synthesis and cell division. In addition, it depletes the T cells of ATP and therefore kills resting T cells. Thus, the net effect of an ADA deficiency is the selective destruction of T cells and a loss of cell-mediated immune responses. T-helper-cell activity is also lost; consequently, antibody production is also impaired. Deoxyadenosine phosphate also damages thymic epithelial cells. A few patients with ADA deficiency have been treated with transfusions of normal erythrocytes as a source of ADA, with encouraging results.

Other forms of CID have been described that are due to a failure of development of lymphoid stem cells or to defects in thymic epithelial function. Treatment of these other

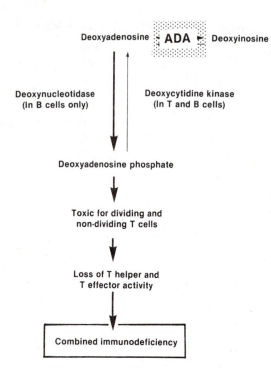

Deoxyadenosine ⋮ ADA ⋮ Deoxyinosine

Deoxynucleotidase
(In B cells only)

Deoxycytidine kinase
(In T and B cells)

Deoxyadenosine phosphate

Toxic for dividing and
non-dividing T cells

Loss of T helper and
T effector activity

Combined immunodeficiency

FIGURE 18–2. The enzyme adenosine deaminase (ADA) normally converts deoxyadenosine to deoxyinosine. In the absence of ADA, deoxyadenosine phosphate accumulates within cells. This compound is toxic for both helper and effector T cells. As a result both arms of the immune response are blocked and a severe combined immunodeficiency results.

forms of CID involves transplantation of stem cells from fetal bone marrow or liver. Graft-versus-host disease (Chap. 19) is the major complication of this therapy, but if it is successfully combatted, encouraging results have been obtained from the transplantation method.

Other major forms of combined immunodeficiency include one associated with short-limbed dwarfism and one in which antibody production is present but very variable. This latter condition is known as Nezelof's syndrome. Combined immunodeficiency inherited as an autosomal recessive trait is an important condition in newborn Arab horses.

Deficiencies of the T-Cell System

If the third and fourth pharyngeal pouches fail to develop, then affected individuals will produce neither thymic epithelium nor parathyroid glands. The resulting disease is characterized by biochemical disturbances due to the absence of parathyroid glands and an absence of T-cell function as a result of thymic aplasia. It may also be associated with cardiac and facial abnormalities and is known as the DiGeorge syndrome.

Because of the absence of functioning T cells, affected individuals fail to thrive and develop infections with the yeast *Candida*, chronic pneumonia, and diarrhea, especially as a result of virus infection. There are few circulating lymphocytes and none with the characteristics of T cells, specifically, Thy-1$^+$ or E-rosetting ability. Immunoglobulin levels and antibody responses are relatively normal implying that B-cell and possibly T-helper function is unimpaired. Possible treatments include the use of thymic hormones or transplantation of thymic epithelial cells, either from a very early fetus or from a cell culture.

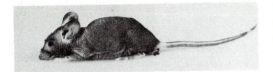

FIGURE 18-3. A nude (nu/nu) mouse: These mice remain healthy if raised apart from other mice in clean surroundings, in spite of an absence of T cells.

Nude mice may be considered to be animal models of a congenital T-cell immuno-deficiency syndrome (Fig. 18-3). Nude mice are a strain of hairless mice that fail to develop a functional thymus although thymic epithelium may develop. Because the T cells fail to develop within the thymus, the nude mice are deficient in mature T cells, but possess a limited number of immature T cells and B cells. As a result, occasional lymphocytes may be found in peripheral blood. Thymic grafts from normal mice, by restoring epithelial-cell function, permit the T cells of nude mice to mature and develop immune competence.

Nude mice are clearly deficient in conventional cell-mediated immune responses, as reflected by prolonged allograft survival and lack of responses to T cell mitogens. Their IgG and IgA levels are commonly also depressed, presumably as a result of a loss of T-helper-cell function.

Although nude mice show an enhanced susceptibility to virus-induced neoplasia, they fail to develop more than the normal level of spontaneous tumors. This observation was, for many years, a major objection to the immunological surveillance theory since, if T cells destroy tumors, then T-cell-deficient animals should suffer from an increased incidence of neoplasia. It has been shown, however, that nude mice possess normal levels of NK cells (Chap. 19).

Purine Nucleoside Phosphorylase (PNP) Deficiency

Purine nucleoside phosphorylase (PNP) has a similar function to adenosine deaminase, in that it cleaves the nucleosides deoxyguanosine and guanosine to guanine. As a result of a PNP deficiency, deoxyguanosine accumulates in the bloodstream, whence it is taken up and phosphorylated by T cells (Fig. 18-4). Thus, deoxyguanosine phosphate accumulates in T cells and inhibits DNA synthesis. This accumulation, however, will only affect dividing T cells. As a result cell-mediated immunity fails to develop, but antibody production is relatively normal, since T helper cells are not required to proliferate in order to promote B-cell function.

Deficiencies of the B-Cell System

A severe hypogammaglobulinemia was the first recognized immunodeficiency disease, being described by Bruton in 1952. There are several different types, an X-linked recessive (the Bruton type), an autosomal recessive, and a sporadic form.

When children are born, they possess IgG acquired by transplacental passage from their mother. This passively acquired maternal IgG provides protection against infection for several months. Normally, as this maternal antibody wanes, children develop their own antibodies. In hypogammaglobulinemic children, these antibodies fail to develop. As a result, the children begin to suffer from severe recurrent infections with organisms, such as *Strep pneumoniae, Strep pyogenes,* and *Hemophilus influenzae,* although they show normal resistance to viruses such as vaccinia, rubella, or mumps. The condition is relatively

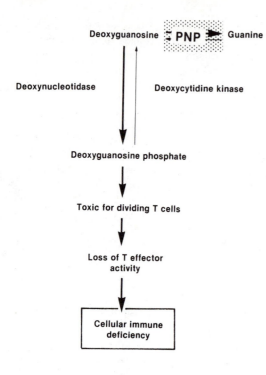

Deoxyguanosine ⇌ PNP → Guanine

Deoxynucleotidase   Deoxycytidine kinase

Deoxyguanosine phosphate

↓

Toxic for dividing T cells

↓

Loss of T effector activity

↓

Cellular immune deficiency

FIGURE 18-4. The enzyme purine nucleoside phosphorylase (PNP) normally converts deoxyguanosine to guanine. In the absence of this enzyme, deoxyguanosine phosphate accumulates. Since this is toxic for dividing T cells only, T-helper-cell activity remains normal, but T effector activity is lost. The result is a cellular immune deficiency while antibody production remains normal.

easily diagnosed by serum electrophoresis (Chap. 7) which demonstrates reduced γ globulin levels. These children usually have no B cells or plasma cells, and their lymphoid organs lack cells in the B-dependent areas. Close analysis shows, however, that these children do have normal numbers of pre-B cells, but they fail to develop to functional maturity. Treatment is through repeated administration of immune serum globulin in an attempt to passively immunize these children against infection.

An immunodeficiency of adults known as common variable immunodeficiency is associated with the absence of plasma cells (B-cell numbers are apparently normal) and very low levels of all immunoglobulin isotypes. The disease appears to be due to an inability of B cells to convert to plasma cells. Some patients with this condition have a deficiency of the enzyme 5′-nucleotidase.

There also exist a variety of congenital immunodeficiency syndromes in which there is a selective deficiency of some but not all of the major immunoglobulin isotypes. These deficiencies may be due to the absence of a specific isotype or, alternatively, to production of "nonfunctional" antibodies. The most common of these dysgammaglobulinemias is a selective IgA deficiency that occurs as a result of the production of T suppressor cells specific for IgA. This disease may be asymptomatic, but, more commonly, it leads to recurrent respiratory and digestive tract infections. IgA deficiency is also associated with severe allergies, since excessive quantities of IgE are commonly produced. It may well be that in the absence of IgA, intact antigens are able to penetrate mucosal surfaces, reach, and stimulate B$_ε$ cells. The condition is diagnosed by demonstrating an absence of IgA in serum and respiratory-tract fluids. Some abnormalities of T-cell function have also been described in these dysgammaglobulinemic individuals.

A selective IgM deficiency has been described in humans, dogs, and horses—affected humans suffer from overwhelming sepsis, and the condition is, therefore, treated with antibiotics. Deficiencies of each of the IgG subclasses have also been described. In many cases, affected individuals suffer from recurrent respiratory-tract infections.

Complex Immunodeficiency Syndromes

The Wiscott-Aldrich syndrome is an X-linked congenital disorder characterized by thrombocytopenia, eczema, and an immunodeficiency reflected by recurrent middle-ear infections (Table 18–1). Serum IgM is usually very low, but IgG and IgA levels are normal or slightly raised while IgE levels may be very high. There is also a T-cell deficiency. This condition may gradually develop over several years as the immunologic defect gradually worsens. Treatment of this complex syndrome is difficult, but encouraging results have been achieved with transfer factor.

Ataxia-telangiectasia is an autosomal recessive condition characterized by cerebellar lesions, telangiectases (dilation of blood vessels) of the skin, recurrent upper-respiratory-tract infections, and endocrine abnormalities. The cerebellar lesions lead to ataxia. The immunodeficiency appears to be associated with an absence of IgG4, IgG2, IgA, and IgE, as well as reduced numbers of T cells and reduced T-cell responses.

A hypergammaglobulin E has been associated with recurrent staphylococcal infections. The abscesses formed in these cases may not elicit normal inflammatory responses. Affected individuals may have defective chemotaxis in their neutrophils and macrophages.

Hyperactivity of the Immune System—Amyloidosis

Amyloid is the name given to an amorphous, eosinophilic, extracellular substance that infiltrates tissues in certain pathological conditions. It may be classified either as immunocytic, if it is associated with a myeloma or other lymphoid tumor, or as reactive, if it is associated with chronic bacterial infections such as arthritis, osteomyelitis (bone-marrow infections), abscesses, or tuberculosis. Reactive amyloidosis is a major cause of death in animals repeatedly immunized for commercial antiserum production. It is also commonly associated with autoimmune disorders. In general, amyloid deposits are usually found in the liver, spleen, and kidneys, particularly within glomeruli (Fig. 18–6). Amyloidosis may be produced in laboratory mice by feeding them a diet rich in casein, or by injecting large or repeated doses of bacterial endotoxin or Freund's complete adjuvant.

On electron microscopy, all forms of amyloid can be shown to consist of a feltlike mass of protein fibrils (Fig. 18–6). By x-ray crystallography, it can be further shown that all amyloid proteins have their polypeptide chains arranged in the form known as β-pleated sheets. This is a uniquely stable molecular conformation that renders the fibrils both extremely insoluble and almost totally resistant to normal proteolytic enzymes. Consequently, once deposited in tissues, they are almost impossible to remove. The accumulation of amyloid in tissues is, therefore, essentially irreversible, leading to gradual cell loss and tissue destruction.

The β-pleated sheet configuration of amyloid also gives it unique staining properties; for example, it stains metachromatically with toluidine blue and binds specifically to Congo red dye.

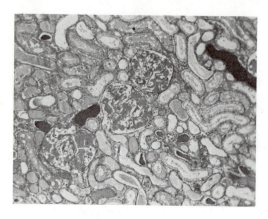

FIGURE 18–5. Amyloidosis of the kidney. Note the amorphous deposits within the glomeruli. These will eventually cause renal failure and death (Congo red stain).

Although all amyloid proteins have the β-pleated sheet configuration, biochemical analysis has shown that most are composed of one of two basic proteins (Fig. 18–7). In immunogenic amyloid and a few cases of reactive amyloid, this protein, known as amyloid L (AL) is a proteolytic digestion product of immunoglobulin light chains. In myelomas, light chains are usually generated in excess, and limited proteolytic digestion of these permits the V_L region to assume a β-pleated configuration. It has been suggested that immunogenic amyloid deposits consist of light chains modified by proteolytic enzymes from cells such as macrophages and deposited in tissues in excessive amounts.

The major protein component of reactive amyloid, known as amyloid A (AA). AA is not immunoglobulin-derived but may be deposited in close association with plasma cells. It is probably derived from proteolytic digestion of an α globulin called serum amyloid A (SAA). SAA is an acute-phase protein found in high concentrations in the serum of humans and animals with experimental or natural amyloidosis and in the serum of patients undergoing chronic immune stimulation or inflammation, as in tuberculosis or rheumatoid arthritis. It is found in low levels in normal serum. Since SAA has been shown to be strongly immunosuppressive in mice, it has been suggested that it normally serves to control the immune response. Under conditions of chronic antigenic stimulation or inflammation,

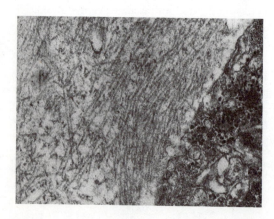

FIGURE 18–6. Amyloid fibrils seen in bundles parallel to a cell membrane: Paired filaments may be distinguished within each fibril. (Courtesy of the late Dr. E. C. Franklin. From Adv. Immunol., *15:* 258, 1972. With permission.)

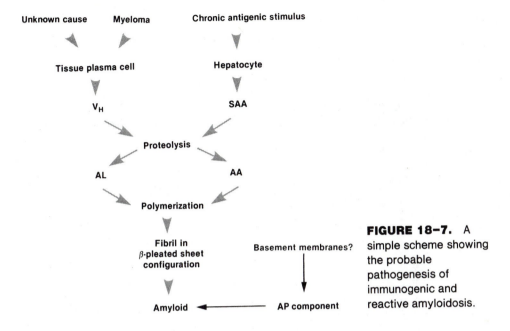

FIGURE 18–7. A simple scheme showing the probable pathogenesis of immunogenic and reactive amyloidosis.

interleukin 1 induces excessive production of SAA by hepatocytes. Its subsequent digestion can lead to the deposition of AA as amyloid in tissues.

Amyloid deposits also contain, in addition to AA, a small quantity of another acute-phase protein derived from hepatocytes known as amyloid P protein (AP), which is related to C-reactive protein (Chap. 6). Although AP is probably unimportant in the pathogenesis of amyloidosis, C-reactive protein is known to be immunosuppressive, and the presence of AP, like that of AA, might be a reflection of an attempt by the body to control excessive immune reactivity.

Although AL and AA are associated with the two major forms of amyloid, it must be emphasized that any protein that can form extensive β-pleated sheets will give rise to amyloid if deposited in tissues. Many of the less common manifestations of amyloidosis may, therefore, be caused by proteins distinct from AL or AA. It has been suggested, therefore, that a more appropriate collective term for the amyloidoses is β *fibrilloses,* since the β-pleated conformational structure is the common feature of all these conditions.

Sources of Additional Information

Baehner, R. L., Nathan, D. G., and Karnovsky, M. L. Correction of metabolic deficiencies in the leukocytes of patients with chronic granulomatous disease. J. Clin. Invest., *49:* 865–870, 1970.

Boxer, L. A., et al. Correction of leukocyte function in Chediak-Higashi syndrome by ascorbate. N. Engl. J. Med., *295:* 1041–1045, 1976.

Carson, D., Kaye, J., and Seegmiller, J. E. Differential sensitivity of human leukemic T cell lines and B cell lines to growth inhibition by deoxyadenosine. J. Immunol., *121:* 1726–1731, 1978.

Glenner, G. G. Amyloid deposits and amyloidosis: The β-fibrilloses. N. Engl. J. Med., *302:* 1283–1292, 1333–1343, 1980.

Gottlieb, M. S., et al. *Pneumocystis carinii* pneumonia and mucosal candidiasis in previously healthy homosexual men. Evidence of a new acquired cellular immunodeficiency. N. Engl. J. Med., *305:* 1425–1431, 1981.

Kennard, J., and Zolla-Pazner, S. Origin and function of suppressor macrophages in myeloma. J. Immunol., *124:* 268–273, 1980.

Koller, L. D. Effect of environmental contaminants on the immune system. Adv. Vet. Sci. Comp. Med., *23:* 267–295, 1979.

Strober, S. T and B cells in immunological diseases. Am. J. Clin. Pathol., *68*(suppl.): 671, 1977.

West, S. One step behind a killer (AIDS). Science 83 *4:* 36–45, 1983.

19

Surveillance and the Elimination of Foreign and Abnormal Cells

Although the immune responses first attracted the attention of scientists by virtue of the body's capacity to recognize and eliminate invading microorganisms, the observation that animals also possess the capacity to reject foreign skin grafts has led to the development of a much broader view of the function of the system as a whole.

In a complex multicellular organism, mechanisms for interaction between cells must exist. These interactions are generally mediated by means of surface structures or receptors through which "signals" are transmitted (see Fig. 10–6). If, for some reason, a cell becomes abnormal and, as a consequence, its surface structure becomes modified, then it is possible for this change to be recognized by other cells. The cell-mediated immune system appears to be designed so that cells with modified surfaces may be identified and then promptly eliminated. The cell-surface structures that function as recognition units in this way are the Class I and II histocompatibility antigens. These antigens are characteristic of an individual animal rather than of particular organs or cell types, although their distribution is not uniform throughout the body. The cells that are capable of recognizing and responding to these altered histocompatibility antigens include T lymphocytes and natural killer (NK) cells.

Terminology

Genetically identical animals are said to be **syngeneic** or **isogeneic.** Genetically dissimilar animals of the same species are **allogeneic.** Animals of different species are **xenogeneic.**

A graft between two locations within the same animal is known as an **autograft.** A graft between two genetically identical animals is an **isograft.** A graft between two genetically dissimilar animals of the same species is an **allograft.** A graft between two animals of differing species is a **xenograft.**

Histocompatibility Antigens and Graft Rejection

The survival of an allograft is directly related to the histocompatibility differences between graft and recipient. Differences at the major histocompatibility locus lead to rapid, irreversible graft rejection. Differences at minor histocompatibility loci provoke slow, easily reversed rejection. The major antigens against which the rejection process is directed are those of the Class I and Class II histocompatibility antigens and the major blood-group antigens.

Class I antigens of the major histocompatibility complex are identifiable by the use of specific antisera and are described as serologically defined (SD) antigens. By using a set of these antisera, it is possible to identify, or "type," each of the antigens on the cells of both the recipient and the potential donors and so select the closest match.

How to Type Class I Histocompatibility Antigens

The usual tests for Class I histocompatibility in man are known as microcytotoxicity tests.

Usually, rabbit complement (preabsorbed or selected for a low level of natural cytotoxicity) is added to a mixture of blood lymphocytes from the person to be tested and antiserum directed against specific histocompatibility antigens. After incubation, the degree of cell killing is estimated by measuring the percentage of cells that take up the vital dyes trypan blue or eosin Y. (These dyes are taken up only by dead cells.)

Antisera of known specificity for individual Class I antigens are derived from a variety of sources. Two of the most usual sources are the blood of multiparous women and the blood of individuals who have received multiple blood transfusions. (Although blood transfusions are always carefully matched to ensure red-blood-cell compatibility, it is not necessary to do the same for white blood cells. As a result, recipients of blood transfusions commonly receive incompatible leukocytes and hence make antibodies to histocompatibility antigens on these cells.) These sera usually have to be carefully absorbed to render them monospecific and suitable for use in histocompatibility testing. More recently, use has been made of highly specific monoclonal antibodies.

Probably of more importance in influencing graft rejection are the Class II antigens found on lymphocytes, macrophages, epidermal cells, and sperm. These antigens are detectable by measuring their ability to stimulate allogeneic lymphocytes to divide in a mixed lymphocyte culture and are, therefore, called lymphocyte-defined (LD) antigens. By using carefully selected cell mixtures, it is possible to type the LD antigens on the periperal blood lymphocytes.

How to Type Class II Histocompatibility Antigens

The usual method used to determine Class II histocompatibility antigens is the mixed-lymphocyte culture (MLC) technique.

Two lymphocyte suspensions from different donors are mixed in a culture tube. As a result of encountering foreign Class II antigens, the cells are stimulated and respond by dividing. This division can be measured by adding tritiated thymidine 4 to 5 days later and measuring the uptake of this by counting the radioactivity of the tritium in a liquid scintillation counter. Only dividing cells take up the thymidine, and the amount of radioactivity is directly related to the degree of cell division. Obviously, if both cell populations are responding simultaneously, the results will be very difficult to interpret. For this reason, one of the cell populations is either irradiated or treated with the drug mitomycin C to prevent it dividing. This population can, therefore, stimulate the other cell population but not respond to it. Low stimulation or absence of stimulation implies compatibility at the Class II locus. The greater the degree of cell proliferation in the MLC, the greater the degree of incompatibility between the stimulating and responding cells.

When dogs are given kidney grafts from donors incompatible at both the SD and the LD loci, they survive for about 7 days (Table 19–1). If, on the other hand, they are compatible at all these loci, graft survival is prolonged to about 40 days. A more impressive result is obtained with canine liver grafts, which survive for about 8 days in unrelated animals, and for 200 to 300 days in DLA (dog leukocyte antigen)-identical recipients. The failure of DLA-compatible grafts to survive indefinitely is due to the cumulative effects of a large number of minor histocompatibility differences.

TABLE 19–1   Mean Survival Times of Canine Tissues Transplanted Between DLA-Incompatible Mongrel Dogs

Organs	Survival Time (Days)
Skin	12.0
Kidney	7.0
Liver	7.7
Pancreas	10.5
Lung	5.8
Small intestine	8.1
Heart	8.4
Tracheal cartilage	250.0
Parathyroids	<14.0

Survival times are usually significantly longer in grafts between DLA-incompatible beagles.

In man, well-matched renal allografts survive for at least two years in 90% of immunosuppressed recipients when derived from related living donors and have a 65% success rate when derived from cadaveric donors (Fig. 19–1). Grafts from donors incompatible at the ABO-blood-group locus are rapidly rejected.

A simple and rapid test for histocompatibility is to take lymphocytes from a potential graft recipient and inject them into the skin of a potential donor. If the injected cells are not compatible with the recipient, the injected lymphocytes will attack and destroy the near-

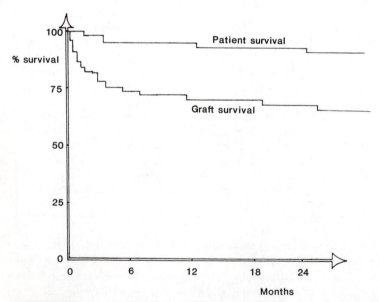

FIGURE 19–1. The survival of 225 renal grafts from dead donors. (From Morris, P. J. Transplant. Proc. *13:* 27, 1980. Reprinted by permission of Grune and Stratton, Inc. and the author.)

est foreign tissue and provoke an inflammatory skin reaction. This reaction is known as the normal lymphocyte transfer test. It measures primarily compatibility at the LD (Class II) loci, since the intensity of the inflammatory response provides an indication of the degree of incompatibility between donor and recipient.

The Allograft Reaction

If a kidney allograft is transplanted between unrelated, untreated individuals, it will survive for about a week. The rejection process is associated with disruption of renal blood vessels, decreased urine production, and cessation of renal function. If a second graft from the same donor is made, it will be rejected by the recipient within one to two days without ever becoming functional. This accelerated reaction to a second graft is known as a second-set reaction and is a form of secondary immune response. The second-set reaction is specific for a graft from the original donor or from a donor syngeneic with the first. It is not restricted to any particular site or to any specific organ, since histocompatibility antigens are present on most nucleated cells.

Histology of Allograft Rejection

The events that take place during graft rejection vary among different types of grafts. For example, if a skin graft is placed on an animal, it takes some time for vascular and lymphatic connections to be established between the graft and the host. Only when these connections are made can host cells penetrate the graft and commence the rejection process. The first indication of this process is a transient neutrophil accumulation around the blood vessels at the base of the graft. This phenomenon is followed by an infiltration of mononuclear cells (lymphocytes and macrophages) that eventually extends throughout the grafted skin. The first signs of tissue damage are observed in the capillaries of the graft, whose endothelium becomes destroyed. As a result, the blood clots and stops flow through these vessels; tissue death follows rapidly. In renal grafts, the blood supply to the transplanted kidney is established at the time of transplantation. The whole organ gradually becomes infiltrated with mononuclear cells (Fig. 19–2), which cause damage to the endothelial lining of small intertubular blood vessels. This vascular damage is progressive, and tubular destruction, stoppage of blood flow, hemorrhage (bleeding), and death of the grafted kidney follow thrombosis (clotting) of these vessels.

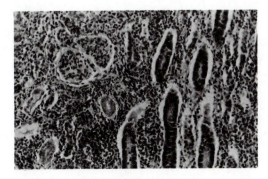

FIGURE 19–2. A section of a canine kidney that had been acutely rejected after 14 days in an allogeneic recipient: Note the extensive mononuclear cell infiltration (original magnification x360). (Specimen kindly provided by Dr. R. G. Thomson. From Tizard, I. Veterinary Immunology, 2nd ed. W. B. Saunders, Philadelphia, 1982. With permission.)

In a second-set reaction, vascularization of skin grafts usually does not have time to occur, since an extensive and destructive mononuclear cell and neutrophil infiltration rapidly occurs in the graft bed. Similarly, the blood vessels of second kidney grafts rapidly become thrombosed as a result of the action of antibodies and complement on the vascular endothelium. Xenografts are usually rejected extremely promptly. For example, porcine renal xenografts transplanted to dogs are rejected in 10 to 20 minutes because of the presence of natural antibodies to pig antigens in dog serum.

The Mechanism of Graft Rejection

As described above, the rejection of grafts is of two general types (Fig. 19–3). In first-set reactions, grafts are rejected in a matter of days. In second-set reactions or xenografts, rejection is a very much more rapid process. Both processes occur as a result of damage to vascular endothelium. The first-set reaction may be divided into two stages. First, information about the antigenic structure of the graft must reach antigen-sensitive cells, usually located in the draining lymph node. Second, effector cells from this lymph node must invade the graft and mediate its destruction.

Sensitization of the Recipient   Information on graft antigens may reach the antigen-sensitive cells of the recipient by two routes. Either graft cells may release soluble histocompatibility antigens or, more important, circulating T cells may, on passing through the blood vessels of the graft, recognize foreign histocompatibility antigens. These T cells may

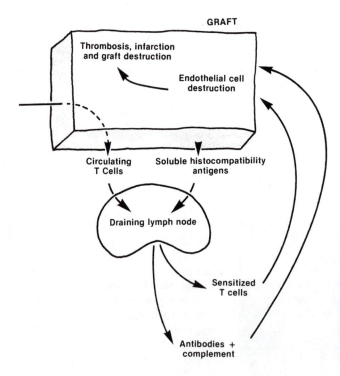

FIGURE 19–3. A schematic diagram showing the major mechanisms of graft rejection. (From Tizard, I. Veterinary Immunology, 2nd ed. W. B. Saunders, Philadelphia, 1982. With permission.)

then pass from the graft in either the lymphatics or the blood vessels and eventually lodge in the draining lymph node as a consequence of local triggering of the lymphocyte "trap" (Chap. 9). It is probable, at least in skin grafts, that the lymphatic route is of most importance, since rejection is considerably delayed if a graft is prevented from developing lymphatic connections with the host.

The cells that recognize the graft as foreign move to the draining lymph node and recruit specific effector T cells within the draining lymph node. The paracortical regions of lymph nodes draining a graft contain increased numbers of cells, among which are clusters of large pyroninophilic lymphoblasts. The numbers of these cells are greatest about six days after grafting and decline rapidly once the graft has been rejected. In addition to these signs of an active T-cell-mediated immune response, it is usual to observe some germinal-center formation in the cortex and plasma-cell accumulation in the medulla, suggesting that a humoral immune response also occurs.

Destruction of the Graft   As a result of the events that occur in the draining lymph node, effector T lymphocytes leave the node in the efferent lymph and eventually reach the graft through the vascular system. When these cells enter the blood vessels of the graft, they bind and destroy the vascular endothelium by direct cytotoxicity. As a result of this damage, hemorrhage, platelet aggregation, thrombosis, and infarction (stoppage of blood flow) occur. The grafted tissue dies because of this failure in its blood supply. There is also evidence to indicate that the intensity of the graft rejection process is related to the number of allogeneic lymphocytes and dendritic cells within the grafted tissue. It has been suggested that a form of graft-versus-host response may contribute significantly to the rejection process.

Although cytotoxic T cells are of most importance in destroying foreign grafted tissues, antibodies also play a significant role in graft destruction (Table 19-2). This is brought about by antibodies, acting in conjunction with complement, and neutrophils or through antibody-dependent cytotoxic cell activity (Chap. 12). It is particularly important in second-set and xenograft reactions.

TABLE 19-2   Some Mechanisms of Cytotoxicity Important in the Destruction of Grafts

Mechanism	Cells Involved	Pathway	Relative Importance in Graft Rejection
Cell-mediated cytotoxicity	T cells	Direct contact	++++
	T cells	Through lymphotoxin	+
	Macrophages	Through SMAF*	+
	Macrophages	Nonspecifically activated	+
Antibodies and cells	Null-lymphocytes Macrophages Neutrophils	Through Fc receptors and antibody	++
Antibodies and complement	—	Complement-mediated cytolysis	+++

*SMAF = specific macrophage-arming factor.

Rejection of Cardiac Allografts

In humans and dogs that have received heart transplants, the pathology of the rejection process is uniquely different. The major lesion observed in these grafts is extensive endothelial cell proliferation in the walls of cardiac blood vessels (Fig. 19–4). The resulting obliteration of the blood-vessel lumen eventually results in cardiac failure and death. A similar lesion is sometimes seen in renal allografts undergoing chronic rejection. About 30 to 60% of cardiac allograft recipients survive for at least two years (Fig. 19–5).

Why Are Allografts Rejected?

The successful surgical transplantation of organs and tissues only became feasible with the development of aseptic surgical techniques. Thus, the process of allotransplantation is entirely artifactual—it has no counterpart in nature and is unlikely to have a physiological role. It has been pointed out previously, however, that the identification and destruction of altered "self" cells, for example, virus-modified or chemically modified cells or tumor cells, is of great potential benefit to an animal.

It has, therefore, been suggested that graft rejection is but a reflection of the existence of a surveillance system whose function is to identify and eliminate any cell that possesses either foreign or modified histocompatibility antigens. But as was discussed in Chapter 12, in order for a cytotoxic T cell to destroy a virus-infected or chemically modified target cell,

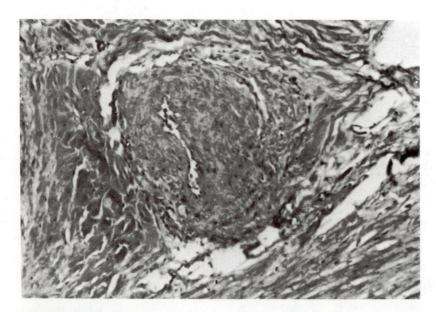

FIGURE 19–4. A section of coronary artery from a canine cardiac allograft showing severe narrowing of the lumen as a result of intimal proliferation (original magnification x100). (From Penn. O. C., et al. Transplantation, *22:* 313, 1976. With permission of Williams and Wilkins.)

STANFORD CARDIAC TRANSPLANTATION

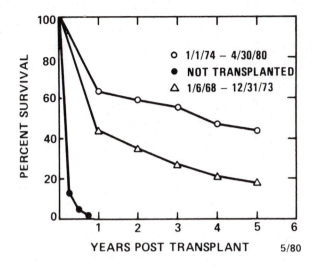

FIGURE 19-5. The survival of cardiac allograft recipients. (From Oyer, P. E., et al. Transplant. Proc., *13:* 203, 1981. Reprinted by permission of Grune & Stratton, Inc. and the author.)

both the target and the cytotoxic cell must be identical at the Class II MHC loci, while in order for an allograft to be rejected, it must be different at the Class I or II loci. This discrepancy has not been fully explained, although it is probable that cytotoxicity against allograft targets may be mediated by a different cell population than that required to destroy modified self targets (see p. 203).

Graft-versus-Host Reaction We have already described the normal lymphocyte transfer reaction, in which lymphocytes from a potential graft recipient are injected into a potential donor animal. These transferred lymphocytes recognize that their new host is foreign and attack nearby cells, as a result a local inflammatory response occurs. In other words, the graft attacks the host! In a normal lymphocyte-transfer reaction, the results of this graft-versus-host (GVH) reaction are usually not serious, since the recipient is capable of destroying the foreign lymphocytes and thus terminates the reaction. If, however, the recipient cannot, for some reason, reject the grafted lymphocytes, then these cells may cause uncontrolled destruction of the host's tissues, and, eventually, death. This type of GVH reaction may occur if the recipient of the lymphoid cells has been immunosuppressed or is immunodeficient. It has been observed, for example, in children that receive bone-marrow or thymus transplants in an attempt to cure congenital immunodeficiencies (Chap. 18). Individuals suffering from a GVH reaction develop lymphocytic infiltration of the intestine, skin, and liver. These lymphocytes result in mucosal destruction and diarrhea, ulcerative skin and mouth lesions, liver destruction, and jaundice. Affected animals show cessation of growth (runting) and eventually die.

Brain Transplants

Although the concept of total brain grafts remains within the realm of science fiction and horror movies, preliminary experiments have shown the feasibility of grafting small

fragments of allogeneic brain tissue. These fragments implanted in brain do not provoke an allograft response (presumably due to the immunologically privileged status
of the brain), but can survive and secrete neurotransmitters.

This procedure might be used for treatment of conditions in which the production
of brain neurotransmitters is defective. For example, Parkinson's disease occurs as a
result of a deficiency of the neurotransmitter dopamine in the caudate nucleus of the
brain. As a result, affected individuals show severe muscular tremor and rigidity of
movement. If fragments of fetal rat brain are implanted into the caudate nucleus of rats
with experimental Parkinson's disease, they secrete sufficient dopamine to cause a
substantial clinical improvement. A single "experiment" of this type in a human patient
failed to change the patient's condition.

Grafts that Are Not Rejected

Privileged Sites   Certain areas of the body, such as the anterior chamber of the eye,
the cornea, and the brain, lack effective lymphatic drainage. Consequently, although antigen derived from grafts made in these sites will reach lymphoid tissue, cytotoxic effector
cells cannot reach the graft, and these grafts survive relatively well. It is for this reason that
corneal allografting is a successful procedure in human and canine surgery.

Sperm   Sperm, of course can successfully and repeatedly penetrate the female reproductive tract without provoking a significant immune response. Seminal plasma, in fact, is very
immunosuppressive, and sperm exposed to this fluid are nonimmunogenic, even after washing. Prostatic fluid, one of the immunosuppressive components of seminal plasma, also
inhibits complement-mediated hemolysis.

Pregnancy   Because the fetus and its placenta possess paternal antigens, they may be
considered as an allograft within the mother. Nevertheless, the fetus is consistently successful in establishing and maintaining itself through pregnancy, in spite of great histocompatibility differences. The reasons for this acceptance of the fetus and its placenta are not
completely understood. It is known, however, that the uterus is not a privileged site, since
grafts of other tissues, such as skin, made in the uterine wall are readily rejected. In fact,
under some circumstances, the mother may make antibodies against fetal blood-group antigens, and these can destroy fetal red blood cells either in utero, as in humans, or following
ingestion of colostrum, as occurs in other mammals (see p. 372).

The immunological destruction of the fetus is prevented by the combined activities of
several different specific and nonspecific immunosuppressive mechanisms (Table 19–3).
First, the fetus is protected from the mother's immune system by the trophoblast (that part
of the placenta in closest contact with maternal tissue). Trophoblast cells have very low
surface concentrations of Class I and Class II histocompatibility antigens and are also covered by a layer of sulfated mucoprotein that is a potent suppressor of allogeneic recognition.

Second, the fetus is a source of immunosuppressive factors. These include the hormones estradiol and progesterone and possibly also chorionic gonadotrophin. The major
protein in fetal serum, α-fetoprotein, is immunosuppressive as a result of its ability to stimulate suppressor cell function. In addition, a number of pregnancy-associated glycoproteins,

TABLE 19-3 Some of the Factors Responsible for the Immunosuppression of Pregnancy

Origin	Factor
Fetus	α-fetoprotein
	Pulmonary surfactant
Trophoblast	Placental interferon
	Chorionic gonadotrophin
Mother	Blocking antibodies
	Suppressor cells
	Progesterone

including α_2-macroglobulin and placental interferon, have immunosuppressive properties, and amniotic fluid is rich in immunosuppressive phospholipids.

Third, both blocking antibody and suppressor cells are produced in response to fetal antigens. These interfere with the maternal antifetal immune response. The blocking antibody coats placental cells, thus preventing their destruction by maternal T cells. This antibody can be eluted from the placenta and shown to be capable of suppressing other cell-mediated immune reactions against paternal antigens, such as graft rejection. Absence of this blocking material has been shown to account for some cases of recurrent abortion in women. (This observation implies that some form of immune response is, in fact, necessary for a successful pregnancy!)

It must not be assumed from the foregoing list of immunosuppressive factors that the pregnant female is grossly immunosuppressed. In fact, the immunosuppression generated by the fetus is very local in nature. Pregnant animals have only minor deficiencies in cell-mediated immune reactivity to nonfetal antigens, showing for example, a slight delay in the rejection of skin grafts, or transient unreactivity to the tuberculin skin test (Chap. 23).

Cultured or Stored Organs   If an organ or tissue is grown in tissue culture or stored frozen, its potential for successful transplantation is greatly enhanced. Thus, if thyroid tissue is grown in an organ culture for about 25 days before transplantation, it will survive in a recipient as if it were an isograft. Uncultured thyroids are rejected in about ten days (Fig. 19-6). If, however, the recipient is first primed by exposure to an uncultured graft, it will then be able to reject a cultured one. Conversely, if an accepted cultured graft is returned to the donor, it will provoke acute rejection.

It is believed that this phenomenon is due to the loss of passenger lymphocytes, macrophages, and dendritic cells from the thyroid tissue during culture. If true, the rejection of a thyroid allograft may be largely due to a reaction between host and donor lymphocytes within the graft. This suggestion is supported by the observation that pretreatment of donors with cytotoxic drugs reduces the subsequent allograft rejection. Similarly, if a kidney is disrupted into its constituent cells and each cell population is tested for its ability to provoke allograft rejection, it is found that by far the most immunogenic components are the "passenger" leukocytes.

Prolonged survival of cultured organs or cells has also been described for islet cells and for ovaries. Freeze-dried pig dermis is very useful in covering extensive wounds, and

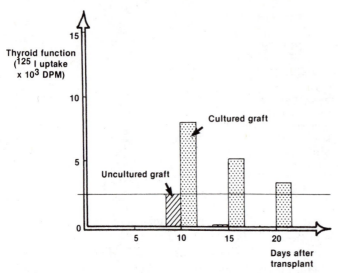

FIGURE 19–6. Thyroid allografts normally function for less than ten days before becoming inactive (less than 2.5×10^3 dpm). If cultured in vitro, however, for several weeks prior to grafting, they show prolonged survival, many functioning for at least 20 days. (From Lafferty, K. J., et al. Science, *188:* 260, 1975. Copyright 1975 by the American Association for the Advancement of Science. With permission.)

there have been reports of successful bone and aortic allografts after storage of the grafts in liquid nitrogen. Treatment of porcine heart valves with glutaraldehyde also renders them immunologically inert so that they can be employed to replace defective valves in humans.

Immunologically Favored Organs On some occasions, individuals that have received a whole liver graft do not appear to mount an allograft response against it, whereas in others, a response may be mounted that is relatively weak and easily suppressed. The liver grafts may, by their presence, be capable of protecting another organ, such as a kidney allograft from the same donor, resulting in its prolonged survival. If recipients are first sensitized and then are given liver allografts, subsequent grafts are retained, the implication being that liver grafting also blocks immunological memory. It is likely that these effects occur in response to the release from the liver of immunosuppressive factors, such as hepatic glycoferroprotein and bilirubin (Chap. 13).

In some circumstances, such as in individuals who have maintained functioning renal allografts for several years, immunosuppressive therapy may be gradually reduced and occasionally be totally discontinued as a graft acceptance becomes complete. This phenomenon may be an example of high dose tolerance—that is, tolerance that results when the amount of antigen is in excess of the capacity of the antigen-sensitive cells to respond to it (Chap. 13). In the case of graft acceptance following immunosuppression, it is believed that antigen-sensitive cells are gradually eliminated by the immunsuppressive agents. Once their numbers are sufficiently low, the relatively large mass of grafted tissue may be sufficient to establish and maintain tolerance. Alternatively, it has been shown in experimental systems that, over time, the graft vascular epithelium may be replaced by cells of host origin. As a result of the formation of this barrier, the graft will be protected against rejection.

Suppression of the Allograft Response

The many techniques available for inhibiting the allograft response may be classified into three general groups. First, the most widely employed techniques involve drugs or radiation that, by inhibiting cell division, serves to reduce the multiplication of antigen-sensitive cells upon encountering antigen. This approach is crude and dangerous, since other rapidly proliferating cell populations, such as intestinal epithelium and bone-marrow cells, may also be destroyed, with disastrous consequences. Second, it is possible to employ techniques that serve to selectively eliminate T cells. This can be done by means of specific anti-T cell serum, by selective drugs or by thoracic-duct drainage. Third, the normal immune responses are well controlled by the body, and although not widely employed at present, manipulation of these natural control mechanisms is likely to provide potentially useful techniques for the control of the allograft response in the future.

Nonspecific Immunosuppression

Radiation   X-radiation exerts its effect on cells by several different mechanisms. The simplest of these is through ionizing rays hitting an essential, unique molecule within the cell. The most important of these molecules are the nucleic acids, particularly DNA. A loss of even one nucleotide entails a permanent mutation of a gene, with potentially lethal effects on the progeny of the affected cell. Another mechanism involves radiation of aqueous solutions, which results in ionization and the formation of highly reactive free hydrogen and hydroxyl radicals. These free radicals can react with dissolved oxygen to form peroxides that have toxic effects on many cell processes. Although x-radiation is of some use in prolonging graft survival in many experimental animals, it is usually necessary to irradiate the recipient for several days prior to grafting. This is impractical in clinical situations since it is not possible to predict when an organ such as a kidney will become available.

Corticosteroids   Corticosteroids are immunosuppressive for several reasons. First, they are highly toxic for some lymphoid cells, particularly those in the thymus, and they diminish B-cell responses to mitogens as well as immunoglobulin synthesis. Second, steroids are capable of stabilizing lysosomal membranes, thus inhibiting the release of lysosomal enzymes and impairing antigen processing. Third, steroids may render macrophages unresponsive to lymphokines, inhibit macrophage expression of Ia, and block the production of IL-1. Steroids are also potent anti-inflammatory agents, since they reduce the release of hydrolytic enzymes from neutrophils and macrophages. Thus, when applied directly to skin grafts, steroids may inhibit rejection without causing systemic immunosuppression.

Cytotoxic Drugs   The major immunosuppressive drugs, having been designed to inhibit cell division, act largely on various stages of nucleic acid synthesis and activity. Thus, many of these drugs are analogues that interfere with nucleic-acid synthesis through competitive blocking of substrate-binding sites on enzymes. For example, azaserine blocks glutamine synthesis; azathioprine, 6-mercaptopurine, and 6-thioguanine block purine synthesis; 5-fluorouracil blocks pyrimidine synthesis; and methotrexate blocks folic-acid synthesis (Fig. 19–7).

The other major group of immunosuppressive drugs comprises the alkylating agents, which act by cross-linking DNA helices, preventing their separation and thus inhibiting template formation. The alkylating agents include cyclophosphamide, chlorambucil, and the antibiotics actinomycin and mitomycin C. The final group of commonly employed cytotoxic drugs are those that inhibit cell division by disrupting microtubule formation. They include drugs such as colchicine and the *Vinca* alkaloids, vincristine and vinblastine.

All these cytotoxic drugs are immunosuppressive by virtue of their ability to interfere with DNA synthesis and thus prevent the replication of antigen-sensitive cells in response to antigen. The relative sensitivity of T cells and B cells to these drugs may vary. Thus, azathioprine, the most commonly used drug in human renal transplantation, tends to inhibit the cell-mediated rejection process in doses that leave the humoral immune response

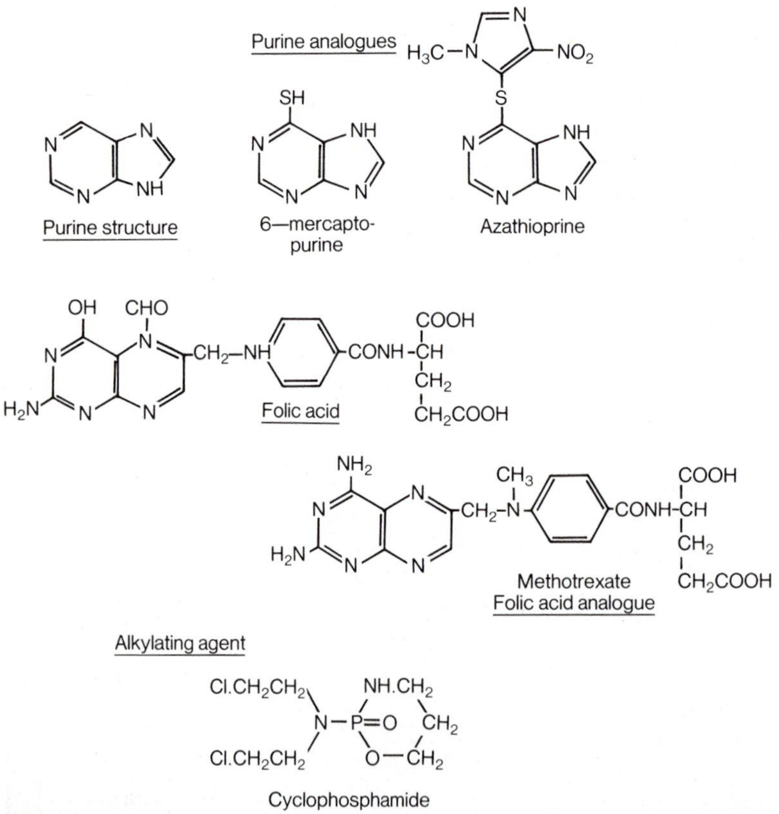

FIGURE 19–7. The structure of some commonly employed immunosuppressive drugs and the normal compounds with which they compete: Cyclophosphamide is an alkylating agent that cross-links DNA chains and hence prevents their separation. (From Tizard, I. Veterinary Immunology, 2nd ed. W. B. Saunders, Philadelphia, 1982. With permission.)

unimpaired, whereas cyclophosphamide tends to selectively prevent B cell responses. Since azathioprine acts at an early stage in the immune response, it can prevent rejection episodes in unsensitized individuals. It is, however, of little use in preventing ongoing rejection.

Specific Methods of Immunosuppression

Depletion of Lymphocytes   Because of the many adverse side effects of the nonspecific immunosuppressive agents (not the least important of which is an increased predisposition to infection), there has been considerable effort made to establish more specific alternative immunosuppressive procedures. One relatively simple experimental technique that largely depletes T cells is cannulation of the thoracic duct. The recirculating lymphocytes that pass through the duct are mainly T cells, and interference with their recirculation in this way can precipitate a dramatic drop in the number of T lymphocytes. Obviously, this procedure does not lend itself readily to routine use; an alternative procedure is to administer an antiserum specific for T lymphocytes. Antilymphocytic serum (ALS) can be made by inoculating a recipient of a different species with a purified lymphocyte suspension. (Horses are commonly employed to make anti-human lymphocyte serum.) The antiserum produced must be refined to ensure that it is specific for lymphocytes. It is usual to attempt to remove antibodies for the other blood elements by repeated absorption. ALS suppresses the cell-mediated immune response and leaves the humoral immune response relatively intact. Theoretically, it is, therefore, a great improvement over other immunosuppressive techniques. In practice, however, ALS has proved to be of variable efficiency. In experiments in mice, ALS-treated animals have been shown to accept rat xenografts, whereas clinical use of ALS in humans has not been universally accepted as being useful. Being a foreign antigen, ALS induces an immune response against itself, a feature that prevents prolonged therapy and increases the risks of anaphylaxis and serum sickness. Finally, since ALS is a suppressor of all cell-mediated immune functions, it may render treated individuals susceptible to virus infections. An attractive alternative to ALS is the use of monoclonal antibodies directed against specific T-cell subsets or even against specific T-cell idiotypes.

Cyclosporin A   Cyclosporin A (CS-A) is a fungal polypeptide containing eleven amino acids arranged in a circular fashion (Fig. 19–8). It acts as a specific suppressor of the T-cell responses by blocking the response of T_H cells to interleukin-1 so that they fail to produce interleukin-2 (Chap. 11). It may also block the response of effector T cells to interleukin-2. The net effect of the action of cyclosporin A is, therefore, the blocking of the T-helper-cell response without affecting either T suppressor cells or nonresponding lymphocytes. CS-A can prevent rejection of kidney, splenic, ovarian, lung, heart, and bone-marrow allografts, especially when administered with steroids. Thus, the combination of cyclosporin A and prednisolone can give essentially 100% survival of renal allografts (Table 19–4). Unfortunately, some patients receiving cyclosporin A have developed B-cell lymphomas. (You may remember how Epstein-Barr virus has the ability to transform B cells into immortal [tumor] cells in culture, but in vivo this is prevented by cytotoxic T cells. Cyclosporin A destroys these cytotoxic T cells and hence permits the malignant B cells to grow in an uncontrolled fashion). If it were not for this and toxicity for the kidney, cyclosporin A would be a perfect immunosuppressive agent.

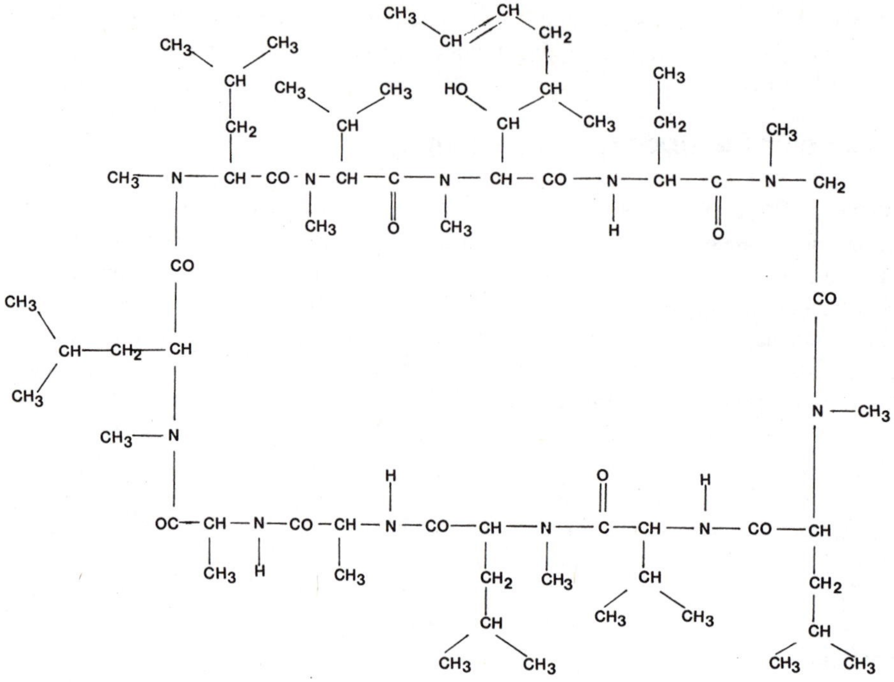

FIGURE 19–8. The structure of cyclosporin A.

Blood Transfusions

For many years, the administration of blood transfusions to potential renal allograft recipients prior to transplantation was discouraged on the grounds that they might sensitize the recipient and so hasten graft rejection. Experience has shown, however, that multiple transfusions given prior to transplantation greatly enhance graft survival.

TABLE 19–4   Transplant Survival Rates 1982–1983

Organ Grafted	Recipient or Graft Survival at 1 Year (%)
Kidneys—living related donor	85–95
Kidneys—nonliving donor	80–85
Heart	70–80
Lung	— *
Liver	70
Bone marrow	30–80
Cornea	95
Pancreas	24

Many of these recent successes are attributable to use of cyclosporin A.

*10 months' survival, maximum

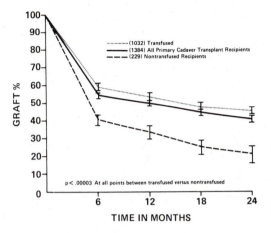

FIGURE 19–9. The effects of blood transfusion on individuals receiving their first transplant from a dead donor. (From Spees, E. K., et al. Transplant. Proc., *13:* 155, 1981. Reprinted by permission of Grune & Stratton Inc. and the author.)

Thus, in one series, pre-renal allograft transfusions changed an 18% survival at one year in controls to 70% survival at one year (Fig. 19–9). In another series, 20% of untransfused recipients showed accelerated rejection as compared with 10% of transfused recipients. The mechanisms involved are unclear, but may be due to stimulation of antibodies directed againt T-cell recognition sites. These antibodies may be detected in patients with successful renal allografts, but not with rejected grafts.

Tumors as Allografts

When organ transplantation became a common and widespread procedure as a result of the development of potent immunosuppressive agents, it was observed that patients with prolonged graft survival and immunosuppressive therapy were about 100 times more likely to develop neoplasia than were nonimmunosuppressed individuals (Table 19–5). It has also been observed that patients with congenital or acquired immunodeficiency syndromes show an enhanced tendency to develop malignant tumors. (For example, AIDS patients may

TABLE 19–5 Incidence of Malignancies in Human Allograft Recipients

	Graft Recipients (%)	General Population (%)
Lymphomas	33	3–4
Prostate carcinoma	17	2
Carcinoma of colon and rectum	14	5
Carcinoma of breast	26	11
Carcinoma of cervix	14	5
Carcinoma of lung in men	22	8

Data derived from Penn, I. Tumor incidence in human allograft recipients. Transplant. Proc., *11:*1047, 1979 1979.

develop Kaposi's sarcoma.) It has, therefore, been suggested that immunocompetent cells are responsible for the prevention of neoplasia. It was from this suggestion that the concept of a surveillance function for the immune system was developed, providing a stimulus for a growing interest in the role of the immune responses in neoplastic diseases.

Experimental evidence has shown that the view of the T-cell system as a system that identifies and destroys tumor cells is no longer completely tenable. One of the most important pieces of evidence to support this is the observation that nude (nu/nu) mice (Chap. 18), although deficient in T cells, are no more susceptible than normal mice to chemically induced or spontaneous tumors (although they are more susceptible to tumors induced by the polyoma virus). The natural resistance of nude mice, and indeed of all normal animals, to tumors is probably dependent upon the various populations of NK cells. Mice deficient in NK cells (beige mice) do show an increased susceptibility to spontaneous tumors.

Thus, although the original surveillance hypothesis has had to be greatly modified, there is good evidence to show that antitumor defense mechanisms do exist and may be enhanced in order to protect an individual against cancer. It should be pointed out, however, that there is a great difference between the strong and effective cell-mediated immune response triggered by allogeneic grafts and the quantitatively much poorer responses to the very weak antigens associated with tumor cells.

Tumor Antigens

Tumor cells that are functionally different from their normal precursors may also be antigenically different, in that they gain or lose antigens. They may, for example, lose histocompatibility or blood-group antigens. Some tumors of the intestine, such as colon carcinomas, may lose the ability to produce mucus. More commonly, tumor cells gain antigens, and some naturally occurring tumors of adult humans are characterized by the production of antigenic proteins normally found only in the fetus. For example, tumors of the gastrointestinal tract may produce a glycoprotein known as carcinoembryonic antigen (CEA), which is commonly found in the fetal intestine. The appearence of CEA in serum may indicate the presence of a colon or rectal adenocarcinoma. Other examples of the generation of a fetal antigen by tumor cells include production of α-fetoprotein by hepatoma cells (α-fetoprotein is normally found only in the fetal liver); also, squamous-cell carcinoma cells may possess antigens also found in normal fetal liver and skin. These **oncofetal antigens** are very poor immunogens and do not, therefore, provoke protective immunity.

Tumors induced by oncogenic viruses tend to gain new antigens characteristic of the inducing virus. These antigens, although coded for by the viral genome, are not part of the virus particle. Examples of this type of antigen include the FOCMA antigens found on the lymphoid cells of cats infected with feline leukemia virus and MATSA (Marek's tumor-specific antigens) found on Marek's-disease tumor cells in chickens. (Both of these are virus-induced, naturally occurring T-cell tumors).

Chemically-induced tumors are different from the virus-induced variety in that they carry surface antigens unique to the tumor and not to the inducing chemical. Tumors induced by a single chemical in different animals of the same species may be antigenically quite unrelated, and even within a single chemically induced tumor mass, it is possible to demonstrate the existence of antigenically distinct subpopulations of cells. As a result, resistance to one chemically induced tumor does not prevent growth of a second tumor induced by the same chemical.

Immune Responses to Tumor Antigens

In general, if tumor cells are antigenically sufficiently different from normal, they will be regarded as foreign and attacked. The major mechanisms of tumor-cell destruction involve NK cells and cytotoxic T cells, although activated macrophages may also participate in this process.

NK Cells and Interferon   As discussed earlier (Chap. 10), a population of large granular lymphocytes possess NK activity insofar as they are able to bind and kill tumor-cell targets without the necessity of prior antigenic stimulation. The cytotoxic activities of NK cells are not restricted to tumor cells. NK cells may also destroy virus-infected cells, fetal cells, and some subpopulations of bone-marrow and thymus cells. The NK cells probably recognize a limited range of antigenic specificities, but NK recognition does not require the expression of MHC determinants on the target cells, and there is no evidence for a memory response.

The mechanisms through which NK cells destroy targets is also unclear. Usually, like T-cell-mediated cytotoxicity, binding to the target is followed by its lysis, but there is some evidence to suggest that the cells produce soluble cytotoxic factors. NK cells produce interferon upon encountering target cells. This interferon acts to enhance NK activity by promoting the rapid differentiation of pre-NK cells. (Remember that interferon also enhances T-cell-mediated cytotoxicity [Chap. 12]).

Most of the evidence that supports a role for NK cells in immunity to tumors is derived from studies on tumor cell lines grown in vitro. Thus, in general, it can be shown that NK cells may destroy cultured tumor cell lines, and that a correlation exists between the level of NK activity measured in vitro and resistance to tumor cells in vivo. Second, it is possible to increase resistance to tumor growth in vivo by passive transfer of NK cells. NK cells will destroy human leukemia, myeloma, and some sarcoma and carcinoma cells in vitro, and this activity is enhanced by interferon. NK cells have also been shown to invade small primary mouse tumors. Patients with Chediak-Higashi syndrome have a selective deficiency of NK cells and a high prevalence of lymphoproliferative diseases. A similar phenomenon is seen in beige (be/be) mice, which are also deficient in some NK cell subpopulations. Some carcinogenic agents, such as urethane, dimethylbenzanthracene, and low doses of radiation can inhibit NK activity. Neutralization of interferon by means of specific antisera can enhance tumor growth in mice, possibly by depressing NK-cell activity. Finally, preliminary studies have suggested that interferon treatment may be useful in human cancer therapy.

TABLE 19–6   Immunosuppressive Factors Released from Tumor Cells

Prostaglandins
α-fetoprotein
Phospholipids
Ill-defined soluble factors that
    block macrophage activation
    block lymphocyte activation
    block antibody production
    induce suppressor T cells
    induce suppressor macrophages

Thus, collectively, it is possible that NK cells acting under the influence of interferon may have an important role in immune surveillance against tumors.

Macrophages   In many experimental tumor systems, macrophages may be shown to exert a major antineoplastic function. This is especially true of macrophages activated by exposure to interferon. These activated macrophages may act in either a specific or non-specific fashion and apparently exert their functions as a result of releasing tumoricidal factors such as arginase and reactive oxygen metabolites. Nonspecific activation of macrophages by bacille Calmette-Guérin (BCG) and *Propionobacterium acnes* have, therefore, been used in attempts to enhance resistance to neoplasia. Unfortunately, macrophages may also exert a proneoplastic effect through the release of immunosuppressive prostaglandins. In addition, many malignant tumors release a heat-stable factor, which inhibits macrophage activation, while the macrophages of tumor-bearing individuals may show defective mobilization and chemotaxis. As a consequence, the results of immunoenhancing therapy have tended to be erratic.

Specific Immunity   It is occasionally possible to detect a cell-mediated response to tumor antigens either by skin testing or by an in vitro test, such as macrophage migration inhibition. It is also possible to show that lymphocytes from tumor-bearing animals may exert a cytotoxic effect on tumor cells cultured in vitro. Antibodies to tumor cells are commonly found in many tumor-bearing animals; for instance, about 50 percent of sera from dogs with lymphosarcomas contain precipitating antitumor antibodies. These antibodies may be of some protective significance, since in conjunction with complement, antibodies may be capable of lysing tumors of dispersed cells. Antibodies do not appear to be effective in lysing solid tumors.

Failure of the Immune Responses to Tumor Cells

The fact that neoplasia are so readily induced in experimental animals and are so relatively common in humans testifies to the inadequacies of the immunological protective mechanisms. Studies of tumor-bearing individuals have indicated the existence of a number of mechanisms by which immune systems fail to reject tumors.

Immunosuppression   It is commonly observed that tumor-bearing animals are severely immunosuppressed. This suppression is most clearly seen in animals bearing lymphoid tumors; in these animals, tumors of B cells appear to suppress antibody formation, whereas tumors of T-cell origin generally suppress the cell-mediated immune responses. The suppression observed in leukemia virus infections is possibly a reflection of a generalized disturbance in the lymphoid-cell system brought about by these viruses. In contrast, immunosuppression observed in animals bearing chemically induced tumors appears to be due, at least in some cases, to the release of immunosuppressive factors, such as prostaglandins, from the tumor cells or from tumor-associated macrophages (Table 19–6). Finally, it should be pointed out that the presence of actively growing tumor cells represents an extremely severe protein drain on an animal. This protein loss may be reflected in an impaired immune response.

Much of the immunosuppression seen in tumor-bearing individuals may, however, clearly be attributed to the development of suppressor cells. Thus, administration of anti-

I-J sera to tumor-bearing mice has been found to inhibit tumor growth as a result of inhibition of suppressor-cell function. Enhanced suppressor-cell activity can be detected in the serum of patients with osteogenic sarcomas, thymomas, myelomas, and Hodgkin's disease, and in many tumor-bearing animals. In most cases, these suppressor cells are undoubtedly T cells generally bearing Fcγ receptors and the T8 antigen. In others, however, the suppressor cell may be macrophagelike, having the ability to bind to surfaces, while in still others, it may have B-cell characteristics.

Conventional cancer therapy may act by influencing suppressor-cell activity. Thus cyclophosphamide is particularly effective in inhibiting suppressor-cell function. On the other hand, that the immunostimulating agents *Propionobacterium acnes,* (*Corynebacterium parvum,*) and BCG (bacille Calmette-Guérin) commonly enhance suppressor-cell activity may account for their relative lack of success.

Inhibitors of the Cell-Mediated Immune Response   Although tumor cells are antigenic and may stimulate a protective cell-mediated immune response, the humoral immune response commonly has an opposite effect. Thus, the serum of tumor-bearing animals, when given to other tumor-bearing animals, may cause the tumor of the second animal to grow even faster—a phenomenon known as **enhancement.** Serum of this type may also effectively inhibit the in vitro cytotoxicity of T cells for tumor cells. The nature of the blocking material that causes tumor enhancement is not clear, but it may be either antigen or an immune complex consisting of antibody complexed to tumor-cell antigen. Certainly, many tumors release large quantities of cell-surface antigen, and this may bind to cytotoxic T cells, saturating their antigen receptors and so blocking their capacity to bind to target cells. Alternatively, blocking antibodies may be produced—non-complement-fixing antitumor antibodies that effectively mask tumor antigens and thus protect the tumor cells from attack by cytotoxic T cells. In general, the presence or absence of these blocking factors correlates well with the state of progression or regression of a tumor.

How Blocking Antibodies Were Discovered

Blocking antibodies were first demonstrated by their ability to reduce the cytotoxic effects of specific immune T cells. Thus, a simple ^{51}chromium release assay was set up where it was anticipated that the cytotoxic T cells would destroy the cancer cells. Serum from a variety of sources, including both normal and tumor-bearing individuals were added to the cultures.

Some of the results obtained are seen in Table 19–7.

Hellstrom, I., et al. Blocking of cell-mediated tumor immunity by sera from patients with growing neoplasms. Int. J. Cancer, 7: 226–237, 1971.

Tumor-Cell Selection   There are two possible mechanisms by which the biological activity of tumor cells might influence their survival. One is "sneaking through," the process by which a tumor may not provide sufficient stimulus to induce an immune response until it has reached a size at which it cannot be controlled by the host. Second, tumor cells that are very different from the host cells will be rapidly identified and eliminated without lead-

TABLE 19-7 Cytotoxicity in the Presence of Serum from Tumor-Bearing Individuals (%)

Tumor	Normal Serum	Serum from Patients with the Same Type of Tumor as Targets	Serum for Patients with Unrelated Tumors
Melanoma	42.4	11.3	45.8
Colon carcinoma	50.3	8.7	45.9
Sarcoma	47.5	20.8	47.5
Breast carcinoma	36.1	10.4	30.4

ing to disease. Those tumors that do develop must, therefore, be selected for their inability to stimulate the host's immune system. For example, some Balb/C mouse myeloma cells become refractory to T-cell-mediated cytotoxicity as a result of a loss of cell-membrane histocompatibility antigens.

Tumor Immunotherapy

Two general approaches have been used in attempts to cure or modify tumor growth through immunotherapy (Table 19-8). The simplest is to nonspecifically stimulate the immune system. Obviously, any improvement in an animal's immune capabilities will tend to enhance its resistance to tumors, although a cure may be expected only if the tumor mass is small or is surgically excised. The most widely used immune stimulant is the attentuated strain of *Mycobacterium bovis,* BCG. This organism, being a facultative intracellular parasite, stimulates T-cell activity and activates macrophages. It may be given systemically, or, more effectively, it may be injected directly into the tumor mass. Most information on the use of BCG has come from studies on patients with melanomas. Direct injection of BCG into skin metastases may cause complete regression, not only of the injected lesion but also, occasionally, of uninjected skin metastases also. However, visceral metastases usually remain unaffected. BCG, however, can cause severe lesions at the site of injection and, occasionally, systemic hypersensitivity. The mode of action of the BCG is unclear, but it probably activates macrophages that then attack the tumor cells.

Other immunostimulants that have been employed, although generally with less success than BCG, include *Propionobacterium acnes,* (*Corynebacterium parvum*), levamisole,

TABLE 19-8 Some Approachess to Tumor Immunotherapy

Nonspecific Stimulation of the Immune System
 BCG, *Corynebacterium parvum,* levamisole, thymic hormones, etc.
Passive Immunization
 a. Transfer-factor therapy
 b. Specific monoclonal antibodies either alone or complexed to isotopes or cytotoxic drugs
Active Immunization
 a. Use of chemically modified cells, e.g., neuraminidase or glutaraldehyde treated
 b. Antiviral vaccination, e.g., Marek's disease, warts

and various mixed bacterial vaccines. A related technique that has been used to treat human skin tumors is to paint them with contact allergen dinitrochlorobenzene. The local hypersensitivity reaction provoked by this compound preferentially damages the tumor cells and so promotes tumor regression.

Specific immunotherapy, the second major approach, has also been attempted by many investigators. This may be achieved by active immunization—that is, vaccinating the animal with tumor cells or antigens. One such technique is to take tumor cells, emulsify them in Freund's complete adjuvant, and reinject the mixture into the host. Because so many tumors can evade the immune response, it is usual to treat the tumor cells in an attempt to enhance their antigenicity. Thus, x-irradiated cells and neuraminidase- or glutaraldehyde-treated cells have been used in tumor vaccines. The results obtained to date with tumor vaccines have been very erratic and usually unsatisfactory.

Adoptive transfer of immune lymphocytes is, at least in theory, a logical method of conferring immunity against a tumor in an animal. In practice, however, this technique is not feasible, although some success has been achieved with transfer factor (Chap. 12) extracted from these cells. Since transfer factor functions across species barriers, it is possible that it may be harvested from domestic animals and used therapeutically in humans. Experimental evidence suggests that some thymic hormones may also be of assistance in tumor therapy in that they promote T-cell function.

Passive immunization using serum from immune animals is generally considered undesirable because of the risk of tumor enhancement through transfer of blocking antibody. Nevertheless, normal cat serum causes rapid regression of feline-leukemia-virus-induced tumors for unknown reasons. At the present time, much emphasis is being placed on the potential use of monoclonal antibodies in tumor therapy. Thus, monoclonal antibodies may be raised against tumor-specific antigens. These antibodies can be used to destroy tumors, either when given alone or when complexed to highly cytotoxic drugs or potent radioisotopes, which they carry directly to the tumor cells. Preliminary experiments using these immunotoxins have given very encouraging results.

Successful Antitumor Vaccines

In contrast to the techniques described above, most of which have met with only partial success, there do exist a number of established successful techniques for vaccination against tumor viruses. The most important of these is the vaccine against Marek's disease, a T-cell tumor of chickens caused by a herpes virus. The immune response evoked by this vaccine has two components, First, humoral and cell-mediated responses act directly on the virus to reduce the quantity available to infect cells. Second, an immune response against antigens generated by the virus on the surface of tumor cells is provoked. These antigens provoke successful antitumor immunity. Both the antiviral and antitumor immune responses act synergistically to protect the birds.

Success has also been achieved with inactivated wart vaccines in animals, probably because non-virion, virus-specific antigens develop on tumor-cell membranes and function as immunogens. In view of this phenomenon, it is perhaps possible to predict that future successes are more likely to be due to the development of vaccines against oncogenic viruses, such as these, rather than to more complex immunological approaches directed toward the destruction of tumor cells.

Sources of Additional Information

Allison, A. C., and Ferluga, J. How lymphocytes kill tumor cells. N. Engl. J. Med., *295:* 165–167, 1976.

Anderson, D. J., and Tarter, T. H. Immunosuppressive effects of mouse seminal plasma components *in vito* and *in vitro.* J. Immunol., *128:* 535–539, 1982.

Barker, C. F., and Billingham, R. E. Immunologically privileged sites. Adv. Immunol., *25:* 1–54, 1977.

Beer, A. E., and Billingham, R. E. Immunoregulatory aspects of pregnancy. Fed. Proc., *37:* 2374–2378, 1978.

Broder, S., and Waldmann, T. A. The suppressor cell network in cancer. N. Engl. J. Med., *299:* 1281–1284, 1335–1341, 1978.

Bumol, T. F., et al. Monoclonal antibody and an antibody-toxin conjugated to a cell surface proteoglycan of melanoma cells suppress *in vivo* tumor growth. Proc. Nat. Acad. Sci. USA., *80:* 529–533, 1983.

Carpenter, C. B., d'Apice, A. J. F., and Abbas, A. K. The role of antibodies in the rejection and enhancement of organ allografts. Adv. Immunol., *22:* 1–65, 1976.

Chism, S. E., Burton, R. C., and Warner, N. L. Immunogenicity of oncofetal antigens: a review. Clin. Immunol. Immunopathol., *11:* 346–373, 1978.

Grebe, S. C., and Streilen, J. W. Graft-versus-host reactions: a review. Adv. Immunol., *221:* 119–221, 1976.

Hellström, K. E., and Hellström, I. Lymphocyte-mediated cytotoxicity and blocking serum activity to tumor antigens. Adv. Immunol., *18:* 209–277, 1974.

Herberman, R. B., and Ortaldo, J. R. Natural killer cells: Their role in defenses against disease. Science, *214:* 24–30, 1981.

Karn, I., and Friedman, H. Immunosuppression and the role of suppressive factors in cancer. Adv. Cancer Res. *25:* 271–321, 1977.

Kiersling, R., et al. Killer cells: a functional companion between natural, immune T cell and antibody-dependent *in vitro* systems. J. Exp. Med., *143:* 772–780, 1976.

Minato, N., Reid, L., and Bloom, R. On the heterogeneity of natural killer cells. J. Exp. Med., *154:* 750–762, 1981.

Oettgen, H. F. Immunotherapy of cancer. N. Engl. J. Med., *297:* 484–491, 1977.

Rowlands, D. T., Hill, G. S., and Zmijewski, C. M. The pathology of renal homograft rejection: a review. Am. J. Pathol. *85:* 774–812, 1976.

20

Type I Hypersensitivity: Allergies and Anaphylaxis

Induction of Type I Hypersensitivity
Mast Cells and Basophils
Release of Biologically Active Agents

Control of Type I Hypersensitivity

Measurement of Type I Hypersensitivity

Clinical Manifestations of Type I Hypersensitivity
Acute Systemic Anaphylaxis (Anaphylactic Shock)
Respiratory Allergy
Food Allergy

Prevention and Treatment of Type I Hypersensitivity

Immunological reactions have been known for many years to provoke inflammatory reactions. If inflammation is viewed as a protective process, then these hypersensitivities can be considered merely as additional protective mechanisms mediated by immune processes. However, in some circumstances, they may be so dramatic, severe, or even life-threatening that they can also be considered pathological.

Although the ways in which hypersensitivity can be induced are many, the simplest way to view these reactions is through the classification scheme of the two British immunologists, Philip Gell and Robin Coombs. They noted that all these reactions fall into one of four classes. (For specific details of this classification, the reader would be well advised to review Chap. 5 before beginning this one).

It is perhaps, appropriate, at this time to point out that the classification scheme of Gell and Coombs is for convenience only. In "real life," multiple different hypersensitivities occur together and "pure" hypersensitivities of a single type are uncommon.

Type I hypersensitivities are inflammatory reactions mediated by certain classes of immunoglobulins, especially IgE, bound to mast cells and basophils; the reactions result from the release of pharmacologically active factors (Fig. 20–1).

Of all the adverse consequences of the immune response, the most dramatic are those of Type I hypersensitivity. These reactions are variously termed immediate hypersensitivity, allergies, or anaphylaxis. Because they cause so much discomfort and distress, any possible beneficial effects are not immediately obvious; nevertheless, certain features of this type of hypersensitivity do give us indications of a beneficial biological function. First, it is probable that the localized acute inflammatory response that occurs in this condition plays a significant role in antigen elimination. Second, this type of hypersensitivity is commonly

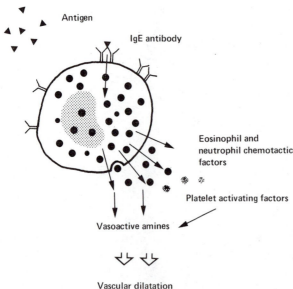

Antigen

IgE antibody

Eosinophil and neutrophil chemotactic factors

Platelet activating factors

Vasoactive amines

Vascular dilatation
Increased vascular permeability
Smooth muscle contraction
Irritation

FIGURE 20–1. Schematic diagram showing the mechanism of type I hypersensitivity. (From Tizard I. Veterinary Immunology, 2nd ed. W. B. Saunders, Philadelphia, 1982. With permission.)

associated with helminth antigens and appears to play a role in resistance to these parasites (Chap. 17). Third, statistical evidence suggests that individuals who suffer from allergies are less likely than unaffected people to die from cancer. The mechanism and significance of this phenomenon are unknown.

Terminology

Before the antibodies that mediate Type I hypersensitivity were characterized as IgE, they were known as **reagins** or **reaginic antibodies.** Because they bind to cells, they are also **cytotropic** or **cytophilic.** If they can bind only to cells of their own species, they are said to be **homocytotropic.** IgE is not, strictly speaking, homocytotropic, since it may bind to cells of several species of animals. The type of reaction that IgE mediates is an **immediate hypersensitivity,** so called because of its prompt occurrence following exposure to antigen. This type of hypersensitivity reaction is also known as **allergy.** Antigens that stimulate allergies may be termed **allergens.** However, many clinicians and laymen use the term allergy to describe any unpleasant reaction of immunological or quasi-immunological origin. If an immediate hypersensitivity reaction is systemic and severe, it is termed **anaphylaxis.** In this chapter, the term Type I hypersensitivity is employed as much as possible, since it has an etiological connotation that many of the other terms now lack.

Induction of Type I Hypersensitivity

Type I hypersensitivity is mediated by antibodies of the IgE class. The conditions under which IgE rather than IgG antibodies are produced are not clear. The antigens that induce IgE antibodies have no discernible unique biochemical features. Certain antigens are, however, potent stimulators of this type of response. These include proteins of pollen grains, some helminth antigens, and some proteins in insect venoms. Freund's complete adjuvant or killed *Bordetella pertussis* organisms may act to preferentially stimulate IgE production in some animals.

In many species, including dogs and humans, some individuals have a greater-than-normal tendency to mount an IgE response. These individuals are said to be **atopic.** Between 10 and 20% of the population of the United States claims to have some type of allergy. It is clear that several factors interact to regulate the expression of allergies. Thus, total-serum IgE levels are influenced by infestations with parasitic helminths. There is a tendency for more males than females to be affected, and the prevalence of allergy rises to peak at about 20 to 24 years before declining gradually. Breast-feeding tends to prevent allergy by minimizing neonatal infection and reducing exposure to foreign antigens.

Probably the most important factors that influence the development of allergies are genetic. There appears to be a major IgE-regulator locus that influences overall IgE production, probably through a T-cell-mediated mechanism. There is also an association between certain HLA haplotypes and the occurrence of atopy. This association implies that the allergic trait may be influenced by a gene or genes within the HLA region—perhaps an immune response gene. Thus, the development of atopy probably depends upon interaction between an IgE-regulator gene and one or more immune-response genes located within the HLA region.

Mast Cells and Basophils

Mast cells are large, round cells (15–20 μm in diameter) distributed throughout the body in connective tissue (Figs. 20–2 and 20–3). Their most characteristic feature is their cytoplasm packed with large granules that stain intensely with dyes such as toluidine blue. The granules usually mask the relatively large, bean-shaped nucleus.

     Mast cells, at least in rodents and humans, fall into two populations differentiated on the bases of their origins and activities. Ordinary connective-tissue mast cells arise from precursors in fetal liver and bone marrow. These cells are found in normal numbers in nude mice. Their numbers increase slowly in tissues, although irritation may cause local proliferation. In contrast, the mast cells found in the epithelial mucosa are apparently derived from thymus-derived precursors, hence are absent from nude mice. They differ from connective-tissue mast cells in several respects. For example, they tend to have fewer granules, and these granules stain differently. They are also relatively short-lived. It has been suggested that these mucosal mast cells respond specifically to nematode antigens. Mast cells carry glycoprotein receptors for the Fc region of IgE, hence are able to bind free IgE molecules. They may have, in addition, receptors for IgG and C3b. Particles coated with either of these proteins may be phagocytosed by mast cells without provoking mediator release.

     No visible change occurs in the structure of the mast cells as a result of their combination with IgE. However, when two cell-bound IgE molecules are linked by antigen, the mast cell responds by abruptly exposing its granules to extracellular fluid. The granules may be expelled from the interior of the cell into the extracellular environment. Alternatively, channels may open in the cell cytoplasm, permitting the extracellular fluid to penetrate to the granules. These mast-cell responses are extremely rapid, occurring only a few

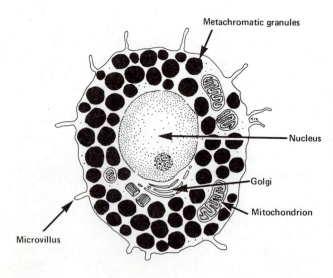

FIGURE 20–2. The principle structural features of a mast cell. (From Tizard, I. Veterinary Immunology, 2nd ed. W. B. Saunders, Philadelphia, 1982. With permission.)

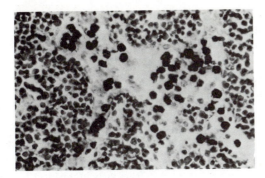

FIGURE 20-3. A section of normal human mesenteric lymph node stained to show mast cells. The metachromatic staining of mast cells is due to the presence of heparin within their cytoplasmic granules. (*Metachromatic* simply means that they stain unusually well with this dye.) (From Tizard, I. Veterinary Immunology, 2nd ed. W. B. Saunders, Philadelphia, 1982. With permission.)

seconds after immune-complex formation on the cell surface (Fig. 20–4). Degranulated mast cells do not die, but they are difficult to identify because of an absence of characteristic morphological features. It is thought that some are identical to the so-called globule leukocytes seen in the intestinal wall of animals after elimination of helminth infections, as a result of the process of "self-cure" (Chap. 17).

Strictly speaking, peripheral-blood basophils should not be considered simply as circulating mast cells. They may, however, be passively sensitized with IgE, and they will respond to antigen in a manner similar to that of mast cells.

Agents that initiate mast-cell degranulation by nonimmunological mechanism include drugs, such as the antibiotic polymyxin B, morphine, and tubocurarine, and the basic polypeptides C3a and C5a released in the complement cascade. These peptides are known as **anaphylatoxins.**

Release of Biologically Active Agents

On exposure to extracellular fluid, mast-cell granules release their vasoactive agents into the surrounding tissue fluid. In addition, the combination of IgE with antigen on the surface

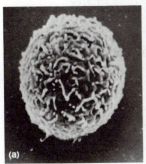
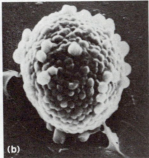
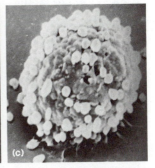

FIGURE 20-4. A scanning electron micrograph of **A**), a normal rat mast cell; **B**) a sensitized mast cell fixed 5 sec. after exposure to antigen, and **C**) a sensitized mast cell fixed 60 sec after exposure to antigen (original magnification x3000). (From Tizard, I. R., and Holmes, W. L. Int. Arch. Allergy. Appl. Immunol., *46:* 867–897, 1974. With permission of S. Karger.)

of mast cells provokes the *de novo* formation of vasoactive substances. It is these agents, both those released preformed from granules and those newly synthesized, that generate the characteristic lesions of Type I hypersensitivity (Table 20–1).

Histamine   Histamine is an amine formed by decarboxylation of the amino-acid histidine and stored, preformed, within the mast-cell granules. Once these granules are exposed to the extracellular fluid, histamine is released through exchange with sodium ions. Histamine possesses a number of biological activities that particularly affect blood vessels and smooth muscle. For example, it dilates and induces increased permeability of small blood vessels so that intradermal inoculation of histamine gives a "wheal and flare" (edema and redness) reaction. Histamine causes smooth-muscle contraction, particularly in the bronchi, gastrointestinal tract, uterus, and bladder. It is a potent stimulator of exocrine secretions, stimulating bronchial mucus secretion, gastric secretion, lacrimination (tear production), and salivation. It also enhances the response of basophils to C5a and promotes the helminthicidal activities of eosinophils.

In small quantities, histamine and its breakdown products are chemotactic for eosinophils, which possessing large quantities of histaminases, can readily break it down.

Serotonin (5-hydroxytryptamine)   Serotonin, a derivative of the amino acid tryptophan, is released from the mast cells of some species of rodents and the large domestic herbivores. It also exists preformed in platelets. It is released from platelets through the activity of a number of factors, including the platelet-activating factors. Serotonin stimulates the heart and causes vasoconstriction that results in a rise in blood pressure. It appears to have little effect on vascular permeability, except in rats and in mice, in which serotonin readily induces wheal-and-flare reactions.

Factors Derived from Arachidonic Acid   Arachidonic acid, an unsaturated long-chain fatty acid, is metabolized by two alternative pathways. Under the influence of

TABLE 20–1   Major Mediators Involved in Type I Hypersensitivity

Mediator	Major Actions
Preformed Mediators	
Histamine	Smooth-muscle contraction, increased vascular permeability, pruritis, increased exocrine secretion
Serotonin	Vasospasm and smooth-muscle contraction
ECF-A	Eosinophil chemotaxis
Platelet-activating factor	Platelet aggregation and secretion
NCF-A	Neutrophil chemotaxis
Mediators Generated *de novo*	
Prostaglandins	Very complex; influence vascular and smooth-muscle tone, platelet aggregation, and immune reactivity
Leukotrienes C and D	Characteristic smooth-muscle contraction and increased vascular permeability
Leukotriene B	Neutrophil and eosinophil chemotaxis
Bradykinin	Smooth-muscle contraction and increased vascular permeability
Serotonin	Smooth-muscle contraction and vasospasm

enzymes known as lipoxygenases, it yields leukotrienes. Under the influence of enzymes known as cyclooxygenases, it yields prostaglandins and thromboxanes.

Leukotrienes   Four major groups of leukotrienes are synthesized by mast cells upon stimulation by antigen. Leukotriene B_4 acts to stimulate neutrophil and eosinophil chemotaxis; indeed, it is the most potent chemotactic factor known. It also stimulates random motility of these cells and enhances their expression of C3b receptors (CR1). The other major leukotrienes, leukotrienes C_4, D_4, and E_4, collectively, may represent what was formerly known as slow-reacting substance of anaphylaxis (SRS-A)—that is, they provoke a slow contraction of smooth muscle (Fig. 20–5). Leukotrienes C_4 and D_4 are up to 20,000 times more potent than histamine in contracting the smooth muscle of bronchioles in certain species. They also increase vascular permeability. Leukotrienes may also be derived from sources other than mast cells, especially macrophages.

Prostaglandins   Prostaglandins are a family of complex lipids with a wide range of activities. Some prostaglandins, such as $PGF_{2\alpha}$ and thromboxane (TxA_2), cause smooth muscle to contract and provoke vasconstriction. Other prostaglandins, such as PGE_1, PGE_2, and prostacyclin (PGI_2) cause smooth muscle relaxation and vasodilation. PGI_2, PGE_1 and $PGF_{2\alpha}$ promote mast-cell-mediator release. As pointed out earlier, the E prostaglandins are potently immunosuppressive.

Since each target tissue may be able to synthesize many different prostaglandins, the ultimate response to prostaglandins represents the algebraic sum of a large number of interactions.

Eosinophil Chemotactic Factor of Anaphylaxis (ECF-A)

There are at least two ECF-A's, both acidic tetrapeptides with molecular weights of less than 1000 daltons, which exist preformed within mast cells. Not only do they attract eosinophils to the site of mast-cell degranulation, they subsequently desensitize them so that the eosinophils can

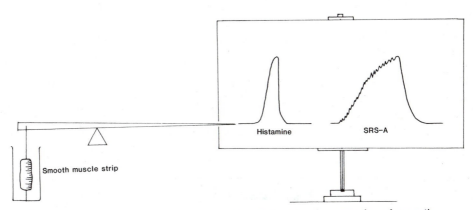

FIGURE 20–5. Histamine causes a rapid and short-lived contraction of smooth muscle. SRS-A causes a prolonged slow contraction and stimulates the spontaneous activity of the muscle. This can be measured by adding these compounds to a strip of smooth muscle (for example, bronchial muscle) in a buffer bath and recording the contraction on a rotating drum.

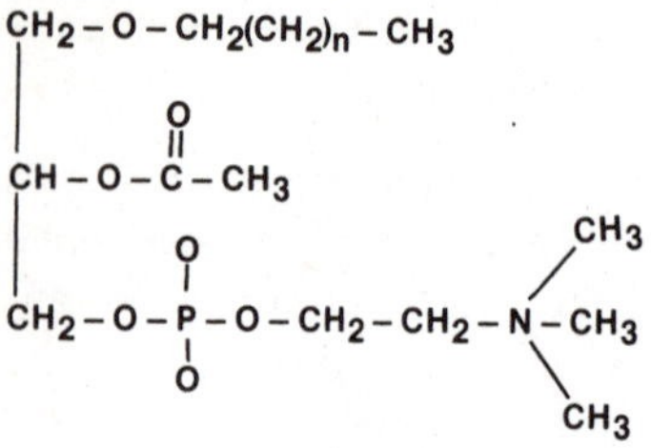

$$CH_2 - O - CH_2(CH_2)_n - CH_3$$

$$CH - O - \overset{\overset{O}{\|}}{C} - CH_3$$

$$CH_2 - O - \overset{\overset{O}{\|}}{\underset{O}{P}} - O - CH_2 - CH_2 - N \overset{CH_3}{\underset{CH_3}{\diagdown}} CH_3$$

FIGURE 20–6.   The structure of platelet activating factor.

move away, and they promote eosinophil superoxide production. These factors account, at least in part, for the eosinophilia so characteristic of Type I hypersensitivity reactions, including helminth infestations.

Platelet-Activating Factor   A phospholipid closely related to lecithin, platelet-activating factor (Fig. 20–6) makes platelets aggregate and release their contents, especially serotonin. It also promotes platelet prostaglandin synthesis and neutrophil aggregation. Platelet-activating factor is inactivated by the enzyme phospholipase D found in eosinophils.

Other Biologically Active Factors   Mast-cell granules appear to be modified lysosomes. Upon phagocytosis of particles by mast cells, the granules fuse with phagosomes to form phagolysosomes. It is, therefore, not surprising that they contain hydrolytic enzymes such as β-hexosaminidase, β-glucuronidase, arylsulfatase, tryptase, kallikreins, and enzymes of the respiratory burst, such as superoxide dismutase. Other factors found in the granules include a neutrophil chemotactic factor (NCF-A) and a neutrophil immobilization factor. The latter factor, as its name suggests, stops the movement of neutrophils after they have been attracted to the area by the chemotactic factor. It does not interfere with the phagocytic activities of the cells.

Heparin is found in connective-tissue mast-cell granules and probably is largely responsible for their metachromatic staining properties. It is released from the granules independently of histamine. Because of the anticoagulant properties of heparin, blood from animals suffering from anaphylaxis may fail to coagulate. Mucosal mast cells do not contain heparin.

Kinins are basic polypeptides, the most important of which is bradykinin. They are derived from kininogens (α globulins) by the activity of the proteolytic enzymes called kallikreins (kinogenases). Kallikreins may be produced directly from mast cells and basophils or indirectly from activated platelets. They may also be produced in plasma by the action of Hageman factor (Factor XII) on an inert prekallikrein (kallikreinogen). Kinins increase vascular permeability and stimulate smooth-muscle contraction.

Control of Type I Hypersensitivity

Regulation of the IgE response   It is well recognized, at least in humans, that not all individuals are equally able to mount an IgE response. The reasons for this, as mentioned previously, are primarily genetic. The ability to mount an IgE response is probably regulated by an IgE-regulator gene and one or more MHC-linked immune-response genes. From studies of the immune system of atopic individuals, it is clear that some individuals either have a deficiency of suppressor cells or have defective suppressor cells. As a result, their IgE-producing B cells can function at a higher rate than normal. It has proved possible to remedy this deficiency of suppressor cells by the use of desensitizing injections of antigens. It is now believed that desensitizing injections mainly act by promoting suppressor-cell activity and, in some way, directly reducing the sensitivity of mast cells to antigen.

In desensitization therapy, antigen is administered in a form designed to stimulate the immune response while reducing, as far as possible, the risks of anaphylactic shock. The first injections contain only a very small quantity of allergen. Over a number of weeks, the dosage is gradually increased. If an allergy is of the seasonal type, the course of injections should be timed to reach completion just prior to the anticipated antigen exposure.

A newer approach to the selective stimulation of suppressor cells is to modify the allergen by attaching it to a nonimmunogenic polymer, such as polyethylene glycol. This molecule can, when bound to an allergen, promote specific suppression of the IgE response by promoting the development of Ts cells.

IgE production is extraordinarily sensitive to regulation by regulatory T cells. There are at least two different populations of suppressor T cells and one of helper T cells that do this. These cells release a soluble factor, which, depending upon its carbohydrate contact, can either inhibit or enhance the IgE response.

Allergy "Shots"

In the early 1900s, it was suggested that hay fever resulted from the activities of a "toxin" in pollen grains. It was argued, therefore, that individuals could be "vaccinated" against this pollen toxin by injection of pollen extracts. When this was attempted, it worked! It was not until the 1930s that the idea of a pollen toxin was disproved and a new hypothesis had to be put forward to account for the effectiveness of allergy "shots." It was, therefore, hypothesized that injection of pollen antigen stimulated "blocking antibody" production. This antibody would then compete with the IgE for any free antigen and thus prevent the antigen from reaching the sensitized mast cells. This hypothesis lasted well into the 1970s and may well be true in part. Current ideas on the subject, however, give most of the credit for the effectiveness of allergy "shots" to suppressor cells.

Regulation of Mast-Cell Degranulation   The release of vasoactive agents from mast cells is modulated by intracellular cyclic nucleotides. Elevation of cyclic AMP or depression of cyclic GMP inhibits mast-cell degranulation, whereas depression of cyclic AMP or elevation of cyclic GMP has a reverse effect. The precise relationship between these two compounds is complex, and the final response depends on the cyclic AMP–cyclic GMP ratio.

On the surface of mast cells, there are two types of receptor for adrenal medullary hormones (adrenoceptors), named α and β. Hormones or drugs, such as norepinephrine and phenylephrine, that stimulate the α adrenoceptor enhance mast-cell degranulation because they depress intracellular cyclic AMP (Table 20–2). Compounds, such as epinephrine and salbutamol, that stimulate the β adrenoceptor have the reverse effect and thus depress mast-cell degranulation. Recently, it has become clear that β adrenoceptor impairment can also contribute to the atopic state. The effects of β adrenoceptor activation can be inhibited by certain respiratory-tract pathogens, such as *B. pertussis* or *Hemophilus influ-*

TABLE 20–2   Effects of Stimulating α and β Adrenoceptors

System	Stimulation of α Adrenoceptor	Stimulation of β Adrenoceptor
Cyclic nucleotides	Lower cAMP	Raise cAMP
	Raise cGMP	Lower cGMP
Mast-cell degranulation	Enhances	Depresses
Smooth muscle	Contracts	Relaxes
Blood vessels	Constrict	Dilate

enzae, or by autoantibodies directed against the β adrenoceptor. Because of this impairment, affected individuals are more susceptible to hypersensitivity conditions, such as chronic asthma.

Regulation of the Response to Mast-Cell-Derived Mediators   The α and β adrenoceptors are found not only on mast cells, but also on secretory and smooth-muscle cells throughout the body. Stimulators of α adrenoceptors mediate vasoconstriction. Consequently, α adrenergic agents may be of use in the treatment of anaphylaxis, reducing edema and raising blood pressure. Stimulators of β adrenoceptors mediate smooth-muscle relaxation and may, therefore, be useful in modulating the severity of smooth-muscle contraction.

Pure α and β stimulants are of only limited use in the treatment of anaphylaxis, because each alone is insufficient to counteract all the effects of mast-cell-derived factors. Epinephrine, on the other hand, has both α and β adrenergic activity and, therefore, its β effects cause smooth muscle to relax. The combination of effects is well suited to combat the vasodilation and smooth-muscle contraction produced by histamine. Ideally, epinephrine (1:1000) solution should be available whenever potential allergens are administered to individuals.

The Destruction of Released Mediators   Eosinophils are attracted to the site of mast-cell degranulation by ECF-A, by leukotriene B, and by histamine and its breakdown products. Once they have arrived, most, if not all, of the various factors released by mast cells are destroyed by eosinophil enzymes (Fig. 20–7). Eosinophils contain histaminases, which break down histamine; proteases and peroxidase, which destroy the leukotrienes; and phospholipase D, which breaks down platelet activating factor. In addition, eosinophils promote the production of prostaglandin E_1, which raises the mast-cell cyclic AMP levels, thus inhibiting degranulation.

It is clear, therefore, that one function of eosinophils is to modulate the inflammatory effects of mast-cell degranulation by destroying the vasoactive factors released by these cells.

Measurement of Type I Hypersensitivity

The term *hypersensitivity* is used to denote a severe reaction that occurs in response to normally harmless material. For example, normal animals do not react to antigens injected

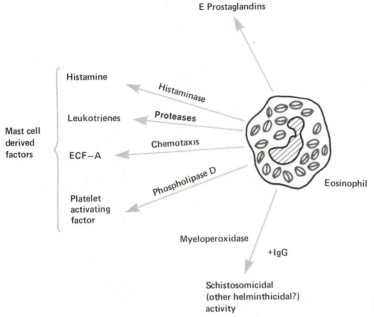

FIGURE 20–7. Some of the activities of eosinophils that serve to inhibit the activity of mast cell-derived factors and thus regulate the inflammatory response in Type I hypersensitivity: Eosinophils are attracted to sites of mast-cell degranulation by ECF-A. The E prostaglandins inhibit further degranulation by stimulating adenyl cyclase and thus elevating cyclic AMP levels. (From Tizard, I. Veterinary Immunology, 2nd ed. W. B. Saunders, Philadelphia, 1982. With permission.)

intradermally. If, however, IgE antibodies are produced to the injected antigen, and if these antibodies bind to skin mast cells, then intradermal inoculation of antigen, even in very dilute solution will provoke a local hypersensitivity reaction. Because of the nature of the mast-cell response, vasoactive agents are released within minutes to produce redness (erythema) as a result of capillary dilation, and circumscribed edema (a wheal) due to increased vascular permeability. The reaction may also involve an erythematous flare due to arteriolar dilation brought about by a local nerve reflex. This type of response to antigen reaches maximal intensity within 30 minutes and tends to fade and disappear within a few hours.

Two other skin-testing techniques may be used to detect reaginic antibodies to specific antigens. One, named the Prausnitz-Kustner or P-K test, is a skin test in which serum from an allergic individual is injected intradermally into a normal individual. After a period of 24 to 48 hours, which allows antibodies to fix to skin mast cells, the antigen is injected at the same site. In a positive reaction, a wheal-and-flare reaction occurs within one to two min. Alternatively, several separate injections of serum at different dilutions may be used, and the antigen solution is then administered intravenously. If positive, each injection site will show an immediate inflammatory response. This test is known as the passive cutaneous anaphylaxis (PCA) test.

An in vitro experimental test of immediate hypersensitivity is the Schultz-Dale technique. In this test, a strip of smooth muscle, such as intestine, is removed from a sensitized animal and washed and suspended in physiological saline. If this tissue is then exposed to specific antigen, degranulation of the mast cells within it will cause it to contract violently. This test may be modified by preincubating the smooth muscle from a normal animal in serum derived from a sensitized one. This passively sensitized muscle may then also contract in response to exposure to specific antigen. Other smooth-muscle-containing tissues, such as the uterus, bronchus, or trachea and certain blood vessels may also be employed to demonstrate Schultz-Dale reactions.

Clinical Manifestations of Type I Hypersensitivity

All the clinical signs of Type I hypersensitivity relate to the release of vasoactive substances from mast cells and basophils. The severity and location of the conditions depend on the number and location of the mast cells stimulated, and this, in turn, is dependent on the amount of antigen and its route of administration. In its most extreme form, antigen administered rapidly and intravenously will cause generalized mast-cell degranulation. If the rate of release of vasoactive agents in this situation is in excess of the body's capacity to respond to the rapid changes in its vascular system, the animal will suffer from anaphylactic shock and may die. If, on the other hand, antigen is administered either locally in small quantities or slowly, then the clinical signs of hypersensitivity will be very much less severe, since the animal will have had an opportunity to compensate for the vascular changes provoked by the mast-cell-derived factors.

Acute Systemic Anaphylaxis (Anaphylactic Shock)

Acute anaphylaxis may be provoked in laboratory animals, especially guinea pigs, by first sensitizing the animal with a single injection of foreign protein given intraperitoneally. After about three weeks, IgE is produced. A dose of antigen given by the intracardiac route will then provoke anaphylaxis. The first signs are restlessness, ruffling of the hair on the neck, sneezing, and pawing at the nose in response to the irritant effect of released histamine. The animal will begin to cough and gasp for air. As the smooth muscle of the gastrointestinal tract and bladder contract, the animal will defecate and urinate. Finally, the interference with respiration leads to asphyxiation and death. On autopsy, the most marked finding is the over-inflation of the lungs. In humans anaphylaxis closely resembles that in the guinea pig. Shortness of breath and increased heart rate precede asphyxiation as a result of bronchial constriction. This bronchial constriction, when less severe, gives rise to an asthmatic attack. In most animals, anaphylaxis involves the respiratory tree, either by causing bronchial constriction as described above or by constricting the pulmonary vein and thus provoking increased pulmonary blood pressure and pulmonary edema.

In the dog, the first species in which anaphylaxis was recorded, the major target organ for anaphylaxis was not the lungs but the hepatic blood vessels. As a result of the constriction of these blood vessels, blood pools in the liver and viscera, and the animal dies from what is essentially a lack of blood.

> **How to Induce Anaphylaxis**
>
> Guinea pigs can be readily sensitized for anaphylaxis by intraperitoneal injection of a foreign protein solution such as egg albumin or horse serum. Only 1 to 5 mg are required and it takes about three weeks for the guinea pigs to become sensitized.
>
> The animal may be shocked by injecting antigen directly into the heart. (Intravenous injections are difficult in the guinea pig). When a shocking dose of about 10 to 15 mg of protein is used, anaphylaxis will develop within a few seconds and the animal will die within 5 min. An autopsy performed immediately will demonstrate that the lungs are grossly inflated and that the blood fails to clot.

Respiratory Allergy

The most important human allergens are pollens and plant spores, animal danders, and mite antigens in house dust. These allergens, suspended in the air, are easily inhaled and thus come into contact with mucus membranes of the eye, nasal tract, and tracheobronchial tree.

In a sensitized individual, exposure to these allergens can give rise to the local allergic reactions known as hay fever (nasolacrimal urticaria) and asthma. In hay fever, the local release of vasoactive factors causes irritation, an increase of vascular permeability leading to a running nose and lacrimation, and inflammation. In the upper-respiratory tract, the local reaction leads to bronchoconstriction and subsequent dyspnea (difficulty in breathing). This dyspnea, or *asthma,* can be very distressing for affected individuals. Because of the mechanics of the pulmonary airways, it is usually possible to inhale air in spite of an inability to exhale it. As a result, the lungs become hyperinflated and emphysema (a breaking down of the walls of the air sacs) may result.

Food Allergy

Allergies to foods constitute another major class of atopic allergies. In this case, the local hypersensitivity reaction in the intestinal walls can lead to discomfort and diarrhea. Absorption of the antigen and local reactions in the skin can give rise to edematous lesions commonly called hives. (These lesions are described as **urticarial** in view of their similarity to the reaction caused by the European "stinging" nettle [*Urtica dioica*].) Respiratory symptoms may also develop. The commonest food allergens include chocolate, cow's milk, wheat and wheat products, strawberries, and fish. Avoidance of these foods is generally the simplest means of controlling these problems.

Prevention and Treatment of Type I Hypersensitivity

In order to prevent Type I hypersensitivity, it is essential that the allergen be identified and removed. This process may be extremely difficult and tedious. Intradermal skin testing using dilute solutions of a vareity of potential allergens may be of assistance. Alternatively (or additionally) in food allergies a change of diet and the readdition of individual components on a test basis may enable the investigator to identify a specific allergen or, more commonly, a group of allergens.

When elimination of the offending allergen is not possible, as, for example, in allergies to pollens, desensitization therapy performed as described previously (see p. 359) may prove effective.

Treatment of Type I hypersensitivity reactions may be accomplished by means of a number of different drugs. One group comprises the sympathomimetic agents, which act as β adrenoceptor stimulants. These include epinephrine and isoprenaline. Salbutamol is a more selective stimulant that causes bronchodilation. Sympathomimetics that act as α adrenoceptor inhibitors include methoxamine and phenylephrine. All have been used extensively in humans.

Another group of drugs widely employed in the treatment of Type I hypersensitivity reactions are the specific pharmacological inhibitors. These drugs, by mimicking the structure of the active mediators, competitively block specific receptors. Thus, antihistamines, such as pyrilamine, promethazine, and diphenhydramine can effectively inhibit the activities of histamine. However, since histamine is but one of a large number of mast-cell-derived mediators, antihistamines possess limited effectiveness in controlling hypersensitivity diseases. The tryptamine antagonist cyproheptadine can block receptors for both serotonin and histamine and may be of assistance in some situations.

Salicylates, such as acetylsalicylic acid and phenylbutazone, are antagonists of the leukotrienes and kinins and are widely used in medicine as anti-inflammatory agents. They may also be very useful in the treatment of acute hypersensitivities.

As an alternative to the specific pharmacological agents described above, considerable use is made of glucocorticosteroids as anti-inflammatory drugs. The corticosteroids can suppress all aspects of inflammation by stabilizing cell and lysosome membranes. Corticosteroids have a palliative effect on chronic Type I hypersensitivities, but it must be borne in mind that these drugs are immunosuppressive and increase an individual's susceptibility to infection.

Two other drugs that may be of assistance in the treatment of Type I hypersensitivity are disodium cromoglycate, which interferes with the release of histamine and leukotrienes from visceral but not mucosal mast cells, and diethylcarbamazine citrate, an anthelmintic with similar pharmacological properties.

Sources of Additional Information

Beaven, M. A. Histamine. N. Engl. J. Med., *294:* 30–36, 320–325, 1976.

Bennich, H. and Johansson, S. G. O. Structure and function of human immunoglobulin E. Adv. Immunol., *13:* 1–55, 1971.

Frankland, W. A. Comprehensive allergy management: The dynamics and state of the art. J. Asthma., *19:* 255–261, 1982.

Goetzl, E. J. Mediators of immediate hypersensitivity derived from arachidonic acid. N. Engl. J. Med., *303:* 822–825, 1980.

Hoffman, D. R., Wood, C. L., and P. Hudson. Demonstration of IgE and IgG antibodies against venoms in the blood of victims of fatal sting anaphylaxis. J. Allergy Clin. Immunol., *71:* 193–196, 1983.

Ishizaka, K. Cellular events in the IgE antibody response. Adv. Immunol., *23:* 1–75, 1971.

Jarrett, E., MacKenzie, S., and Bennich, H. Parasite-induced non-specific IgE does not protect against allergic reactions. Nature, *283:* 302–304, 1980.

Katz, D. H. Recent studies on the regulation of IgE antibody synthesis in experimental animals and man. Immunology, *41:* 1–24, 1980.

Kay, A. B. The role of the eosinophil. J. Allerg. Clin. Immunol. *64:* 90–104, 1979.

Larrick, J. W., et al. Does hyperimmunoglobulin E protect tropical populations from allergic disease? J. Allerg. Clin. Immunol., *71:* 184–188, 1983.

Ventner, J. C., Frazer, C. M., and Harrison, L. C. Autoantibodies to β_2-adrenergic receptors: a possible cause of adrenergic hyporesponsiveness in allergic rhinitis and asthma. Science, *207:* 1361–1363, 1980.

21

Type II Hypersensitivity: Blood Groups and Blood Transfusions

Erythrocytes, like nucleated cells, possess characteristic cell-surface antigens. Unlike the histocompatibility antigens of nucleated cells, however, erythrocyte-surface antigens do not appear to be intimately linked to an animal's capacity to mount an immune response, although they do influence graft rejection (grafts between individuals incompatible in the major blood groups are rejected rapidly).

Except in the case of the M-L antigens of sheep erythrocytes, which are associated with the membrane potassium pump, the exact functions of these antigens are unknown. Most erythrocyte-surface antigens are either carbohydrate or protein in nature and appear to be integral components of the cell membrane. However, some blood-group antigens, although found on erythrocytes, are synthesized at other sites within the body. These antigens are found free in serum, saliva, and other body fluids and are passively absorbed onto erythrocyte surfaces. Examples of such antigens include the Lewis antigen and the C4-related antigens—Chido and Rogers of Man (Chap. 14).

If normal erythrocytes are administered to an allogeneic recipient, their surface antigens will stimulate an immune response. The transfused erythrocytes are rapidly eliminated through intravascular hemolysis mediated by antibody and complement and through extravascular destruction occurring as a result of opsonization and clearance by the cells of the mononuclear-phagocytic system. Cell destruction mediated by antibodies in this way is classified as a Type II hypersensitivity reaction.

Blood Groups

The antigens found on the surface of erythrocytes are termed blood-group antigens. There are many different blood-group antigens on the surface of an individual's red blood cells. They vary in their antigenicity, some being of greater importance than others. The expression of these blood-group antigens is controlled by genes and inherited in simple mendelian fashion. For each blood-group system, there exists a variable number of alternative alleles. (If blood-group alleles are invariably inherited together in groups of two or more, they are known as **phenogroups**). The alleles or phenogroups control in turn a variable number of erythrocyte-cell membrane antigens.

In addition to possessing blood-group antigens on their cells, normal animals may also possess serum antibodies directed against foreign blood-group antigens. For example A-negative humans carry antibodies to the A carbohydrate in their sera. These natural isoantibodies are thought to be derived not from contact with group-A red blood cells but as a consequence of exposure to similar antigenic determinants (heterophile antigens) that occur commonly in nature. Many blood-group antigens, for example, are common structural components of a wide range of organisms including plants, bacteria, protozoa, and helminths. The occurrence of these natural isoantibodies is not, however, a uniform phenomenon, and not all blood-group factors are accompanied by the production of natural isoantibodies to their alternative alleles.

Blood Transfusion and Consequences of Incompatible Transfusions

Red blood cells can be readily transfused from one animal to another. If the donor erythrocytes carry antigens identical to those found on the recipient's erythrocytes, no immune response will result. If, however, the recipient possesses natural isoantibodies to antigens on donor erythrocytes, they will be subject to immediate attack. Natural isoantibodies are usually (but not always) of the IgM class. When these antibodies combine with foreign erythrocyte antigens, they may cause agglutination, immune hemolysis, opsonization, and phagocytosis of the transfused cells. In the absence of naturally occurring antibodies, allogeneic erythrocytes stimulate an immune response in the recipient. The transfused cells then circulate for a period of time before antibody production takes place and immune elimination occurs. A second transfusion with identical allogeneic cells results in their immediate destruction.

Although the body is able to eliminate small numbers of aged red blood cells on a continuing basis, the rapid destruction of large numbers of foreign red blood cells can lead to the development of severe pathological reactions. The signs of this destructive process are referable to massive intravascular hemolysis. Treatment of these transfusion reactions consists of stopping the transfusion and maintaining urine flow with a diuretic, since accumulation of hemoglobin within the kidney may result in renal tubular destruction. Recovery follows elimination of all foreign erythrocytes.

Blood Groups of Man

ABO and Lewis Systems

In 1901, the German immunologist Karl Landsteiner first demonstrated the existence of blood-group antigens on human red blood cells as well as natural isoantibodies directed against those antigens in human sera. He did this quite simply by collecting blood from members of his laboratory staff. He separated the red blood cells from the serum and then he studied the results of mixing serum and red blood cells from different individuals. He found that the sera of some individuals could agglutinate the red blood cells of some individuals but not others. In analyzing the results he found he could group individuals. One group, group A, possessed an antigenic determinant, A, on their red blood cells and antibodies to a determinant, B, in their serum. Another group, group B, possessed determinant B on their red blood cells and antibodies to determinant A in their sera. A third group had neither A nor B on their red blood cells but had both anti-A and anti-B in their sera. This group was called group O. Some time later, individuals were described who had both A and B determinants on their red blood cells but neither anti-A nor anti-B in their sera. This group was called AB. Clearly, coexistence of blood-group antigen and its specific antibody never occurred since in vivo hemagglutination would interfere with the blood circulation and destroy that individual's red blood cells.

The blood group designations A, B, AB, and O indicate the phenotype of an individual's red blood cells. These antigens are inherited according to a simple Mendelian system involving three allelic genes called, A, B, and O. The A gene controls the formation of A substance, the B gene controls the B substance, while the O gene is not expressed. A and B genes are dominant over O. Thus, an AB person is heterozygous, having inherited an A gene from one parent and a B gene from the other. An O person must be homozygous for O, while persons in groups A and B must be either homozygous (AA or BB) or heterozygous (AO or BO) (Table 21–1).

Individuals of blood group O, in fact, produce an antigen called H antigen, which is

TABLE 21-1   The Inheritance of the ABO Blood-Group System

Genotype	Phenotype (Blood Group)	Antibodies in Serum
AA		
AO	A	anti-B
BB		
BO	B	anti-A
AB	AB	neither anti-A nor anti-B
OO	O	anti-A and anti-B

a precursor of the A and B substances. The H gene is found at a locus separate from the ABO locus. This locus controls the production of H substance that, in the presence of A or B genes, is converted to A, B, or AB substance.

In North America, approximately 45% of the population are of group O, 42% A, 10% B and 3% AB. However, these values vary between ethnic groups so that in blacks, for example, the distribution is 49% O, 28% A, 20% B, and 3% AB.

In addition to the A, B, and H substances, two other blood-group specificities also belong to this group. These are the Le^a (Lewis a) and Le^b (Lewis b) antigens inherited at a different locus.

The three loci, ABO, H, and Le all code for glycosyl transferases that determine the structure of the blood-group substances. The glycosyl transferases each act on two precursor oligosaccharide molecules. These consist of alternating units of galactose-N-acetyl D-glucosamine-galactose-N-acetyl-D galactosamine. In the Type 1 precursor, the terminal galactose is bound by a β-1,3 linkage while in the Type 2 precursor it is bound by a β-1,4 linkage (Fig. 21-1).

The glycosyl transferase coded for by the H gene adds a fucose molecule to the terminal galactose residue to both precursor molecules to form H substance. If an individual is of blood group O, then no further reactions occur and H substance may therefore be found on the erythrocytes of O individuals. However, individuals possessing the A gene have a glycosyl transferase that links N-acetyl-D-galactosamine to the terminal galactose of H substance to create A substance. On the other hand, if the individual possesses a B gene, then another glycosyl transferase (D-galactosyl transferase) will add an additional galactose residue to the terminal galactose of H substance and so produce B substance. Possession of both A and B genes ensures that both A and B substances are produced.

Le^a substance is produced from precursor 1 through the Le gene by linking a fucose molecule to the N-acetyl glucosamine residue. Le^b substance is produced from Le^a through the actions of the H glycosyl transferase, which adds another fucose molecule to the terminal galactose residue. Le^b substance may also be linked to an N-acetyl galactosamine by the A glycosyl transferase or to a galactose by the B glycosyl transferase to produce structures with A or B antigenic determinants respectively (Fig. 21-1).

How to Determine an Individual's ABO Status

In order to determine the ABO blood group of an individual, specific antisera are required. Anti-A is usually obtained from human volunteers of blood group B. Their nat-

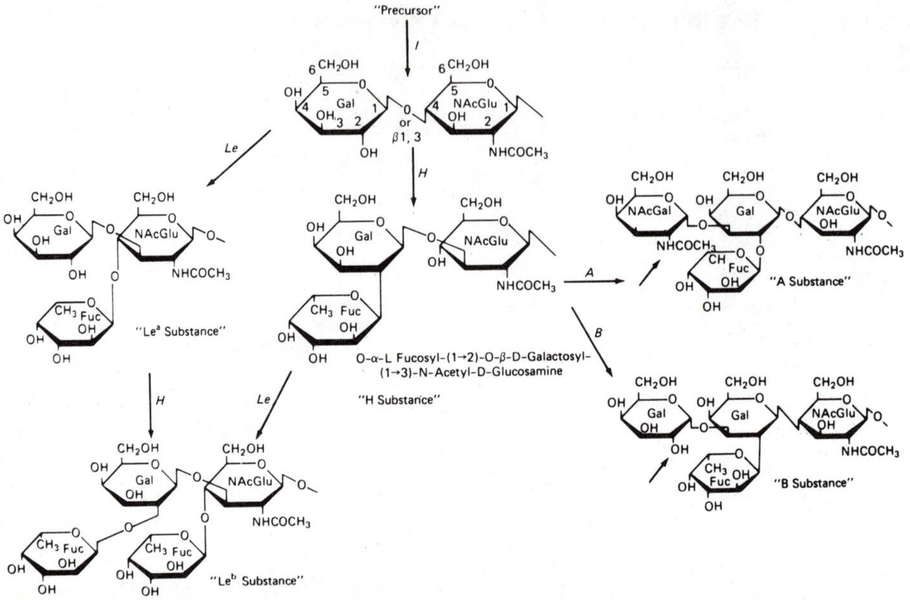

FIGURE 21-1. The synthesis of the ABO and Lewis blood-group substances. Sugars are added in sequence to a precursor glycoprotein by glycosyl transferases controlled by the I, H, Le, A, and B blood-group genes. There are two forms of precursor. One, with a $\beta1,3$ linkage is the precursor of Le^a and Le^b. The other, with a $\beta1,4$ linkage is the precursor of A and B. (Reprinted by permission of the publisher from Comprehensive Immunogenetics, by W. H. Hildeman, E. A. Clark, and R. L. Raison. Copyright 1981 by Elsevier Science Publishing Co., Inc.)

ural anti-A is commonly boosted by injection of pure A substance derived from pigs. Commercial anti-A is usually dyed blue. Anti-B is similarly obtained from group-A volunteers and it is usually dyed yellow.

For rapid testing, whole blood is used as a source of cell, and two drops of blood are mixed on a slide with a drop of anti-A and a drop of anti-B. When testing blood for compatibility in transfusion, it is usual to separate it into cells and serum. The cells, after washing, are suspended in saline at 2 to 5%, mixed with the different antisera in a tube, and examined for agglutination after centrifugation. Similarly, the serum is tested against cells of known specificity.

Generally, the results of the two tests should confirm one another—that is, the results of testing the cells should be compatible with the results of testing the serum. Obviously, if discrepancies occur, the testing must be repeated and the blood not used for transfusion until the cause is known.

Secretors and Nonsecretors

In about 75% of humans, the A and B substances may be found not only bound to cell membranes but also free in body secretions such as serum, urine, and saliva. On cell membranes, the blood-group substances are attached to glycoproteins. This trait is controlled by

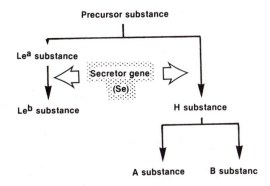

Precursor substance

Le^a substance

Secretor gene (Se)

Le^b substance

H substance

A substance   B substanc

FIGURE 21–2. The mode of action of the secretor (Se) gene. In the absence of this gene, A, B, and H substances bind strongly to cells and are not found free in body fluids. The gene probably acts on H precursor substance to reduce cell binding. The Se gene is also required for the synthesis of Le^b substance. Thus, Le^{b+} individuals must possess the Se gene in either the homozygous or heterozygous states.

a secretor (Se) gene. The Se gene acts to permit binding to glycoproteins when it is present (that is, in homozygous [SeSe] or heterozygous [Sese] individuals). In the homozygous recessive state (sese), glycoprotein binding fails to occur and, as a result, ABH subtances are absent from body fluids (Fig. 21–2).

The process is complicated by the fact that the glycosyl-transferases of the Lewis system only work in Se^+ individuals. Thus, Lewis antigens are only found bound to glycoproteins, which are then passively adsorbed to cells.

The Rhesus System

In 1940, Landsteiner and Wiener showed that antibodies produced against Rhesus monkey erythrocytes agglutinated the red blood cells of 85% of a human population. The antibodies were directed against a molecule called the Rhesus (Rh) antigen and individuals possessing it were called Rh positive. The remaining 15% who did not carry it were called Rh negative. Natural isoagglutinins against the Rh antigens do not occur.

Since that time, the Rh system has been shown to be immensely complicated, and approximately 30 different antigenic types have been identified. The inheritance of these is complex, and two theories have been put forward to account for it. One theory proposed by Fisher and Race proposes that the system consists of six antigenic determinants (C,D,E,c,[d],e), the products of three closely linked loci. The most important of these loci is called D and is responsible for the production of the D antigen, the most important of the Rh antigens. There may be an alternative allele to D called d; however, this has never been demonstrated to exist. Thus d denotes the absence of D. A person is Rh positive who inherits D from either parent. A homozygous parent will transmit D to all his or her children. A heterozygous parent will only transmit it to half his or her children.

An alternative theory has been put forward by Wiener, who has suggested that a single locus is responsible for the generation of several allelic antigenic determinants. In this system Rh_o corresponds to D, the major Rhesus antigen, Rh' corresponds to C, and rh'' corresponds to E.

Other Human Blood-Group Systems

Humans possess a large number of other blood-group systems (Table 21–2). Some are relatively simple—for example, the Kidd group, which consists of two alternative alleles.

TABLE 21–2 Some of the Major Human Blood-Group Systems

System	Total Number of Antigens Recognized
Rh	38
MNS	29
Lutheran	20
Kell	19
ABO	9
Duffy	5
I	5
Lewis	4
P	3
Kidd	2
Diego	2
Cartright	2
Vel	2
Xg	1

Others are very complex—for example, the MN system with 29 identified allelic antigens. Some antigens are found on red blood cells of individuals but are not grouped. One group, the Xg system, is sex-linked.

Blood Groups and Disease

It has already been pointed out how certain histocompatibility antigens are closely associated with disease prevalence or susceptibility (Table 3–2). This association is generally accounted for by the actions of MHC-linked immune-response genes. Since blood-group antigens are not necessarily linked to the MHC, there is no *a priori* reason why they should be linked to specific disease conditions. Nevertheless, there is a clear association between peptic ulceration and nonsecretors of blood group O. In contrast, cancer of the stomach and pernicious anemia are commoner in individuals of blood group A.

Of much more importance than these associations is the direct role of blood-group antigens in hemolytic disease of the newborn.

Hemolytic Disease of the Newborn

Hemolytic disease of the newborn usually occurs as a result of Rhesus-incompatibility. It develops when an Rh-negative mother carries an Rh-positive fetus (Fig. 21–3). Normally, of course, the fetal red blood cells are separated from the mother's circulation by the intact trophoblast. However, during the last trimester of pregnancy, and especially during the process of childbirth, the fetal red blood cells may escape into the maternal circulation. (They can be detected by selective staining of a maternal blood smear). Once these cells reach maternal circulation they are, of course perceived as foreign and, therefore, provoke an antibody response.

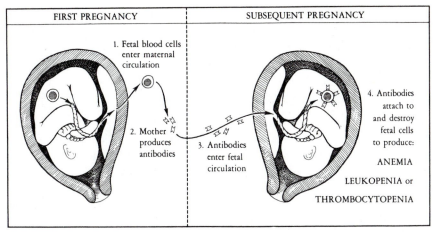

FIRST PREGNANCY | SUBSEQUENT PREGNANCY

1. Fetal blood cells enter maternal circulation

2. Mother produces antibodies

3. Antibodies enter fetal circulation

4. Antibodies attach to and destroy fetal cells to produce:

ANEMIA

LEUKOPENIA or

THROMBOCYTOPENIA

FIGURE 21–3. Schematic representation of isoimmunization due to fetomaternal incompatibility. (From Bellanti, J. A. Immunology II. W. B. Saunders, Philadelphia, 1979. With permission.)

Antibodies to fetal red blood cells are not usually made prior to the first childbirth. Repeated pregnancies may, however, eventually provoke high antibody levels in the mother. Maternal IgG antibodies provoked in this way can cross the placental barrier and reach the fetal circulation where they react with the fetal red blood cells and cause their destruction. This red-blood-cell destruction may be so severe that it results in the death of the fetus. Alternatively, the fetus may survive to be born in a jaundiced or anemic state. The fetus may attempt to compensate for the loss of red blood cells by releasing immature erythrocytes (erythroblasts) from its bone marrow. (Hemolytic disease of the newborn [HDN] is also called erythroblastosis fetalis). The destruction of the fetal erythrocytes can release toxic quantities of bilirubin into the bloodstream. Because of the immature state of the fetal liver, this bilirubin may accumulate, be deposited in brain cells, and cause severe brain damage.

The Diagnosis of Hemolytic Disease

It is usual to blood-type the erythrocytes of pregnant women. If an expectant mother is Rh-negative and the father is Rh-positive, then a physician will be in a position to anticipate HDN. HDN, however, does not occur in all cases of rhesus incompatibility. Thus, not all Rh-positive fathers are homozygous, and, in theory therefore, incompatibility will only occur in 75% of pregnancies between an Rh-positive father and a negative mother. Second, fetal red blood cells only reach the maternal circulation in 20 to 70% of cases. Third, the risks of the disease occurring are very low at the time of first parturition, but increase with each subsequent pregnancy. Thus, as a result of all these factors, HDN develops in one in every 200 to 400 births, unless steps are taken to prevent it.

In pregnancies with a high probability of HDN, prenatal diagnosis can be made by detecting hemoglobin degradation products in amniotic fluid. After birth, diagnosis is made on the basis of clinical signs, but it must be confirmed by demonstrating the presence of antibodies directed against the fetal red blood cells. These antibodies are not able to cause direct agglutination, but can be detected by means of a direct antiglobulin or Coomb's test (Chap. 7). It is also possible to screen maternal serum during pregnancy for a rise in titer to antigen D (Rh_o).

Prevention of Hemolytic Disease

When the factors that influence the development of HDN were studied, it was noticed that the disease tended not to occur if the parents were incompatible at the ABO locus. This is because any fetal red blood cells entering the maternal circulation in ABO-incompatible pregnancies are immediately destroyed by the natural isoantibodies and will not, therefore, provoke an immune response. These natural isoantibodies rarely cause hemolytic disease themselves since they are of the IgM class and thus cannot cross the placenta to reach the fetal circulation.

On the basis of this observation, it was predicted that pre-existing anti-Rh antibodies might destroy any Rh-positive erythrocytes entering the maternal circulation and hence prevent sensitization. This prediction has been amply confirmed. Thus, passively administered anti-D (Rh_o) is given within 72 hours of any delivery at which the mother might be sensitized (Fig. 21–4). (This anti-D is produced in male volunteers.) As a result of this treatment, sensitization is effectively prevented, and the prevalence of HDN reduced to 1 in every 20,000 deliveries.

If hemolytic disease does occur, the usual method of treatment is exchange transfusion, which corrects the anemia and at the same time removes sensitized red blood cells, antibodies, and bilirubin.

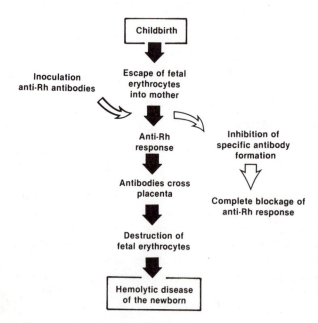

FIGURE 21–4. The prevention of hemolytic disease in human infants. Anti-Rh antibodies, if given to mothers within 72 hours after birth, effectively prevent sensitization at that time by specifically inhibiting the mother's own anti-Rh response.

Blood Groups and Hemolytic Disease of Animals

All animals tested have been shown to possess blood groups similar to those seen in man. Some are relatively simple, while some are enormously complex. Thus the B system of cattle contains over 1000 different alleles, and it has been suggested that there are sufficient alternative combinations to provide a unique blood group for each bovine in the world.

HDN is also recorded in animals. In the major domestic animals, however, the placenta is impermeable to antibodies. As a result, these animals must obtain maternal antibody through the first milk or colostrum. Consequently, hemolytic disease does not develop in utero but follows immediately after a young animal suckles for the first time. The clinical signs of these diseases are very similar to the condition in humans, but prevention is relatively simple—namely, preventing the young animal from suckling.

One other interesting feature of hemolytic disease in cattle is that it is entirely man-made. Fetal red blood cells do not cross the placenta in cattle, and, as a result, cows are never naturally sensitized to fetal red blood cells. There are, however, some antiparasitic vaccines that commonly contain bovine erythrocytes. Administration of these vaccines, therefore, effectively sensitizes cows to other cattle blood-group antigens and can lead to the development of hemolytic disease in calves.

Parentage Testing

Under some circumstances, disputes may arise over the precise father of a child. By using analysis of inherited factors, such as blood groups, it is possible with a high degree of probability to eliminate an incorrectly designated father. There are two rules that govern such decisions.

1. Since blood-group factors are inherited, they must be present on the erythrocytes of one or both parents. Thus, if a blood-group factor is present in a child but absent from both its putative parents, then parentage must be reassigned (Table 21–3).

TABLE 21–3 Parentage Testing: A Simple Example

	Phenotype	Genotype
Blood group of child	O	OO
Blood group of mother	A	AO or AA
Blood group of putative father 1	AB	AB
Blood group of putative father 2	B	BO or BB

The mother must have the AO genotype since her child is homozygous for O.

Putative father 1 could not be the father of this child since he must pass on either A or B to his children.

The paternity of putative father 2 is not excluded. This finding emphasizes an important rule: Blood-group testing such as this can only exclude paternity, not confirm it.

2. If one parent is known to be homozygous for a particular blood-group factor, then this factor must, of necessity, appear in the offspring.

By means of a combination of blood-group testing, histocompatibility analysis, and isoenzyme analysis it is now possible to assign parentage with a very high degree of accuracy. Nevertheless, it must be emphasized that parentage can never be proven absolutely. It can only be excluded.

Sources of Additional Information

This science of immunohematology has reached such a sophisticated level that it really warrants its own text. In this chapter, we have reviewed the subject very superficially. Three basic texts that go into the subject in detail are:

Frigoletto, F. C., Jewett, J. F., and Konugres, A. A., eds. Rh Hemolytic Disease: New Strategy for Eradication. G.K. Hall Medical Publishers, Boston, 1982.
Mourant, A. E., Kopec, A. C., and Domaniewska-Sobczak, K. Blood Groups and Diseases. Oxford University Press, Oxford, 1978.
Race, R. R., and Sanger, R. Blood Groups in Man, ed 6. Blackwell Scientific Publications, Oxford, 1975.

The major journal that publishes papers encompassing this topic is *Vox Sanguinis,* the official journal of the International Society of Blood Transfusion.

22

Type III Hypersensitivity: Pathological Consequences of Immune-Complex Deposition

The formation of immune complexes through the combination of antibody with antigen is the initiating step in a number of biological processes. One of the most significant of these processes is the complement cascade. When complement-fixing immune complexes are deposited in tissues, the subsequent generation of chemotactic factors leads to a local accumulation of neutrophils. These neutrophils release hydrolytic enzymes normally contained within lysosomes, and these enzymes in turn cause local tissue destruction. Lesions generated in this fashion are classified as Type III or immune-complex-mediated hypersensitivity reactions.

Classification of Type III Hypersensitivity Reactions

The severity and significance of Type III hypersensitivity reactions depends, as might be expected, upon the amount and site of deposition of immune complexes. In general, two major types of reaction are recognized. One is known as the Arthus reaction, named after the biologist who first described it. The Arthus reaction occurs when immune complexes are deposited locally within tissues. Arthus reactions may be induced in any tissue into which antigen can be deposited.

A second form of Type III hypersensitivity reaction results from the formation of large quantities of immune complexes within the circulation, as may occur when antigen is administered intravenously to a hyperimmune recipient. Complexes generated in this way tend to be deposited in the walls of blood vessels. Local activation of complement then leads to neutrophil accumulation and the development of inflammation (vasculitis). Circulating immune complexes are also deposited within glomeruli, and the occurrence of a glomerulonephritis is also, therefore, characteristic of this type of hypersensitivity. If the complexes bind to blood cells, anemia, leukopenia, or thrombocytopenia may occur.

It might reasonably be pointed out that the combination of antigen with antibody inevitably results in the generation of immune complexes. It seems, however, that the occurrence of clinically significant Type III hypersensitivity reactions is related to the formation of very large amounts of immune complexes. For instance, several grams of antigen may be needed to sensitize an animal, such as a rabbit, in order to produce experimental Arthus reactions or generalized immune-complex disease. In addition, it is becoming apparent that minor immune-complex-mediated lesions arise relatively frequently following the normal immune responses to many antigens, without giving rise to clinically significant disease.

Local Type III Hypersensitivity Reactions

The Arthus Reaction

If antigen is injected subcutaneously into an animal that possesses circulating antibody capable of precipitating that antigen, then an acute inflammatory reaction will develop within several hours at the site of injection. The reaction starts as an erythematous, edematous swelling; eventually, local hemorrhage and thrombosis occur and, if severe, culminate in tissue death (necrosis).

Histologically, the first changes observed following antigen injection are neutrophil adherence to vascular endothelium, followed by emigration through the walls of small blood vessels, particularly venules. By six to eight hours, when the reaction has reached maximal intensity, the injection site is densely infiltrated by very large numbers of these cells (Fig. 22–1). As the reaction progresses, destruction of blood-vessel walls occurs, resulting in edema and hemorrhage. Platelet aggregation and thrombosis are also associated with this vascular destruction. By 8 hours, mononuclear cells may be observed within the lesion, and by 24 hours or later, depending on the amount of antigen injected, they become the predominant cell type. Eosinophil infiltration is not a significant feature of this type of hypersensitivity.

The fate of the injected antigen may be determined by means of a technique such as the direct fluorescent antibody test (Chap. 7). It can be shown that antigen diffuses away from the injection site through tissue spaces. When small blood vessels are encountered, the antigen will diffuse into the vessel walls, where it comes into contact with circulating antibody. Consequently, immune complexes are generated and deposited between and beneath endothelial cells. If these immune complexes fix complement, a number of events follow, the most important of which is neutrophil chemotaxis and accumulation (Fig. 22–2).

Neutrophils are attracted by C5a and C567, products of the complement cascade. In addition, the neutrophils of some species have a C3 receptor and so will adhere to immune complexes containing this component. Neutrophils that encounter immune complexes promptly phagocytose and destroy them. However, during this process, large quantities of active hydrolytic enzymes are released into the tissues. These enzymes mediate the tissue damage seen in the Arthus reaction.

Neutrophil hydrolytic enzymes are normally stored within lysosomes. They may be

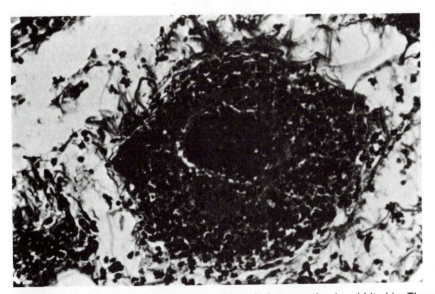

FIGURE 22–1. A histological section of an Arthus reaction in rabbit skin: The vessel is thrombosed and perivascular neutrophil accumulation is extensive. (From Thomson, R. G. General Veterinary Pathology. W. B. Saunders, Philadelphia, 1978. With permission.)

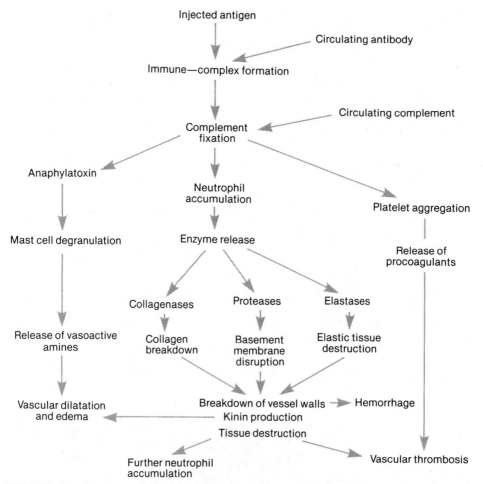

FIGURE 22–2. A schematic diagram showing the major mechanisms of the Arthus reaction. (From Tizard, I. Veterinary Immunology, 2nd ed. W. B. Saunders, Philadelphia, 1982. With permission.)

released into tissue through a number of processes, the most obvious of which is cell death; other release mechanisms, however, are probably of greater importance in the Arthus reaction. For example, when neutrophils attempt to phagocytose immune complexes attached to a nonphagocytosable structure, such as a basement membrane, they secrete their lysosomal contents directly into the surrounding medium. Similarly, they may release lysosomal enzymes into the phagosome before immune complexes are completely enclosed so that the enzymes escape into the surrounding tissues. C5a also stimulates neutrophil degranulation and enzyme release.

The lysosomal enzymes released in this way are primarily hydrolytic (see Table 4–1). They include collagenases that disrupt collagen fibers, neutral proteases that destroy ground substances and basement membranes, and elastases that destroy elastic tissue. Neutrophil proteases also act on C5 to generate C5a and thus promote further neutrophil accumulation and degranulation. Other enzymes released by neutrophils may degranulate mast cells or generate kinins and reactive oxygen metabolites. As a result of all this enzyme release, destruction of tissues, especially of blood-vessel walls occurs, resulting in the development of the edema, vasculitis, and hemorrhage characteristic of the Arthus reaction.

In addition to causing neutrophil accumulation, complement activated by immune complexes may also cause platelets to clump and release procoagulants (Chap. 14). This factor, in conjunction with the severe vascular damage, may result in extensive thrombosis. Finally, the production of anaphylatoxins (C3a and C5a) and of the C2 kinin and the release of kininogens from neutrophils and vasoactive amines from neutrophils, platelets, and mast cells all contribute to the development of a severe local inflammatory response.

The antibodies involved in the Arthus reaction must be both precipitating and complement-fixing and are, therefore, usually of the IgG class.

Although the "classical" direct Arthus reaction is produced by local administration of antigen to hyperimmunized animals, any technique that permits immune complexes to be deposited in tissues will stimulate a similar response. A reversed Arthus reaction can, therefore be produced if antibody is administered intradermally to an animal with a high level of circulating antigen. Injected preformed immune complexes, particularly those containing a moderate excess of antigen, will provoke a similar reaction, although, as might be anticipated, there is less involvement of blood-vessel walls and the reaction is less severe. A passive Arthus reaction can be produced by giving antibody intravenously to a nonsensitized animal followed by an intradermal injection of antigen. Real enthusiasts can produce a reversed passive Arthus reaction by giving antibody intradermally followed by intravenous antigen.

How to Induce an Arthus Reaction

Monsieur Arthus produced his reaction originally by injecting a rabbit with horse serum daily for several weeks. It is not absolutely necessary to induce the reaction this way. All that need be done is to immunize a rabbit against an antigen so that high-titered precipitating antibodies are produced. When a small quantity (about 1 mg) of antigen is injected subcutaneously or intradermally into such an animal, a diffuse reddened swelling starts about two hours later. Small hemorrhages develop, and edema and erythema progressively increase. Eventually, frank hemorrhage and necrosis may develop at the injection site.

Farmer's Lung

Farmer's lung is a naturally occurring Type III hypersensitivity reaction in the lungs of farmers who inhale dust from moldy hay. Normally, dust particles are relatively large and are thus trapped in the upper respiratory tract by mucus and eliminated. If, however, hay is stored when damp, the growth of organisms will result in a local rise in temperature. This heating may permit the selective growth of organisms known as thermophilic actinomycetes to grow. One of the most important of these thermophilic actinomycetes is *Micropolyspora faeni*, an organism that produces huge quantities of very small spores, which, on inhalation, can penetrate as far as the alveoli.

Repeated inhalation of these spores will result in sensitization and in the development of high-titered precipitating serum antibodies to *M. faeni* antigens. Inhaled spores will therefore encounter antibody within alveolar walls, and the resulting deposition of immune complexes and complement activation may result in the development of severe pneumonia, the basis of which is massive neutrophil accumulation and tissue damage as a result of a Type III hypersensitivity reaction (Fig. 22–3). Clinically, farmer's lung is associated with difficulty in breathing (dyspnea) occurring 5 to 10 hours after exposure to grossly moldy hay.

Many other syndromes in man have an identical pathogenesis and are usually named after the source of the offending antigen. Thus "pigeon-breeder's lung" arises following exposure to the dust from pigeon feces, "mushroom-grower's disease" is due to hypersensitivity to inhaled spores from actinomycetes in the soil used for growing mushrooms, and "librarian's lung" results from inhalation of dusts from old books and so forth.

Although hypersensitivity pneumonitis as an entity occurs in response to inhaled antigens, it should be remembered that the immune response to pneumonia-causing microorganisms such as *Strep pneumoniae* may also contribute to the development of pathological lesions through a Type III hypersensitivity reaction.

Generalized Type III Hypersensitivity Reactions

If antigen is administered intravenously to animals with a high level of circulating antibodies, then immune complexes form within the circulation. Most of these complexes, especially the large ones, are removed by the cells of the mononuclear-phagocytic system. Some complexes, however, particularly those formed with excess antigen, are soluble, hence poorly phagocytosed. In addition, alternate-pathway complement components are capable of inserting themselves into and solubilizing large immune complexes. These soluble complexes may fix complement and stimulate platelet aggregation and the release of vasoactive amines, thus affecting the properties of the vascular endothelium. Consequently, immune complexes may be deposited in the walls of blood vessels, particularly medium-sized arteries and in vessels where there is physiological effusion of fluid—for example, glomeruli, synovia, and the choroid plexus (Fig. 22–4).

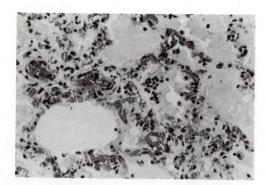

FIGURE 22–3. A histological section of the lung from an acute case of hypersensitivity pneumonitis due to inhalation of actinomycete spores. (Courtesy of Dr. B. N. Wilkie. From Tizard, I. Veterinary Immunology, 2nd ed. W. B. Saunders, Philadelphia, 1982. With permission.)

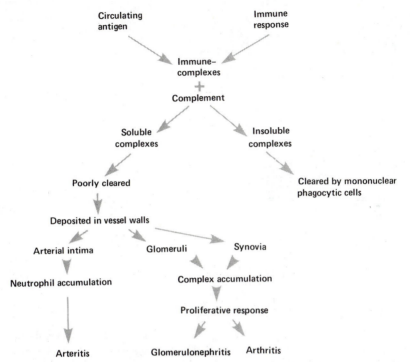

FIGURE 22–4. The major features of the pathogenesis of serum sickness. (From Tizard, I. Veterinary Immunology, 2nd ed. W. B. Saunders, Philadelphia, 1982. With permission.)

Acute Serum Sickness

Many years ago, when the use of antisera for passive immunization was in its infancy, it was observed that individuals who had received a very large single dose of foreign (horse) serum showed a characteristic series of side effects about ten days later. These side effects consisted of a generalized vasculitis with erythema, edema, urticaria of the skin, neutropenia, lymph-node enlargement, joint swelling, and proteinuria. The reaction was usually of short duration, subsiding within a few days, and was known as serum sickness. A similar reaction can be produced experimentally in rabbits by a single high dose of antigen given intravenously. Its occurrence can be shown to coincide with the presence of large quantities of immune complexes in the circulation as a result of the immune response to circulating antigen (Fig. 22–5).

Histologically, two types of lesion may be seen. First, there is a transient glomerulonephritis, the nature of which tends to vary with the size and avidity of immune complexes involved. Thus, relatively large complexes in slight antigen excess appear to penetrate the vascular endothelium but not the basement membrane, and so become deposited in the subendothelial region, where they stimulate endothelial swelling and proliferation (Fig. 22–6). In contrast, if very small and poorly avid complexes are formed, as occurs in gross antigen excess, then these can penetrate both the vascular endothelium and the base-

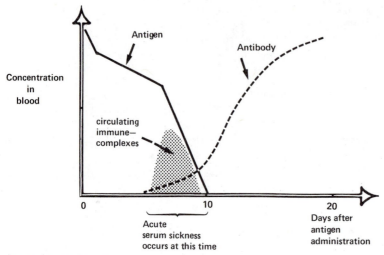

FIGURE 22–5. The time relationships of acute serum sickness. (From Tizard, I. Veterinary Immunology, 2nd ed. W. B. Saunders, Philadelphia, 1982. With permission.)

ment membrane and stimulate epithelial swelling and proliferation. Neutrophils do not normally accumulate within these glomeruli; nevertheless, damage does occur as a result of the vasoactive properties of fixed complement and leads to proteinuria.

Second, widespread arterial lesions develop. The most important of these is an Arthus-type lesion: neutrophil infiltration, disruption of the internal elastic membrane, and medial necrosis that occurs in medium-sized muscular arteries, presumably due to local deposition of immune complexes. Although the mechanisms of this deposition are not clear, it is probable that a transient Type-I-hypersensitivity reaction may be required to initiate the arteritis.

Chronic Serum Sickness

If, instead of a single high dose of antigen, an animal such as a rabbit is given repeated injections of small doses of antigen, then two other types of glomerular lesions may develop (Fig. 22–6). Continued deposition of subepithelial immune complexes may lead to an apparent increase in the thickness of the glomerular basement membrane, forming the so-called wire-loop lesion (membranous glomerulopathy). Alternatively, these immune complexes, especially if the antibody affinity is high, may be deposited in the mesangial region of glomeruli. Mesangial cells are probably a form of mononuclear phagocyte; as such, they possess receptors for immune complexes and complement, as well as being phagocytic. They respond to these immune complexes by proliferation (Fig. 22–7). Normally, such proliferation scarcely affects glomerular function unless the mesangial cells expand to completely surround the glomerular capillaries. By immunofluorescence, it can be shown that "lumpy-bumpy" aggregates of immune complexes are deposited in capillary walls and on the epithelial side of the glomerular basement membrane (Fig. 22–8). Arteritis is not a significant feature of experimental chronic serum sickness.

Chronic immune-complex-mediated lesions are, however, not restricted to the capil-

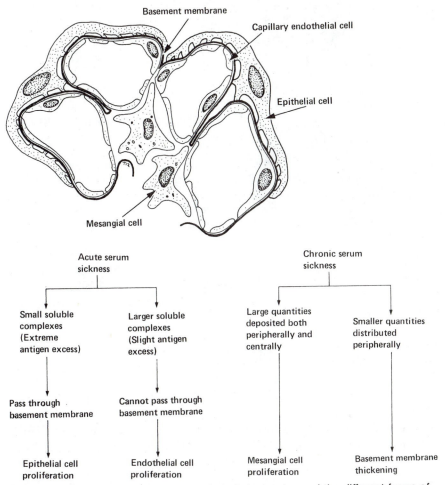

FIGURE 22-6. The structure of a normal glomerulus and the different forms of immune-complex-induced glomerulonephritis. (From Tizard, I. Veterinary Immunology, 2nd ed. W. B. Saunders, Philadelphia, 1982. With permission.)

laries of the glomeruli. Physiological effusion of fluid is also a feature of the capillaries of the choroid plexus of the brain and of the capillaries of joint synovia. Deposition of immune complexes in the walls of these vessels can also lead to the development of significant inflammatory lesions.

Immune-Complex-Mediated Diseases

A number of important clinical syndromes are associated with the development of immune-complex-mediated lesions in man and animals. All are associated with the persistence of antigen in the bloodstream in the presence of antibodies. Glomerulonephritis is, therefore, characteristically associated with chronic viral and autoimmune diseases.

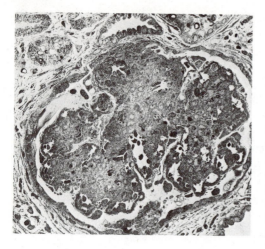

FIGURE 22–7. A thin section of a glomerulus with immune-complex lesions. There is dramatic mesangial-cell proliferation and basement-membrane thickening. (With permission from Angus, K. W., et al. J. Comp. Pathol., *84:* 319–330, 1974. Copyright: Academic Press Inc. (London) Ltd.)

Examples of chronic virus diseases associated with chronic immune complex lesions include Aleutian disease of mink and equine infectious anemia. A glomerulonephritis has also been associated with lymphocytic choriomeningitis in mice and was, for a long time, assumed to be due to deposition of virus–antibody complexes in the glomeruli. The development of these lesions, however, is inhibited by anti-interferon serum, while pure interferon itself can also induce a severe glomerulonephritis in mice.

Immune-complex-mediated glomerulonephritis occurs in systemic lupus erythematosus in man and in the autoimmune disorders of New Zealand Black/New Zealand White (NZB/NZW) hybrid mice. The immune complexes in these animals consists largely of DNA/anti-DNA complexes. In rheumatoid arthritis, the local inflammatory joint lesion is probably also immune-complex-mediated. The offending complexes probably consist of normal immunoglobulin complexed to an autoantiglobulin known as rheumatoid factor. Poststreptococcal glomerulonephritis of man may be an example of a lesion mediated by complexes formed between antibodies and bacterial antigens.

One of the commonest causes of renal failure in humans is a condition known as IgA nephropathy or Berger's disease. In this condition, whose origin is unknown, massive IgA

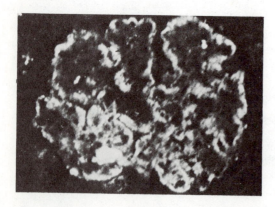

FIGURE 22–8 A fluorescent photomicrograph of a glomerulus with mesangiocapillary glomerulonephritis. The fluorescent antiglobulin reveal "lumpy-bumpy" deposits characteristic of immune-complex deposition. (With permission from Angus, K. W., et al. J. Comp. Pathol., *84:* 319–330, 1974. Copyright: Academic Press Inc. (London) Ltd.)

and IgE deposits are found in the glomerular mesangia. Affected individuals have increased numbers of IgA$^+$ lymphocytes and depressed suppressor cells for IgA production.

How to Detect and Measure Immune Complexes

If a Type III hypersensitivity mechanism is suspected of being involved in a disease, it may be desirable to detect and measure the immune complexes.

In general, tissue-bound immune complexes may be detected by direct immunofluorescence staining, using either labelled anti-immunoglobulin or anti-C3.

There are a number of different techniques available to measure circulating immune complexes within the bloodstream. None are entirely satisfactory, and their clinical significance may not be entirely clear. Most techniques make use of the principle that binding of immunoglobulin to antigen causes a change in the Fc region that activates C1q and permits binding to Fc receptors on cells. Thus, the immune complexes can be bound to C1q fixed to plastic tubes and, after washing, the bound immunoglobulin, may be detected by means of an enzyme- or isotope-labeled antiglobulin. Alternatively, the C1q may be first radiolabelled and, after binding to immune complexes, the complexes may be precipitated and the radioactivity measured.

The Raji cell line is a cultured lymphoid cell line that possesses Fc and C3b receptors. After immune complexes are permitted to bind to these cells, they may be measured using a radiolabelled antiglobulin serum.

A third approach is to make use of the large size of immune complexes and selectively precipitate them with polyethylene glycol. The level of the immunoglobulin in the precipitate can then be measured using radial immunodiffusion or laser nephelometry.

Sources of Additional Information

Cochrane, C.G., and Koffler, D. Immune complex disease in experimental animals and man. Adv. Immunol. *16:* 185–224, 1973.

Germuth, F.C., and Rodriguez, E. Immunopathology of the Renal Glomerulus: Immune Complex Deposition and Anti-basement membrane disease. Little, Brown and Co., Boston, 1973.

Holdsworth, S.R. Fc dependence of macrophage accumulation and subsequent injury in experimental glomerulonephritis. J. Immunol., *130:* 735–739, 1983.

Oldstone, M.B.A., Tishon, A., and Buchmeier, M.J. Virus-induced immune-complex disease: Genetic control of C1q binding complexes in the circulation of mice persistently infected with lymphocytic choriomeningitis virus. J. Immunol., *130:* 912–918, 1983.

Schatz, M., Patterson, R., and Fink, J. Immunologic lung disease. N. Engl. J. Med., *300:* 1310–1320, 1979.

Smith, R.J., Iden, S.S., and Rohloff, N.A. A model of Arthus pleurisy: modulation by various pharmacologic and therapeutic agents. Clin. Immunol. Immunopathol. *26:* 24–34, 1973.

Theofilopoulos, A.N., and Dixon, F.J. The biology and detection of immune complexes. Adv. Immunol., *28:* 89–220, 1979.

Weissman, G., Smolen, J.E., and Korchak, H.M. Release of inflammatory mediators from stimulated neutrophils. N. Engl. J. Med., *303:* 27–34. 1980.

23

Cell–Mediated (Type IV) Hypersensitivity

When certain antigens are injected into the skin of sensitized animals, an inflammatory response, taking many hours to develop, may occur at the injection site. Since this delayed-hypersensitivity reaction cannot be transferred from sensitized to normal animals by serum, but only through lymphocytes, it is apparently cell-mediated. Delayed-hypersensitivity reactions of this sort are classified as Type IV hypersensitivity reactions and occur as a result of the interaction between the injected antigen and sensitized T lymphocytes. An important example of a delayed hypersensitivity reaction is the tuberculin response, the reaction mediated in a tuberculous animal as a result of an intradermal injection of tuberculin—an antigenic extract derived from the tubercle bacillus *(Mycobacterium tuberculosis)*.

The Tuberculin Reaction—A Classic Type IV Reaction

Tuberculin is the name given to extracts of *Mycobacterium tuberculosis* (or the closely related *Mycobacterium bovis* or *Mycobacterium avium*), which are employed as antigens in the skin-testing of humans or animals in an effort to identify those with tuberculosis. Several types of tuberculin have been employed for this purpose, the most important of which is purified-protein-derivative (PPD) tuberculin, which is prepared by growing organisms in synthetic medium, killing them with steam and filtering. The PPD tuberculin is precipitated from this filtrate with trichloracetic acid, washed, and finally resuspended in buffer ready for use.

When PPD tuberculin is injected intradermally into a normal individual, there is no significant local inflammatory response. On the other hand, if it is injected into a person sensitized by infection with the tubercle bacillus, a delayed-hypersensitivity response will occur. Following injection of tuberculin into such an individual, no changes are detectable either grossly or histologically for several hours. By 24 hours, however, vasodilation and increased vascular permeability occur, as a result of which erythema and swelling are observed. This swelling is charactertistically indurated (hard). On histological examination, the lesion is observed to differ from the classic acute inflammatory response in that the infiltrating cell population consists largely of mononuclear cells (macrophages and lymphocytes) (Fig. 23–1), although a transient neutrophil accumulation also occurs in the early stages of the reaction. The reaction reaches its greatest intensity by 24 to 72 hours after injection and may persist for several weeks before gradually fading. In very severe reactions, necrosis may occur at the injection site.

The tuberculin reaction is an immunologically specific reaction mediated by T cells. The antigen is first taken up by Langerhans cells. It is believed that circulating antigen-sensitive T cells encounter this cell-bound antigen and respond by recruiting other lymphocytes and by dividing, differentiating, and releasing lymphokines (Fig. 23–2). The lymphokines involved and the order in which they act are unclear, but it is thought that macrophages accumulate at the site through the release of macrophage chemotactic factors and that their emigration from this site is then inhibited by migration inhibitory factors. The vascular changes are probably mediated through the release of skin-reactive factors and lysosomal enzymes from macrophages. These macrophage enzymes may also provoke local fibrin deposition and thrombosis. The macrophages ingest and eventually destroy the

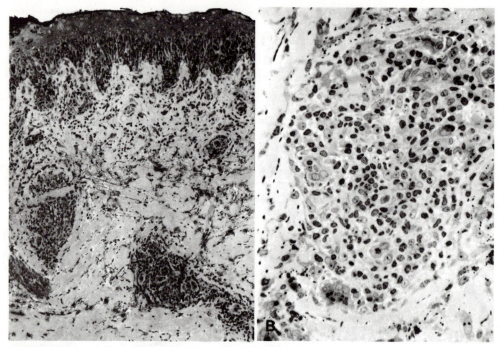

FIGURE 23–1.   Forty-eight-hour tuberculin reaction elicited in a PPD-sensitive individual: Massive perivascular mononuclear aggregates are seen in the deep dermis, and a more diffuse infiltrate in the papillary dermis. Epon thin section (1 μm) stained with Giemsa (original magnifications: **A** × 110, **B** × 400). (From Parker, C. W., ed. Clinical Immunology. W. B. Saunders, Philadelphia, 1980. With permission.)

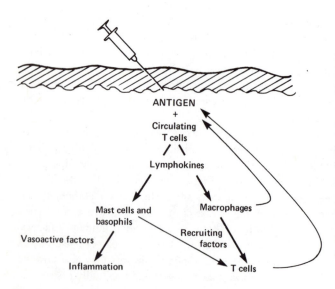

FIGURE 23–2. Schematic diagram depicting the pathogenesis of the delayed hypersensitivity reaction: This is essentially an inflammatory reaction in which both macrophages and T cells participate in order to eliminate the inducing antigen. (From Tizard, I. Veterinary Immunology, 2nd ed. W. B. Saunders, Philadelphia, 1982. With permission.)

injected antigen, so that its elimination removes the stimulus for further lymphokine production, permitting the tissues to return to normal.

The initial T-cell response also generates a lymphokine that attracts basophils and causes local mast cells to degranulate. Serotonin in rodents and histamine in humans derived from these cells enhance the migration of mononuclear cells into the lesion.

Cutaneous Basophil Hypersensitivity

Some antigens may elicit a different form of delayed inflammatory response in skin. In these cases, the lesion is infiltrated with large numbers of basophils as well as mononuclear cells. This reaction, called cutaneous basophil hypersensitivity (CBH), can be transferred between animals with antibody, with purified B cells, or with T cells. It is, therefore, a very heterogeneous phenomenon that probably arises through a number of different mechanisms. CBH is observed in chickens in response to intradermal Rous sarcoma virus, in rabbits in response to schistosomes, and in humans in allergic contact dermatitis and renal allograft rejection.

The Delayed-Hypersensitivity Cell

It has been suggested that a specific type of T cell, the delayed-hypersensitivity cell (T_{DH}) may be directly responsible for Type IV hypersensitivity reactions. Studies show, however, that the T-cell types involved are clearly heterogeneous. Thus, many are Lyt 1^+23^-, but some are Lyt 1^-23^+. Some are Ia$^+$, while others are Ia$^-$. Notwithstanding this fact, the cells that mediate delayed hypersensitivity are susceptible to regulation by T_H and T_S cells.

Pathological Consequences of Type IV Hypersensitivity

Although the intradermal tuberculin reaction is artificial in that antigen is administered by injection, a similar host response occurs, if living tubercle bacilli lodge in tissues. *M. tuberculosis*, however, is resistant to intracellular destruction until a cell-mediated immune response has developed (Chap. 12), and dead organisms are very slowly removed because they contain large quantities of poorly metabolized waxes. As a result, the delayed-hypersensitivity reaction to whole organisms tends to be prolonged, and, consequently, macrophages accumulate in very large numbers. Many of these macrophages attempt to ingest the bacteria and die in the process, whereas others fuse to form multinucleated giant cells. The lesion that develops around invading tubercle bacilli, therefore, consists of a mass of necrotic material containing both living and dead organisms and is surrounded by a layer of macrophages, which in this location are known as epithelioid cells (Chap. 4). The entire lesion is known as a tubercle. Persistent tubercles may become relatively well organized and fibrosed, resulting in the formation of a granuloma. (Interleukin 1 may stimulate collagen production by fibroblasts and hence contribute to this process). Granuloma formation is a frequent consequence of local persistent inflammation. Thus, small granulomas will form if tuberculin is bound to polyacrylamide beads are injected subcutaneously. This inflammation may be of immunological origin, as in tuberculosis or brucellosis in some species, but it may also occur as a result of the presence in tissues of other chronic irritants. Granulomas, for example, may arise in response to the prolonged irritation caused by talc, asbestos particles, or schistosoma eggs (Fig. 5–10).

Allergic Contact Dermatitis

Under some circumstances, exposure of tissues to reactive chemicals leads to the formation of protein–chemical complexes. If these complexes are recognized in association with histocompatibility antigens and so are regarded as foreign, affected cells may be destroyed through a cell-mediated immune response. If this reaction occurs in the skin, it gives rise to a condition known as allergic contact dermatitis.

The chemicals that induce allergic contact dermatitis are usually relatively simple; they include such compounds as formaldehyde, picric acid, aniline dyes, plant resins, organophosphates, and salts of metals, such as nickel and beryllium (Fig. 23–3). Thus, allergic contact dermatitis can occur on pathologists' fingers as a result of exposure to formaldehyde, on parts of the body exposed to the resins (urushiol) of the poison-ivy plant *(Rhus radicans)*, and around the necks of animals as a result of exposure to dichlorvos (2,2-dichlorovinyldimethyl phosphate) in flea collars.

The lesions of allergic contact dermatitis generally vary greatly in severity, ranging from a mild erythema to severe inflammation and blister formation. (Fig. 23–4). Histologically, the lesion is marked by a mononuclear cell-infiltration and vacuolation of skin cells under attack by cytotoxic T cells (Fig. 23–5).

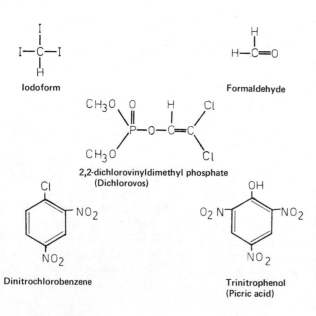

FIGURE 23–3. Some of the simple chemicals that can cause allergic contact dermatitis. (From Tizard, I. Veterinary Immunology, 2nd ed. W. B. Saunders, Philadelphia, 1982. With permission.)

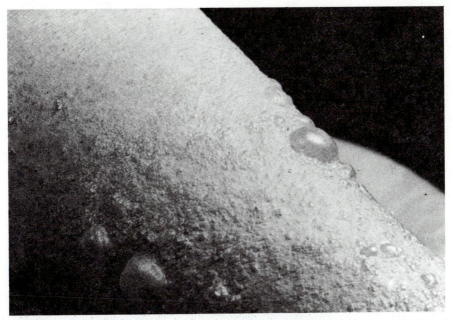

FIGURE 23–4. Acute allergic contact dermatitis. (From Parker, C. W., ed. Clinical Immunology. W. B. Saunders, Philadelphia, 1980. With permission.)

The Measurement of Cell-Mediated Immunity

Although diagnostic immunology is based largely upon the detection of antibodies, measurement of cell-mediated immune responsiveness in man or animals may be necessary under some circumstances. Currently, three major groups of techniques are widely used.

The simplest is the intradermal skin test described earlier in this chapter. The resulting inflammatory response may be considered cell-mediated, provided that it has the characteristic time course and histology of a Type IV reaction. Intradermal skin tests are not always convenient, and injection of antigen into an animal may effectively sensitize it. For these reasons, in vitro tests may be more appropriate. The in vitro tests are designed to measure either the proliferation of T lymphocytes in response to antigen or their production of lymphokines.

In order to measure T-cell proliferation in response to antigen, a suspension of purified peripheral blood lymphocytes from the animal to be tested is mixed with antigen and cultured for 48 to 96 hours. Twelve hours before harvesting, thymidine labelled with the radioactive isotope tritium is added to the cultures. Normal, nondividing lymphocytes do not take up thymidine, but dividing cells do, because they are actively synthesizing DNA. Thus, if the T cells are proliferating, they will take up the tritiated thymidine, and the radioactivity of the washed cells will provide a measure of the degree of proliferation. The greater the response of the cells to antigen, the greater the radioactivity. The ratio of the radioactivity in the stimulated cultures to the radioactivity in the controls is the stimulation index.

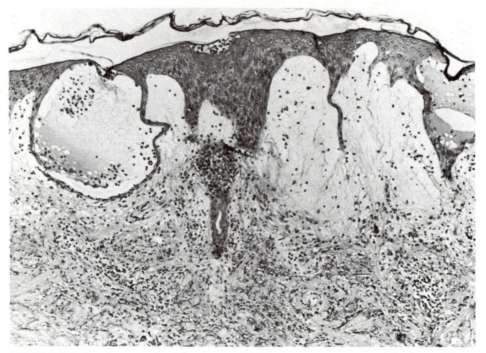

FIGURE 23-5. Multilocular bullae and mononuclear infiltration in acute allergic contact dermatitis. (From Parker, C. W., ed. Clinical Immunology. W. B. Saunders, Philadelphia, 1980. With permission.)

The measurement of lymphokine release by T cells is a much more complicated procedure. One of the commonest techniques involves incubating a purified lymphocyte suspension with antigen. After 24 to 48 hours, the supernatant fluid of the culture is removed and assayed for migration-inhibitory-factor (MIF) activity. This may be done by measuring the ability of the supernatant to inhibit the migration of macrophages out of a capillary tube (See Fig. 12-4).

It is sometimes useful to measure the ability of an animal to mount cell-mediated immune responses in general. One way to do this is to surgically graft the animal with allogeneic skin and measure its survival time. A much simpler technique is to paint the animal's skin with a sensitizing chemical, such as dinitrochlorobenzene. The intensity of the resulting contact dermatitis provides a rough estimate of the animal's ability to mount a cell-mediated immune response.

An alternative in vitro technique is to measure the response of lymphocytes to mitogenic lectins, such as phytohemagglutinin, concanavalin A, or pokeweed mitogen (Chap. 10). The intensity of the lymphocyte proliferative response, as measured by tritiated thymidine uptake, provides an estimate of the reactivity of an animal's lymphocytes.

None of the currently available techniques that measure cell-mediated immunity, with the possible exception of intradermal testing, lends itself readily to use by any but investigators in well-equipped laboratories. The measurement of cell-mediated immunity has become an increasingly important feature of the analysis of immune reactivity, however, and refined and much simpler techniques are expected to become available in the future.

Sources of Additional Information

Adams, D.O. The granulomatous inflammatory response: A review. Am. J. Pathol., *84:* 164–191, 1976.

Callaghan, J.D., et al. Delayed hypersensitivity to mumps antigen in humans. Clin. Immunol. Immunopathol., *26:*, 102–110, 1983.

Gershon, R.K., Askenase, P.W., and Gershon, M.D. Requirement for vasoactive amines for production of delayed-type hypersensitivity skin reactions. J. Exp. Med.; *142:* 732–747, 1975.

Godfrey, M.P., Phillips, M.E., and Askenase, P.W. Histopathology of delayed-onset hypersensitivities in contact-sensitive guinea pigs. Int. Arch. Allerg. Appl. Immunol., *70:* 50–58, 1983.

Repo, H., Kostiala, A., and Kosunen, T.V. Cellular hypersensitivity to tuberculin in BCG-revaccinated persons studied by skin reactivity, leukocyte migration inhibition and lymphocyte proliferation. Clin. Exp. Immunol., *39:* 442–448, 1980.

Toews, G.B., et al. Epidermal Langerhans cell density determines whether contact hypersensitivity or unresponsiveness follows skin painting with DNFD. J. Immunol., *124:* 445–453, 1980.

Turk, J.L. Delayed Hypersensitivity, ed. 2. American Elsevier, New York, 1975.

24

Autoimmunity: Breakdown in Self–Tolerance

It was believed for many years that normal healthy animals lacked the ability to mount any immune response against self-antigens as a result of self-tolerance. It is now clear, however, that a degree of immune reactivity against normal body constitutents is physiological. Thus, a small number of lymphocytes, reactive to normal-tissue antigens, are always present in the spleen. Stimulation of these cells by nonspecific stimulants (such as bacterial endotoxin) will provoke a transient appearance of antibodies in serum; these antibodies can react with normal tissue but have no adverse effects. A good demonstration of this phenomenon is seen when mice are injected with a suspension of rat erythrocytes. As a result, they not only make antibodies to the rat cells, they also develop a self-limiting and transient response to their own red blood cells that can be detected by means of an antiglobulin test. This transient autoimmune response is normally rapidly controlled by suppressor cells. If, however, suppressor-cell activity in mice is suppressed, as, for example, occurs in NZB mice, then the red blood cells are destroyed and the anemia provoked may be quite severe. Normally, however, these self-reactive cells are suppressed and do not make significant quantities of antibody.

In other situations, some responses to self-antigens (autoimmune responses) play a physiological role. For example, naturally occurring anti-idiotype antibodies appear to serve as physiological regulators of the immune system, and it has been claimed that venomous snakes possess neutralizing antibodies to their own venom. The recognition of self-histocompatibility antigens leading to MHC restriction of cell interactions also reflects an ability to recognize "self." On occasion, the suppression of the autoreactive cells may break down. When this happens, clones of normally quiescent lymphocytes will grow and generate very large quantities of autoantibodies or autoreactive T cells. As a result, the immune responses against normal cells or tissue may cause disease—autoimmune disease.

Mechanisms of Breakdown

Exposure of Previously Hidden Antigens

There are a number of ways in which immunological unreactivity to normal body components may be overcome. For example, some antigens may exist in locations where they do not normally encounter circulating lymphocytes. These locations, which include central nervous tissue and testicular tissue, are usually not drained directly by the lymphatic circulation. If the brain or testes are injured, either by trauma or by infection, then the resulting breakdown in vascular barriers may permit antigens released by damaged cells to reach the general circulation, encounter antigen-sensitive cells, and stimulate an immune response. Similar considerations apply to antigens that are normally found only within cells. After myocardial infarction, for example, autoantibodies may be produced against intracellular components, such as mitochondria, although myocardial infarction is manifestly not an autoimmune disease.

Development of New Antigenic Determinants

The formation of autoantibodies may be provoked by the development of new antigenic determinants on normal proteins. Two examples of autoantibodies generated in this fashion are rheumatoid factors and immunoconglutinins.

Rheumatoid factors (RF) are antibodies (largely IgM) that are directed against antigenic determinants on other immunoglobulins. When an immunoglobulin binds to antigen, the Fab regions of the molecule are stabilized in such a way that new antigenic determinants are exposed in the Fc region. These new determinants stimulate rheumatoid-factor formation. Rheumatoid factors are found, therefore, in diseases in which large quantities of immune complexes are generated, such as in the non-organ-specific immune disorders, rheumatoid arthritis, and systemic lupus erythematosus.

Immunoconglutinins (abbreviated IK, after the German spelling) are antibodies directed against antigenic determinants on the activated complement components C2, C4, and C3. The most important of these is the IK directed against C3b. The antigenic determinants that stimulate IK formation are sites on the complement components newly revealed by complement activation. The level of IK in serum is a measure of the amount of complement activation occurring; this amount, in turn, is a measure of the degree of antigenic stimulation to which an animal is subjected. IK levels may, therefore, be employed as nonspecific indicators of the prevalence of infectious disease within a population.

Minor antigenic changes in normal body components may also be generated artificially. Chemically modified thyroglobulin, for example, can be used to stimulate the production of autoantibodies against normal thyroglobulin. It is also possible to render normal tissues antigenic by incorporating them into Freund's complete adjuvant.

Cross-Reactivity with Microorganisms

The organism *Trypanosoma cruzi,* the cause of Chagas' disease in man, possesses antigens that cross-react with mammalian neurons and cardiac muscle. It is, probably, no accident that Chagas' disease is commonly associated with nervous disorders and myocarditis. It has been suggested that the heart lesions that develop in rheumatic fever in children arise as a result of the production of antibodies to group-A streptococci, which cross-react with myocardium. Recent evidence has, however, shown major flaws in the experimental evidence for this theory, and the myocardial lesions are very different from those associated with destruction by autoantibodies. Nevertheless, lymphocytes sensitized by exposure to streptococcal antigens may attack cardiac myofibers.

Development of Previously Suppressed Immunologically Competent Cells

Most autoimmune disorders probably occur as a consequence of the development of cells that had previously been suppressed by the normal control mechanisms of the body. For example, it can be shown that the severity of autoimmune thyroiditis in the OS strain of chickens is increased after neonatal thymectomy. It has been suggested that this increase is due to the removal of suppressor T cells, which normally prevent the development of an immune response to normal thyroid antigens.

It is not uncommon to find autoimmune disease associated with lymphoid tumors. For example, myasthenia gravis may be associated with the presence of a thymoma. In humans, there is a fourfold increase in the incidence of rheumatoid disease in patients with malignant lymphoid tumors, and there is evidence for a similar association in other animals. The reasons are poorly understood, but since many lymphoid tumors may arise as a consequence of a failure in immunological control mechanisms, a simultaneous failure in self-tolerance may also occur. Alternatively, some tumors may represent the development of a "forbidden clone" of cells producing autoantibodies. One other possibility that should be considered is that lymphoid tumors may arise as a consequence of the prolonged stimulation of the immune systems by autoantigens.

Viruses as Inducers of Autoimmunity

A growing body of evidence has served to link many diseases currently considered to be autoimmune to virus infections, and it has been suggested that viruses, particularly those that infect lymphoid tissues, may be capable of interfering with immunological control mechanisms and so permit autoimmunity to occur. Thus, in New Zealand Black (NZB) mice, persistent infection with a Type C retrovirus may be the cause of the development of autoantibodies against nucleic acids and erythrocytes. Systemic lupus erythematosus (SLE) of dogs and humans is a similar condition in which the presence of autoantibodies to many different organs is possibly associated with either a Type C retrovirus or paramyxovirus infection. Reovirus Type 1 infection in mice can provoke autoimmune responses against pancreatic islet cells, anterior pituitary cells, growth hormone, gastric mucosal cells, and nuclei. Affected mice develop mild diabetes and retarded growth.

Clinical Associations between Autoimmune Diseases

It is not uncommon for more than one autoimmune disease to occur simultaneously in the same individual. Autoimmune thyroiditis, for example, is commonly associated with pernicious anemia and occasionally linked with Addison's disease. This clinical association is emphasized by a significant serological overlap between these conditions. Thus, up to a third of patients with autoimmune thyroiditis may also have autoantibodies to gastric parietal cells, while half of the patients with pernicious anemia have antithyroid antibodies (this is not due to immunological cross-reactivity).

The simultaneous occurrence of multiple autoimmune disorders is even more marked in systemic lupus erythematosus in which hemolytic anemia, thrombocytopenia, rheumatoid factors, and Sjögren's syndrome (see p. 406) are all occasionally reported.

Genetic Influences

There is a tendency for some autoimmune diseases to run in families. Thus, the relatives of patients with Hashimoto's disease (see p. 401) commonly have antithyroid antibodies and may also develop thyrotoxicosis. A similar phenomenon is seen in pernicious anemia.

There are very close links between possession of certain histocompatibility antigens and autoimmune disease. Thus, thyrotoxicosis is associated with possession of D3, and insulin-dependent diabetes is associated with an absence of Dw2, but with possession of Bw3 or 4. Systemic lupus is associated with possession of B8, DRw2, and DRw3, rheumatoid arthritis with Dw4 and DRw4, DRw7 and DRw10 (see Table 3–4).

Certain inbred lines of animals have been developed that spontaneously develop autoimmune disease. Thus, chickens of the OS strain develop an autoimmune thyroiditis; an inbred line of dogs has been used for studies on SLE, and it is interesting to note that it was in this colony that the first reported cases of canine Sjögren's syndrome were described.

Inbred New Zealand Black (NZB) mice spontaneously develop a syndrome that bears a striking resemblance to systemic lupus erythematosus (SLE) (p. 407). Thus, they develop an immune-complex type of glomerulonephritis associated with a positive LE cell test. They become hypergammaglobulinemic and hypocomplementemic, and they develop an autoimmune hemolytic anemia. Some mice also develop lymphoid-cell tumors. A large variety of autoantibodies develop in these mice directed against several nucleic-acid antigens, erythrocytes, and T cells, while their B cells are polyclonally activated.

New Zealand White (NZW) mice are phenotypically normal, but the F1 cross between NZW and NZB mice give offspring that have an even more severe SLE-like syndrome. Thus, in these animals, renal disease is more severe and is associated with higher titers of antinuclear antibodies. Studies on the inheritance of these traits in mice suggests that they are controlled by a small number of unlinked major genes and a large number of minor genes. Each autoimmune trait is under the separate control of a distinct gene.

Mechanisms of Tissue Damage

Autoimmune Reactions Involving Type I Hypersensitivity   Milk allergy in cattle is an autoimmune disorder in which milk α casein, normally found only in the mammary gland, gains access to the general circulation and so stimulates an immune response. This happens when milking is delayed and intramammary pressure forces milk proteins into the circulation. For some reason, the immune response stimulated by casein is of the IgE type, and affected cows show clinical signs of acute systemic anaphylaxis. Although antibodies to milk proteins are commonly found in human serum after rapid weaning, Type I hypersensitivity is not a usual sequel.

Autoimmune Reactions Involving Type II Hypersensitivity   Autoantibodies directed against cell-surface antigens may cause lysis with the assistance of either complement or cytotoxic cells. If the autoantibodies are directed against erythrocytes, then autoimmune hemolytic anemia may result. If directed against platelets, thrombocytopenia will occur; if against thyroid cells, thyroiditis will result, and so forth.

Autoimmune Reactions Involving Type III Hypersensitivity   Autoantibodies will form immune complexes when bound to antigen, and these complexes may participate in Type III hypersensitivity reactions. This occurs, for example, in systemic lupus erythematosus, a disease in which a wide variety of autoantibodies are produced, the most significant of which are those directed against nucleic acids. DNA–antibody complexes are formed in affected animals and are deposited in glomeruli to provoke the development of a membraneous glomerulonephritis (Chap. 22). Similarly, in rheumatoid arthritis, immune complexes formed between rheumatoid factor (the antibody) and antigen-bound IgG (the antigen) are deposited in joint tissues and, by fixing complement, contribute to the local inflammatory response.

Autoimmune Reactions Involving Type IV Hypersensitivity Many lesions in autoimmune conditions are heavily infiltrated with mononuclear cells, and it is probable, therefore, that autosensitized T lymphocytes may contribute to the pathogenesis of disease of this type. Examples of such disease include autoimmune thyroiditis, in which thyroid antigens may be shown to cause macrophage-migration inhibition; experimental allergic encephalitis, in which cytotoxic T cells can cause demyelination; and ulcerative colitis, in which cytotoxic T cells may destroy colon cells growing in culture. Another example of a disease that may, in some cases, be due to a cell-mediated autoimmune response is insulin-dependent diabetes mellitus in humans. In some of these cases, lymphocytes from diabetics have been shown to be cytotoxic for pancreatic islet cells.

Autoimmune Disorders Affecting Receptor Function A growing number of autoimmune disorders have been identified in which autoantibodies are directed against specific cell-membrane receptors. These include thyrotoxicosis, in which autoantibodies are directed against thyroid-stimulating hormone receptors; insulin-resistant diabetes mellitus, where they are directed against insulin receptors; and myasthenia gravis, in which they are directed against acetylcholine receptors. The effects on these receptors are variable. Antibodies to thyroid-stimulating hormone receptor stimulate the receptor by mimicking the hormone. Antibodies to insulin receptor have the opposite effect and block the activities of insulin. Antibodies to the acetylcholine receptor on skeletal-muscle cells promote their rapid degradation and thus block neurotransmission.

In Chapter 20, autoantibodies to β adrenoceptors were mentioned. These have been detected in some patients with asthma. By blocking β receptors, these antibodies render the airways highly irritable and, thus, prone to severe asthmatic attacks.

Some Selected Autoimmune Diseases

Autoimmune Thyroiditis

Humans, dogs, and chickens all suffer from naturally occurring autoimmune thyroiditis (Fig. 24–1). In humans, two major forms occur. In one, Hashimoto's thyroiditis, the auto-

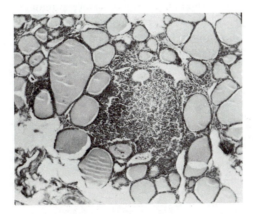

FIGURE 24-1. A lymphocytic nodule in the thyroid of a beagle suffering from an autoimmune thyroiditis (original magnification X100). (Specimen provided by Dr. B. N. Wilkie. From Tizard, I. Veterinary Immunology, 2nd ed. W. B. Saunders, Philadelphia, 1982. With permission.)

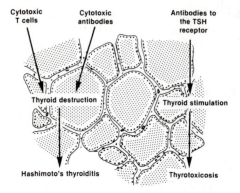

FIGURE 24–2.   The two ways by which autoimmune reactions may influence the thyroid and produce very dissimilar results.

antibodies formed are complement-fixing. As a result, these antibodies, with complement are cytotoxic for thyroid cells. This fact probably does not account entirely for the lesions of Hashimoto's thyroiditis, since thyroid-tissue fragments can grow well in the presence of these cytotoxic antibodies. Because thyroid extracts can inhibit macrophage migration, it may well be that a T-cell-mediated process is also involved.

Thyrotoxicosis (Graves' disease) in contrast to Hashimoto's thyroiditis, is associated with thyroid hyperactivity (Fig. 24–2). The autoantibodies formed in thyrotoxicosis can bind to the same receptor as thyroid-stimulating hormone (TSH) and enhance thyroid activity by reducing cAMP. The children of women with thyrotoxicosis may be born with evidence of thyroid hyperactivity. This phenomenon is apparently due to the passage of thyroid stimulating antibodies across the placenta. It is interesting to note that some patients may develop both cytotoxic antibodies and thyroid-stimulating antibodies and thus develop "hashitoxicosis."

Autoimmune thyroiditis occurs naturally in the OS (obese) strain of white Leghorn chickens. The thyroid of these birds is heavily infiltrated by lymphocytes and plasma cells, which may organize to form germinal centers. Autoantibodies are directed against the thyroglobulin, and affected birds are hypothyroid. This thyroiditis appears to be the result of several interacting genetic lesions. First, the B cells of these chickens make antithyroglobulin, a trait linked to the major histocompatibility complex. Second, these chickens possess a thymic abnormality that results in unusually early maturation of the T-cell system and a failure to mobilize suppressor cells. As a result, autoimmune responses are stimulated before they can be prevented by suppressor cells. Third, these chickens have defective thyroid function in that they are refractory to thyroid-stimulating hormone and are thus more susceptible than normal to thyroid damage. Neonatal thymectomy prevents the development of lesions, but adult thymectomy may increase its severity by removing suppressor T cells, which presumably moderate the disease.

Insulin-Dependent Diabetes Mellitus

Diabetes mellitus is a disease of young adults that is probably due to immune destruction of islets of Langerhans beta cells. It is associated with possession of certain histocompatibility antigens and is probably provoked by certain strains of Coxsackie-B virus. Patholog-

H – Gly – Ser – Leu – Pro – Glu – Lys – Ala – Glu – Arg – Pro – Glu – Asp – Glu – Asn – OH

FIGURE 24–3. The structure of the encephalitogenic peptide derived from myelin: Administration of this peptide in Freund's complete adjuvant provokes autoantibody formation against myelin and leads to experimental allergic encephalitis in animals.

ically, it is associated with lymphocyte infiltration of the islets, and cytotoxic T cells directed against beta cells have been described. Affected individuals, however, also have IgG antibodies directed against islet-cell cytoplasm, which has been shown to destroy islet cells in vitro.

Insulin-Resistant Diabetes Mellitus

Some patients with insulin-resistant diabetes have autoantibodies directed against the insulin receptor. As a result, these individuals may have to be given up to 1000 times the normal dose of insulin in order to prevent hyperglycemia.

Autoimmune Encephalitis and Neuritis

Because brain antigens are normally sequestered behind the "blood–brain" barrier, it is relatively easy to induce an autoimmune encephalitis. Known as experimental allergic encephalomyelitis (EAE), this condition may be produced in animals by inoculating them with brain tissue emulsified in Freund's complete adjuvant. After a few weeks, animals treated in this way show a progressive focal encephalitis and myelitis, usually with paralysis, and the brain lesions consist of focal vasculitis, mononuclear (lymphocyte and macrophage) infiltration associated with perivascular demyelination, and some axon damage. It is possible to detect antibodies to brain tissue in the serum of these animals by means of a complement fixation test, although the lesion itself develops primarily as a result of a cell-mediated autoimmune response. The causal antigen is known as myelin basic protein—a rather small protein, the major antigen component of which is a peptide containing only fourteen amino acid residues (Fig. 24-3).

A clinically significant encephalitis, identical in many features to EAE, occurred following administration of older types of rabies vaccines containing phenolized brain tissue. The clinical signs of this postvaccinal encephalitis appeared between 4 and 15 days after vaccination. For this reason, suckling-mouse brain tissue taken prior to myelination is now used in the production of some rabies vaccines.

If nerve tissue, such as that of the sciatic nerve, is used to immunize experimental animals, it may lead to the development of an experimental allergic neuritis (EAN) (Fig. 24-4). Like EAE, there is a latent period of 6 to 14 days before an ascending polyneuritis and gradual paralysis develop. EAN somewhat resembles idiopathic polyneuritis (Guillain-Barré syndrome) in humans. It is possible, therefore, but not proved, that this condition may also be an autoimmune disorder.

Autoimmune Reproductive Disorders

Inflammation of the testes (orchitis) may be produced in animals by inoculation with testicular extracts emulsified in Freund's complete adjuvant. Autoantibodies to sperm may

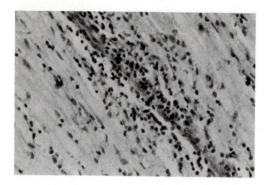

FIGURE 24-4. A section of rat sciatic nerve showing a mononuclear cell infiltration: This is the lesion of experimental allergic neuritis produced by inoculation of rat sciatic nerve in Freund's complete adjuvant. The rat from which this tissue was taken showed complete posterior paralysis. (Courtesy of Dr. B.N. Wilkie. From Tizard, I. Veterinary Immunology, 2nd ed. W.B. Saunders, Philadelphia, 1982. With permission.)

also be detected in the serum of some animals, particularly following injury to the testes or long-standing obstruction of the seminiferous ducts. Blockage of the ducts, such as occurs in vasectomized men, can lead to an increase in seminal pressure and leakage of sperm antigens into the circulation. Thus, 73 percent of vasectomized men will have demonstrable sperm agglutinins within a year. When attempts are made to reverse vasectomy, the presence of these antibodies may effectively prevent the return of fertility by making the sperm agglutinate. Some infertile women may develop autoantibodies to the zona pellucida of the ovum. These will also prevent successful conception.

Autoimmune Nephritis

There are two immunopathogenic types of glomerulonephritis. In the immune-complex type, immune complexes containing complement are deposited in a lumpy, granular fashion on glomerular basement membranes (GBM) (See Fig. 22–8). In contrast, if autoantibodies are produced against GBM antigens, they become deposited in a smooth, linear fashion. These anti-GBM antibodies may be produced experimentally in animals; however, they may arise spontaneously in man in a condition known as Goodpasture's syndrome. In this condition, the autoantibodies react not only with the GBM but also with the basement membrane of pulmonary alveolar septae and capillaries and cause lung hemorrhage.

Pernicious Anemia

Autoantibodies to gastric mucosal intrinsic factor can block the absorption of vitamin B12 into the body. As a result, a severe anemia results. In order to be effective, the autoantibodies must be present in the gastrointestinal lumen, since high serum antibody levels alone are ineffective in provoking disease.

Autoimmune Hemolytic Anemia

Autoantibodies to erythrocytes will provoke erythrocyte destruction and thus cause an autoimmune hemolytic anemia (AIHA). This destruction is due either to intravascular hemolysis mediated through complement or, much more commonly, to removal of antibody-coated erythrocytes by the macrophages of the spleen and liver.

Autoimmune hemolytic anemias may be divided into two major groups depending upon whether the autoantibody is of the IgG or IgM class.

AIHA Mediated by IgG Antibodies

Most cases of AIHA are caused by IgG antibodies, which react optimally with red blood cells at 37°C. Since IgG antibodies are relatively small, they are usually unable to overcome the zeta potential of the red blood cells and, therefore, will not cause direct agglutination. Since IgG does not fix complement efficiently, intravascular hemolysis does not occur but the red blood cells are destroyed by phagocytosis in the spleen. In very severe cases, a blood smear may show leukocytes with ingested erythrocytes. IgG-mediated AIHA is diagnosed by demonstrating the presence of antibodies on the red blood cells. This is done by means of direct antiglobulin or Coombs' test (Chap. 7). The erythrocytes of the affected individual are first washed to remove free serum and then exposed to an antiglobulin serum. Erythrocytes coated with autoantibody will be agglutinated.

AIHA Mediated by IgM Antibodies

IgM autoantibodies mediate a different type of disease from that caused by IgG. Some IgM antibodies that act at 37°C activate complement and thus provoke intravascular hemolysis. Other IgM antibodies cannot agglutinate red blood cells at body temperature, but agglutinate them when the blood is chilled. These are called cold agglutinins. As blood circulates through the extremities (toes, ears, etc.) it may be cooled significantly, and, as a result, erythrocyte agglutination may occur within capillaries. This agglutination can block blood vessels and so lead to vascular stasis and tissue destruction.

Immune Suppression of Hematopoiesis

It has been demonstrated in humans that autoimmune responses may be directed against hematopoietic stem cells. For example, autoantibodies to erythyroid precursors may give rise to red-blood-cell aplasia, and autoantibodies to myeloid precursors may provoke an immune neutropenia. These conditions can be diagnosed only by demonstrating these autoantibodies by immunofluorescence on bone-marrow smears.

Sjögren's Syndrome

In Sjögren's syndrome, which has been described in both humans and dogs, autoimmunity develops against exocrine glands, most notably the lacrimal and salivary glands. As a result, the secretion of these glands is greatly reduced, and affected individuals suffer from corneal and mouth dryness. Sjögren's syndrome is often associated with rheumatoid arthritis, systemic lupus erythematosus, polymyositis and autoimmune thyroiditis.

Myasthenia Gravis

Myasthenia gravis, a disease of humans, dogs, and cats, is a disorder to skeletal muscle characterized by the occurrence of abnormal fatigue and extreme weakness after relatively mild exercise. An individual with myasthenia gravis, for example, will collapse exhausted after walking for only a few yards. The muscles holding up the eyelids tire, and it is difficult for affected individuals to keep their eyes open. The muscles of the esophagus relax and swallowing is difficult. Myasthenia gravis occurs as a result of destruction of acetylcholine receptors on the motor end plates of striated muscle. This destruction stems from the development of autoantibodies against the acetylcholine receptor. These autoantibodies may fix complement, they can participate in ADCC, and they can provoke endocytosis of receptors. Because the number of effective acetylcholine receptors is reduced, the end-plate potentials induced at the neuromuscular junctions fall below threshold levels and, therefore, fail to trigger muscle contraction (Fig. 24–5). Repeating the stimulus is ineffective, since all available receptors are saturated with acetylcholine.

In some individuals with myasthenia gravis, the thymus may show medullary hyperplasia or germinal-center formation or even develop thymic tumors (thymomas). Since normal thymus tissue contains a population of myoid cells (striated muscle cells that possess acetyl choline receptors of their own), it is possible that the thymic changes result from immunological attack on myoid cells. Alternatively, since the thymic hormone thymopoietin is capable of neuromuscular blocking activity, thymoma-associated myasthenia may be secondary to excessive thymopoietin production. This hypothesis is supported by the observation in humans that thymectomy usually, but not always, leads to significant remission of myasthenia gravis.

Diseases of Wide Organ Specificity Associated with Autoimmune Components

In addition to the organ-specific autoimmune conditions discussed so far, there exist a number of diseases that involve many organs throughout the body and that have a major autoimmune component.

Systemic Lupus Erythematosus

Systemic lupus erythematosus (SLE) is a generalized immunologic disorder that has been described in humans, mice, dogs, and cats. About 90% of the human cases occur in females.

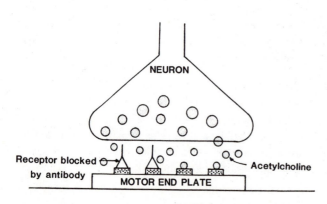

FIGURE 24–5. A schematic diagram showing the pathogenesis of myasthenia gravis: Blockage of receptors by antibody effectively reduces the amount of acetylcholine able to stimulate the motor end plate. Anticholinesterase drugs will, by preventing acetylcholine destruction, enhance the stimulation of the motor end plate.

SLE occurs as a result of a loss of control of the B-cell system. In some, but not all cases this loss has been associated with defective suppressor-cell function. As a result of this loss of control, affected individuals make autoantibodies against a great range of antigens found in normal organs and tissues. These multiple autoantibodies, in turn, give rise to a wide spectrum of pathological lesions and clinical manifestations.

One consistent feature of SLE is the development of autoantibodies against nucleic acids. Several different antinuclear antibody systems have been described in the disease, the most important of which are antibodies to DNA. These autoantibodies cause tissue damage by several mechanisms. They can combine with free DNA to form DNA–anti-DNA immune complexes, which may then be deposited in glomeruli (Chap. 22), causing a membranous glomerulonephritis. The complexes may also be deposited in arteriolar walls, where they result in local tissue destruction and fibrosis, or in synovia, where they provoke arthritis. Antinuclear antibodies also bind to the nuclei of degenerating cells. These "opsonized" nuclei may be phagocytosed, giving rise to structures known as lupus erythematosus (LE) cells (Fig. 24–6). LE cells are found mainly in bone marrow and, less commonly, in blood.

Although antibodies to nucleic acids are characteristic of SLE, a great variety of other autoantibodies are also produced. Autoantibodies to red blood cells, for example, give rise to an antiglobulin-positive hemolytic anemia. Antibodies to platelets give rise to an immunologically mediated thrombocytopenia. Antilymphocyte antibodies may be present, and it is suggested that they may selectively destroy suppressor cells, thus enhancing the excessive immune reactivity. Antimuscle antibodies may provoke myositis, and antimyocardial antibodies may provoke myocarditis or endocarditis. Antibodies to skin components give rise to a characteristic bilaterally symmetrical dermatitis, the lesions of which are commonly restricted to the bridge of the nose and the area around the eyes. This grossly excessive immune reactivity is also reflected in a polyclonal hypergammaglobulinemia, enlargement of lymph nodes with medullary disruption, and thymic enlargement with germinal-center formation.

Pathogenesis of SLE (Fig 24–7)   Although it is clear that SLE involves a loss of control of the specificity of the B-cell response with resulting multiple autoimmune disorders, the initiating causes remain obscure. There is good evidence for a genetic predispo-

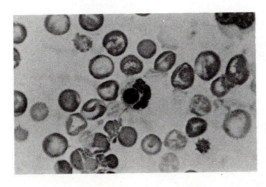

FIGURE 24–6. An LE cell from a case of systemic lupus erythematosus. (Courtesy of Dr. B.N. Wilkie. From Tizard, I. Veterinary Immunology, 2nd ed. W.B. Saunders, Philadelphia, 1982.)

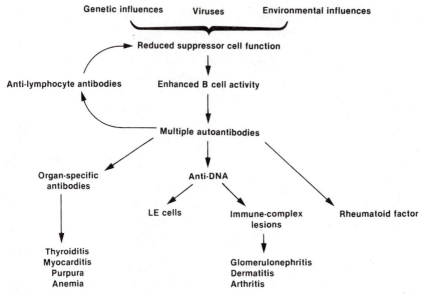

FIGURE 25–7.   A speculative scheme for the pathogenesis of SLE.

in humans and mice. SLE is associated with an increased familial incidence and the presence of certain histocompatibility antigens in man. The bulk of the present evidence suggests that virus infections may be directly responsible for initiation of the condition. Various viruses have been implicated. Thus, individuals with SLE commonly have high-titered antibodies to parainfluenza 1 and measles. Myxoviruslike structures have been observed within renal endothelial cells from SLE patients. Similarly, certain Type C retroviruses have been isolated from SLE patients and associated with the disease.

When dogs affected by SLE are bred, the number of affected offspring is higher than can be accounted for genetically, suggesting that the condition can be vertically transmitted. Cell-free filtrates from asymptomatic but LE-cell-positive dogs, when administered to newborn mice, have been reported to provoke the appearance of antinuclear antibodies and the development of some lymphoid tumors. Type C viruses have been isolated from these tumors, and antisera to these viruses may be used to demonstrate viral antigen on the lymphocytes and in the glomeruli of humans with SLE. Cell-free filtrates of these tumors have also been reported to induce the formation of antinuclear antibodies and the production of LE cells in newborn puppies.

Rheumatoid Arthritis

Rheumatoid arthritis is a common, crippling disease in humans that is also seen in domestic animals, especially dogs. Although, as its name suggests, it typically involves the joints, other body systems are commonly affected. The disease commences as synovitis characterized by extensive infiltration by neutrophils. As the disease progress, the synovia swell and begin to proliferate (Fig. 24–8). Outgrowths of these proliferating synovia extend into the

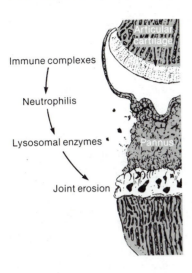

Immune complexes

Neutrophilis

Lysosomal enzymes

Joint erosion

Articular cartilage

Pannus

FIGURE 24-8. The pathogenesis of rheumatoid arthritis. Proliferative inflammatory tissue known as pannus develops in the synovial membrane as a result of immune complex deposition. The subsequent release of proteolytic enzymes results in erosion of articular cartilage.

joint cavities, where they are known as pannus. Pannus consists of fibrous, vascular tissue, that, as it invades the joint cavity, releases proteolytic enzymes that erode the articular cartilage and the neighboring bony structures. As the arthritis progresses, the infiltrating neutrophils may be partially replaced by lymphocytes, which can form lymphoid nodules and germinal centers. Another feature of rheumatoid arthritis that is commonly encountered is the development of subcutaneous nodules—necrotic foci surrounded by fibrous connective tissue containing lymphocytes and plasma cells. In addition, amyloidosis, disseminated arteritis, glomerulonephritis, and lymphatic hyperplasia are occasional complications.

The immediate cause of rheumatoid arthritis is unknown. Several investigators have proposed that the initiating cause is a microorganism. While none of these theories have been confirmed, recent evidence suggests that Epstein-Barr virus (EBV) may be implicated in some way. EBV can promote polyclonal B-cell expansion which, if not fully controlled, may give rise to multiple autoantibody production. The direct pathogenesis of rheumatoid arthritis is probably due to the chronic deposition of immune complexes in synovia. These immune complexes provoke prostaglandin, collagenase, and plasminogen production and joint destruction through the release of neutrophil hydrolytic enzymes. Development of autoantibodies to IgG is characteristic of rheumatoid arthritis. These autoantibodies, called rheumatoid factors, are of the IgM class and are directed against determinants in the C_{H2} regions of antigen-found IgG. Rheumatoid factors are found not only in rheumatoid arthritis but also in SLE and other conditions in which extensive immune-complex formation occurs. Rheumatoid arthritis and SLE patients may also have autoantibodies to IgD. It is conceivable that this may have a significant effect on the regulation of the immune system in these individuals.

Other Conditions Involving Autoimmunity

Although, theoretically, autoimmune disorders may involve any tissue in the body, and, in practice, many can be experimentally induced, the range of naturally occurring autoimmune disorders in animals is not wide. As has been pointed out, the presence of autoantibodies is insufficient by itself to identify a disease as autoimmune. For example, autoantibodies commonly arise following tissue damage. Thus, antibodies directed against mitochondrial antigens develop in animals suffering from liver or heart damage. In diseases such as trypanosomiasis or tuberculosis, in which widespread tissue damage occurs, auto-antibodies to a wide range of tissue antigens may be detected at low titers in serum.

The late Ernest Witebsky proposed a series of conditions that must be met in order for a disease to be identified as autoimmune: 1) the disease process must be demonstrated to occur as a consequence of the autoimmune response; 2) the autoantibodies should be detectable in all cases of the disease; 3) the disease should be experimentally reproducible by some form of immunization with the antigen; and 4) the disease should be transferrable from an affected animal to a normal animal by means of either serum or living lymphoid cells.

Left-Handedness and Autoimmune Disorders

There is a final twist to the story of autoimmune disorders. It has been noticed that left-handed individuals are more likely to develop autoimmune disorders than right-handed individuals. Thus, in one study 11% of left-handed individuals and 4% of right-handed individuals had autoimmune conditions—mainly Hashimoto's disease, ulcerative colitis, and celiac disease. The reasons are very obscure indeed. However, it has been hypothesized that left-handedness and immune malfunction may both develop as a result of abnormal endocrine influences on the fetus.

Sources of Additional Information

Cooke, A., Hutchings, P., and Playfair, J. Suppressor T cells in experimental autoimmune hemolytic anemia. Nature, *273:* 154–155, 1978

Drachman, D.B. Myasthenia gravis. N. Engl. J. Med., *298:* 136–142, 186–193, 1978.

Dumonde, D.C., ed. Infection and Immunology in the Rheumatic Diseases. Blackwell Scientific Publications, Oxford, 1976.

Fauci, A.S. Immunoregulation in autoimmunity. J. Allerg. Clin. Immunol. *66:* 5–17, 1980.

Gibofsky, A., et al. Disease associations of the Ig-like human alloantigens. Contrasting patterns in rheumatoid arthritis and systemic lupus erythematosus. J. Exp. Med., *148:* 1728–1732, 1978.

Golub, E.S. Know thyself: Autoreactivity in the immune response. Cell, *21:* 603–604, 1980.

Kae, I., and Drachman, D.B. Thymic muscle cells, bear acetylcholine receptors: possible relation to myasthenia gravis. Science, *195:* 74–75, 1977.

Kahn, R. Autoimmunity and the aetiology of insulin-dependent diabetes mellitus. Nature, 299: 15–16, 1982.

Kirkland, H.H., Mohler, D.N., and Horwitz, D.A. Methyldopa inhibition of suppressor-lymphocyte function: a proposed cause of autoimmune hemolytic anemia. N. Engl. J. Med., *302:* 825–832, 1980.

Schwartz, R.S. Viruses and systemic lupus erythematosus. N. Engl. J. Med., *293:* 132–136, 1975.

Strakosch, C.R., et al. Immunology of autoimmune thyroid diseases. N. Engl. J. Med., *307:* 1499–1507, 1982.

Stuart, J.M., et al. Type II collagen-induced arthritis in rats. Passive transfer with serum and evidence that IgG anticollagen antibodies can cause arthritis. J. Exp. Med., *155:* 1–16, 1982.

Index/Glossary

A blood group substance, 370

AA protein, 324–325

Ablastin, 306

ABO blood group system, 368–370

Acetylcholine receptor(s), 401, 406

Acetylethyleneimine, 276

Acetylsalicylic acid, 364

Acquired Immune Deficiency Syndrome (AIDS), 218, 304, 317–318, 343

Actinomycin, 340

Active immunization, 271–272, 274

Acute inflammation, 65

Acute lymphoblastic leukemia(s), 218

Acute phase protein(s). Proteins, synthesized by the liver, whose level in serum rises rapidly in response to acute inflammation and tissue damage, 75, 187

ADCC. *See* Antibody-dependent cellular cytotoxicity.

Addison's disease, 399

Adenosine deaminase, immunodeficiency due to absence of, 170, 319

Adenosine monophosphate, cyclic, 68, 167, 211, 215, 222, 359

Adjuvant. Material that enhances the normal immune response, 26–28

Adjuvant(s), 26, 160, 162, 223, 280
  Freund's complete, 27, 203, 228, 323, 349, 353, 403
  in vaccines, 280

Adrenoceptor(s), 359–360, 364
  autoantibodies to, 401

Aerosol vaccine(s), 280

Affinity. A measure of the binding strength between an antibody-binding site and an antigenic determinant, 108–112

Affinity (*cont.*)
  constant, 108
  labelling, 111
  maturation, 112, 195, 223

African swine fever, 303

Agammaglobulinemia, Bruton type, 254, 300

Agglutination. The clumping of particulate antigen by antibody, 126, 368

AIDS. *See* Acquired Immune Deficiency Syndrome (AIDS).

AIHA. *See* Hemolytic anemia, autoimmune.

Albumin(s). Serum proteins that remain in solution in the presence of half saturated ammonium sulfate, 13, 14, 20, 21, 80

Aleutian disease of mink, 271, 303, 386

Alexine, 242

Alkaline phosphatase, 118

Alkylating agent(s), 276

Allele. An alternative form of a gene. Only one allele of a gene can be expressed at any one time in a haploid invidilual, 33

Allelic exclusion. The phenomenon in which any given B lymphocyte from an individual heterozygous for allotype genes will produce immunoglobulin molecules of a single allotype, 101

Allergen(s). An antigen that stimulates the production of reaginic antibodies, 353, 359, 363

Allergic contact dermatitis, 20, 391–394

Allergic encephalitis, 225, 284

Allergic neuritis, 403

Allergy. A reaction mediated through immediate (Type 1) hypersensitivity mechanisms, 352,
  to foods, 363
  to inhaled antigens, 363

411

Cell-mediated immunity. Immune responses mediated by lymphocytes in the absence of antibodies
cellular basis of, 201–216
measurement of, 393–394
to facultative intracellular parasites, 211, 291
to helminths, 312–313
to viruses, 300
transfer of, 5, 216–217
Ceruloplasmin, 77
CH_{50} unit(s), 241
Chagas' disease, 398
Chamberland, Charles, 3
Chediak-Higashi syndrome, 60, 62, 345
Chemotactic factor(s), 55, 66, 68, 209
Chemotaxis. The movement of cells or organisms under the influence of an external chemical stimulus, 44, 60, 252
Chicken pox, 274
Chido antigen, 40, 244, 254, 367
Chimera. An animal that has been successfully populated by allogeneic cells, 182, 224, 225
Chlorambucil, 340
Cholera, 267, 271, 281
Choroid plexus, 385
Chromium release, 216
Chromosome marker(s), 182
Chronic granulomatous disease, 60
Class I and II antigen(s). *See* Histocompatibility antigen(s).
Class switch, 190
Classical complement pathway. That set of reactions of the complement cascade initiated by antigen-antigen complexes, 241, 243
Clonal selection theory, 181, 189, 228
Clonotype. A clone of cells synthesizing a single gene product such as an immunoglobulin, 189
Clostridium chauveoi, 118
Clostridium tetani, 5, 272
Clotting system, and complement, 240
Colchicine, 215, 340
Cold agglutinin(s), 405
Collagenase(s), 58, 74, 380
Colostrum, 262, 268, 375
Combined immunodeficiency syndrome, 319, 320
Combined variable immunodeficiency, 322
Competitive radioimmunoassay, 113, 114
Complement fixation test, 255
Complement system. A complex linked enzyme and aggregating protein system that is activated by factors such as the combination of antigen and antibody and results in a variety of biological consequences, 32, 39, 55, 93, 129, 194, 211, 261, 288, 291, 400, 405
activation of, 91, 113, 243

Complement system (*cont.*)
cascade reaction of, 241–242
chemotaxis mediated by, 253, 254
components of, 58, 246, 254, 292
cytolysis mediated by, 252
deficiencies of, 254–255
detection of, 241
genes coding for, 254
immune regulation by, 233, 249, 252
in Arthus reaction, 379–380
in clotting process, 254
in inflammation, 253
in resistance to viruses, 299
inhibitors of, 249–250
opsonization by, 252
pathways of, 243–249
receptors for. *See* Receptor(s), complement.
secretion mediated by, 252
Concanavalin A, 171, 185, 222, 234, 235, 394
Conformational determinant(s), 229
Conglutinin. A bovine serum protein that combines with the fixed third component of complement, 251
Congo-red dye, 323
Constant regions of immunoglobulin(s), 88, 89, 136, 141
Contact dermatitis, allergic, 20, 391–394
Contrasuppressor cell(s), 237
Coombs, Robin, 352
Coombs test. *See* Antiglobulin test(s).
Copy insertion, 138
Cornea, allografts, 336
Cortex, bursal, 153
lymph node, 155, 158
thymus, 149
Corticosteroid(s), 287, 364
Corynebacterium parvum. See Propionibacterium acnes.
Counter immunoelectrophoresis, 125, 126
C-reactive protein, 75, 77, 93, 237, 245, 325
Cross reaction(s). The reaction of an antibody with apparently unrelated antigens as a result of their possessing antigenic determinants in common, 21, 228, 398
Cutaneous basophil hypersensitivity. An inflammatory skin reaction characterized by extensive basophil infiltration induced by injection of antigen, 214, 391
Cyclic neutropenia, 60
Cyclic nucleotide(s) (cyclic AMP and cyclic GMP), 68, 167, 211, 215, 222, 359
Cyclooxygenase(s), 68, 357
Cyclophosphamide, 226, 340, 341, 347
Cyclosporin A, 305, 341–342
Cyproheptadine, 364